Nutrition for today

NUTRITION for today

Thora J. Runyan
Iowa State University

Harper & Row, Publishers
New York Hagerstown San Francisco London

Sponsoring Editor: John A. Woods
Project Editor: Richard T. Viggiano
Designer: Gayle Jaeger
Production Supervisor: Stefania J. Taflinska
Compositor: Ruttle, Shaw & Wetherill, Inc.
Printer: The Murray Printing Company
Binder: Halliday Lithograph Corporation
Art Studio: Eric G. Hieber Associates, Inc.

Library of Congress Cataloging in Publication Data

Runyan, Thora J.
Nutrition for today.

Bibliography: p.
Includes index.
1. Nutrition. I. Title. [DNLM: 1. Nutrition. QU145 R943n]
TX354.R86 613.2 75-37645
ISBN 0-06-045682-5

contents

preface

While writing NUTRITION FOR TODAY, I necessarily spent a good deal of time thinking about my topic, nutrition. But I spent as much time considering an equally important subject: you, the reader. So before discussing the book, I would like to talk about how I have imagined you.

Most people who read textbooks are college students in a specific curriculum. We all realize, though, that college courses are not the only source of information. So at times I have also thought of my potential readers as people who have chosen to learn by their own methods, perhaps reading this book on their own time, and perhaps motivated by personal and professional interests rather than by any degree requirements.

Whatever type of student you are, you surely have many interests and activities other than academics. Quite naturally, many of your concerns center on your own life and on the people you know. I suspect, though, that you are too well-read and too well-informed to confine yourself to strictly personal matters. Students, like many young adults today, are now generally less self-seeking than those in previous generations. I am speaking from my own experience, which has given me the privilege of knowing many young people both inside and outside the classroom.

On the basis of this experience, I feel quite certain that you do not want to have your mind made up for you. You prefer to accept or reject conclusions and decisions on the basis of the facts. You quite rightly reserve for yourself the prerogative of deciding which principles and practices are best for you, and you certainly reject rigid declarations of what you should or should not do.

How are these convictions of yours related to the subject of this book? Well, you have undoubtedly heard or read a good deal about nutrition that could apply to you, to the people you know, or to the world population. You may have noticed, and wondered about, conflicts between one statement and another. How could it be otherwise when, for example, a newspaper may print a glowing prediction of ample food for a future population many times larger than that of today—and in the same edition forebode catastrophic food shortages before the end of this decade?

No writer can resolve conflicts such as this for you. I have tried, though, to give you the essential facts of nutrition that can help you resolve some issues to your own satisfaction. As much as possible I have omitted details that I thought you do not want or do not need, and that would probably soon be forgotten even if memorized. I have, however, included basic facts of biology and chemistry that you will need for understanding how foods and nutrients interact with life. In short, I have assumed that, although authors cannot do the learning for the reader, they can at least make it as easy as possible for people to learn by teaching themselves.

The people who have reviewed the manuscript have been both tactfully accurate in correcting my errors and as generous with praise as any writer could hope for. Among those who commented extensively on the text were Professors Ercel Eppright, Kay Mitchell, Howard Appledorf, Frances Lafont, Helen West, Jane Lewis, and Eleanor Whitney.

The many helpful suggestions of these reviewers were valuable to me in two ways. First, they helped me to improve the content of this book. Second, and just as importantly, they reinforced my belief that viewpoints can be accepted even though they differ somewhat from those of other textbook authors. I am positive that a great many students have benefited from the tolerance and modern approach that came through to me in these reviews.

Working with these people and others (my family, colleagues, and students), I have written what I hope is a book that will meet your needs. You are probably already motivated to learn about nutrition if you are involved in one of the many areas obviously related to the subject. Human development, biology, ecology, education, nursing, medicine, and agriculture are just a few. The relevance of the material may also become apparent if you are interested in psychology, sociology, economics, or some other field that might at first glance appear only slightly related to nutrition. But whatever your interests—personal, academic, or professional—I have tried to write what would be both interesting and useful to you. For the subject I have had in mind is not nutrition alone; it is nutrition and you.

Thora J. Runyan

1

nutrition: an introduction

Can people lose weight rapidly despite an unlimited high-calorie food intake, as books on "diet revolutions" and "modern nutrition breakthroughs" claim? Nutritionists and physicians, experienced in the treatment of overweight, persistently attempt to convince people that such methods are not only ineffective but potentially dangerous. Is it possible to overcome fatigue, delay the aging process, and enhance physical beauty by swallowing a daily dose of brand X? Government agencies strive to fulfill their responsibility to control the false and misleading advertising of products which make such claims. Is the American food supply a "chemical feast," "nonfood," "junk," as alarmists describe it? Nutritionists and government sources insist that the quality of our food supply is better than ever before. Should food be raised with organic fertilizers and untouched by pesticides in order to be safe and of high nutritional value? The Food and Drug Administration has repeatedly presented evidence that foods raised in this manner are in no way superior to ordinary foods.

Faced with these conflicting claims, how is the average person to separate fact from fallacy? Most people will react in one of the following ways:

A large group of people will continue to eat as they always have; they are unaware of controversies regarding nutrition, or uninterested in them. Some of these people are already eating well and would have little to gain by changing their diets, whereas others would benefit by changing at least certain aspects of their present eating habits.

Other people will be interested enough in nutrition to examine their own present eating patterns, and fortunate enough to be guided by reliable sources of information. This group can benefit by becoming better able to control their weight, meet their nutrient needs, and avoid wasting money on unnecessary products which they may have believed to be essential for health. They will also benefit by having sound practices reinforced as well as incorrect practices modified.

A third group will be misled by incorrect information. At best, these people will waste time, money, and energy which could better be spent on other needs. At worst, they may end up in poorer health as a result of following extreme diets which are advocated by certain self-styled nutrition experts.

Why is there a problem of getting reliable information to the public? A major reason is that sensational information and "wonder" products are highly lucrative. A totally unreliable book, which promises perfect health, peace of mind, and a long life span, can become a best seller, although books which make more modest and realistic claims for nutrition have little appeal to the hidden hypochondriac in most of us. A food product which is touted as a "health food" obviously has greater appeal to some people than a food which is claimed to be no more than a useful part of a generally well-balanced diet. The public demand for nutritional miracles, then, is one basis for the abundant supply of quack information and products (Figure 1–1).

Another reason is that nutrition is a science (Figure 1–2). The development of nutrition has depended upon development of other disciplines such as chemistry, physics, biology, and the social sciences. Most people find it difficult to plow through textbooks of science in order to gain the background necessary to evaluate the conflicting claims in the field of nutrition. Fortunately, however, a slight acquaintance rather than an intimate knowledge of the principal generalizations of various related sciences is enough to provide most people with the basic information they actually need.

Nutrition is, after all, simply *the science of nourishing living systems.* What is science? What is involved in the process of nourishing? What is a living system? Most of us are so familiar with these terms that we assume we know exactly what they mean, as well as what they do not mean. However, even advanced students of nutrition sometimes find that their understanding has been hampered by an incomplete understanding of one or more of these very basic concepts. For this reason, a discussion of each of these terms is a logical beginning to the study of nutrition.

WHAT IS SCIENCE?

To many, scientists are modern miracle workers; they mix chemicals, crossbreed animals, inject a drug, study the behavior of rats or humans, and observe a result that nobody has observed before. The scientist then calls up a reporter, who interviews him or her and writes a story about the scientific breakthrough in the *New York Times.* A month later, the scientist is informed that he or she has won the Nobel Prize.

Scientists would be delighted if this process actually occurred. More commonly, however, scientific knowledge is gained as follows:

To begin with, a scientific question is posed. The scientist might ask, for example: How many different kinds of plants are growing in that meadow, forest, or back yard; how would a change in the number of plants affect the ecological balance? How long does it take the average rat to learn to run through a given maze in order to get the food or other reward at the end? What happens to people if they have too little (or too much) of a certain vitamin, of a drug, or of space in which to exist?

A scientist or anyone else may, of course, consider issues that are *not* scientific questions: How many angels can dance upon the point of a pin? Do invisible, undetectable spirit creatures inhabit the outer reaches of the universe?

These problems are not scientific questions because they cannot be

FIGURE 1–1

Do the titles suggest that these nutrition books are too good to be true? Maybe it is because they contain useless and even dangerous misinformation.

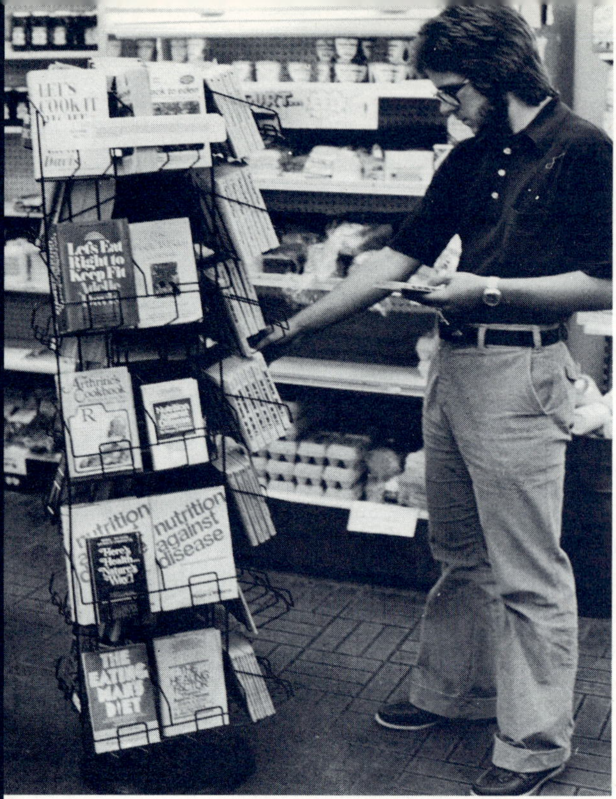

FIGURE 1–2

Nutrition is a science, related to many other areas of knowledge: physical, biological, and social sciences.

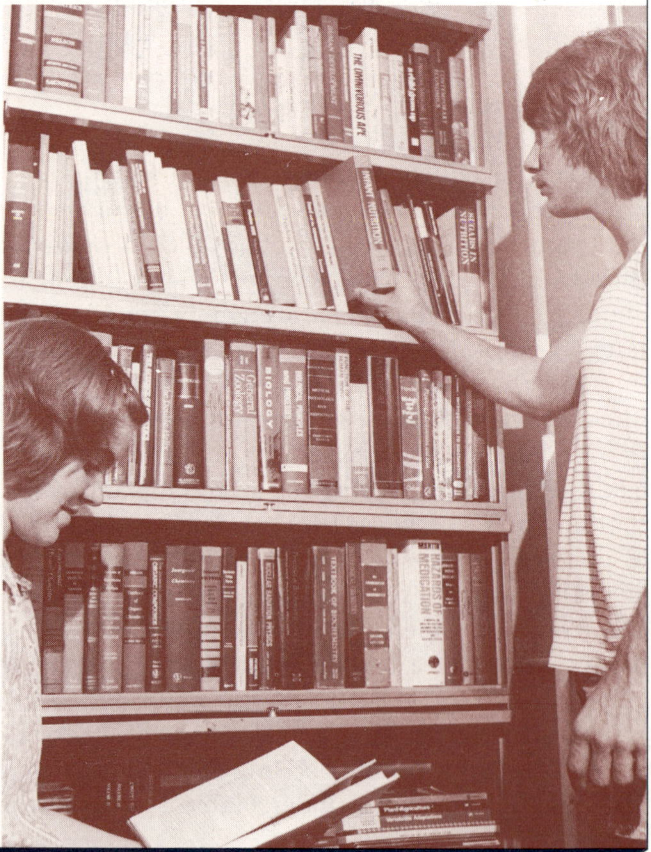

resolved by the two general methods of the scientific quest for answers: observation and experiment.

Observation

In the question regarding the number of kinds of plants growing in a certain area, no elaborate experiments need be performed; the investigator simply counts the number of plants as they naturally occur. He or she recognizes, of course, that the results could be modified by deliberately flooding the area or by spraying weed-killer on the plants. However, the results would then not answer the original question. Instead, they would be answering further questions: How are these plants affected by flooding or by chemicals? Which ones will survive and which will perish? Why will some survive and some not? What effects might this have on soil erosion and water pollution? Answering these questions will require an approach other than simple observation.

Experimentation

In an experiment, a test is made. Let us consider the question regarding the time necessary for the average rat to learn its way through a given maze. Observation of a situation as it occurs in nature cannot answer this question, for rats in a state of nature do not run through mazes. The experimenter must therefore set up a test, and this involves manipulating one or more factors in the rats' environment. In order to get reliable results, the experimenter must be certain that the conditions of the experiment are *controlled.* That is, all factors must remain unchanged except the factor that is being studied. For example, if rats studied on Tuesday proved to be much faster in learning a maze than rats studied on Friday, one might conclude that Tuesday, in some mysterious way, is a better day for learning than is Friday. However, if it is later found that the rats tested on Tuesday had not been fed for 24 hours before the trial, whereas the rats tested on Friday were fed just before the test, a more logical explanation becomes obvious: Hungry rats are more highly motivated to seek food than are nonhungry rats. Although this is a perfectly good conclusion, it does not answer the original question about the *average* rat; the experiment was not properly controlled.

Many scientific problems can be studied by either observation or experiment. The question of what happens to people if they have too little of a certain vitamin is an example. This question could be answered in both of the following ways:

1. Investigators could observe a population in which the usual food supply is known to contain too little of the vitamin to meet the minimum needs of people. They might choose to observe the general health of the people, the death rates, the growth of the children, the ability of the women to produce healthy babies, or many other factors which can be affected by severe vitamin deficiencies.

2. Experimenters could set up a controlled test using human volunteers. Obviously, this raises serious moral questions. Do the volunteers understand the possible consequences of the vitamin deficiency which is to be produced in them? Are they mature enough and intelligent enough to give their informed consent to the study? Are they willing to risk detrimental effects in order to help obtain information that may benefit others? Because a conscientious investigator must answer these questions before beginning work on human subjects, nonhuman species are used in most experiments, and human subjects are generally used only in studies that cannot be done otherwise.

After an investigator has obtained certain results from the observations or experiments, he or she makes a value judgment regarding them. In some cases, the only honest decision that can be made is that the findings are of no particular interest or use. Sometimes, however, the results point to some previously undiscovered fact or previously unrecognized relationship between facts. If this is the case, they are incorporated into a written report and published in a scientific journal.

At this point, the new knowledge, including all the details (how the study was done, what discovery was made, how the new findings are related to other facts and theories in the scientific world), is made available to other scientists. They are then able either to repeat the study, thereby confirming it, or to show that it cannot be repeated, thereby rejecting it. If the finding is confirmed, it may, along with many other findings, become part of a *hypothesis*, which is a conjecture that accounts, within a framework of ideas, for a set of facts that can be used for further investigation. If further studies bring forth findings which make the hypothesis more certain, the hypothesis becomes part of a *theory*. Although in popular usage the word *theory* is sometimes used as if it meant a mere guess (e.g., "Some people believe in vampires, but that's only a theory"), this use of the word is entirely incorrect. A theory is a system of knowledge which can be used to analyze, predict, or explain the nature of a set of phenomena. Whether the theory is retained or discarded depends upon whether it is supported or contradicted by the new knowledge that is continuously being discovered.

Scientific laws, facts, and certainty

If the same result is always obtained when an observation or experiment is repeated many times, it is incorporated into a *law* and is accepted as a *fact*. It is a law of physics, for example, that one form of energy can be converted into another form, but that energy cannot be created or destroyed in chemical reactions; it is a fact that a stone dropped from a cliff falls rather than rises. The word *fact*, however, is often used far too lightly. It is not a fact that vitamin E capsules are good for you just because your neighbor reports that she "feels better" since taking them. Laws and facts represent statements of a very high degree of certainty. Absolute certainty is, of course, rarely attained.

It must be remembered that evidence is never complete, that knowledge of truth is always partial and that to seek certainty is to await eternity.

–J. Bowlby, "Maternal Care and Mental Health Monograph Series No. 2," *World Health Organization*, 1951.

Meanwhile, what of average people? They do not read scientific journals. Indeed, even if they had access to them, it would be impossible to read them all. In addition to the reports published in the several scores of nutrition journals, reports on nutrition research are published in the thousands of professional journals of other disciplines such as biological sciences, social sciences, medicine, biochemistry, food technology, agriculture, education, and home economics. How, then, can the average person become aware of the latest scientific findings?

One way is through popular media such as magazines, newspapers, radio, and television. The information transmitted through these media may be highly accurate, differing from the information in scientific journals only in that it is expressed in terms understandable to the nonscientist. Unfortunately, in other cases, the process of translating scientific discoveries into ordinary language results in a distortion of the original meaning. Learning of new findings through popular media cannot, therefore, be recommended without qualification.

An even less reliable method of obtaining information is through the books, magazines, and advertising of the faddist with a method or product to sell. It is in this area that nutrition is unique among the sciences. Certainly there are quack treatments and crackpot ideas in disciplines such as physics, chemistry, psychology, and economics. In none of these areas, however, is quackery and faddism the big business that it is in the field of nutrition. Food is a basic human need, with deep psychological and social implications. A vast market therefore exists, ready-made for those who seek to profit by exploiting the public's lack of understanding of the science of nutrition and its relationship to health.

WHAT IS NOURISHING?

The second term to be examined in the definition of nutrition as "the science of nourishing living systems" is the word *nourishing*. Broadly, it means to sustain, promote, or foster the development of something, as "Egypt was nourished by the labor of slaves." In nutrition, the word is used in the literal sense of supplying substances, specifically nutrients, necessary for life. It should be emphasized that not everything needed for life is a nutrient. Oxygen, for example, is necessary for life in animals, but is not considered a nutrient because it is obtained by breathing air rather than by ingestion of foods.

The statement that nourishing consists of providing food substances in the necessary kinds and amounts may seem to imply that nutrition is merely a branch of chemistry, in which certain chemicals called nutrients are studied. Certainly an understanding of basic concepts of chemistry is a prerequisite to an understanding of nutrition. However, human nutrition is also intimately related to other areas of knowledge, and it is therefore important that people's patterns of nourishing themselves be seen as the result of many intertwined factors.

WHAT IS A LIVING SYSTEM?

A living system—that which has life—has unique characteristics which distinguish it from dead organisms or from inanimate objects which never possessed life. Essentially these characteristics are functions such as growth, reproduction, response to stimuli, and metabolism. Superficially, a crystal or rock might appear to be alive because it can "grow" (that is, become larger) by addition of material to its outer surface. In fact, however, this type of growth is entirely distinct from the real growth seen in the living world. Living things grow by incorporating environmental materials into their bodies and using these materials to grow from within. The first step in nourishing a living system, then, is to incorporate other living things into itself. How it does this depends on a variety of factors, more or less complex depending upon the kind of life involved.

FACTORS AFFECTING HUMAN FOOD HABITS

Patterns of eating, like other behavior patterns, develop over a period of time as a result of many complex and sometimes intangible influences. The need for food is based on three broad categories of human needs (Figure 1–3).

1 **Biological needs.** Certain amounts and kinds of food materials are necessary to sustain physical life itself.
2 **Psychological needs.** Food is used to provide personal emotional satisfaction.
3 **Social needs.** The sharing and trading of food contributes to the relationships between people in groups ranging in size from small families to nations.

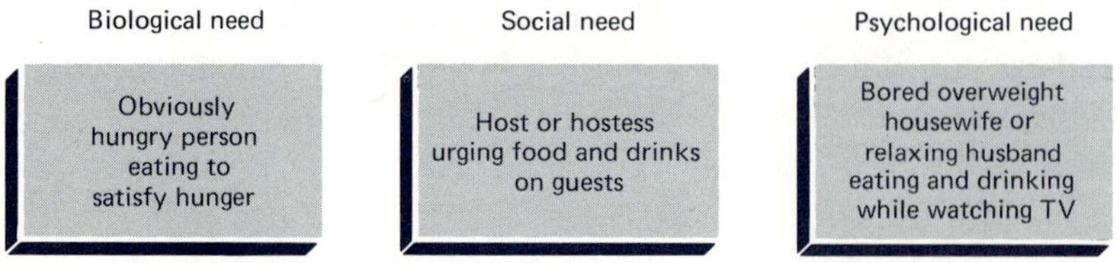

FIGURE 1–3. Food is a biological need that also plays important psychological and social roles in people's lives.

In many cases, these categories may overlap. For example, a liking for sugar appears to be instinctive, hence biological, in nature; young infants who have not yet been exposed to cultural influences readily accept sweet tastes. Psychologically, sweets are also commonly used for obtaining personal pleasure; the bored, overweight woman who comforts herself with a box of chocolates after a quarrel with her neighbor or husband is certainly not meeting a bodily need by her actions. Socially, sweet foods are used in many ways: children are rewarded with desserts, and men give candy to their wives as birthday and anniversary gifts, for example.

The preference of various people for different amounts of salt is also based on all three categories of human needs. Although there appears to be an instinctive biological drive to obtain salt, the ability of different individuals to respond to the chemical stimulus of a given amount of salt varies tremendously; in typical studies, the absolute detection threshold (the lowest level of salt which can be tasted) varies over an eighty-fold range. Interestingly, women have an innately higher sensitivity than men for salty or sweet tastes, although not for sour taste. In addition to these biological factors, many learned or conditioned factors influence the use of salt: a family habit of salting everything before tasting it, the mother's cooking practices, the belief that the use of large amounts of salt is necessary in hot weather, or the opposite belief that salt harms the heart or kidneys.

Psychological and social meanings of food

People like and accept certain foods and not others for many reasons, and these often are based more on the feelings of the person than on the qualities of the food itself. Foods may be particularly liked, for example, primarily because they are associated with pleasant personal experiences or satisfying social relationships. A few examples might be:

1 An adult may have long forgotten, at least at the conscious level, that his mother always pampered him with chicken noodle soup when he was sick during childhood. He may still like chicken noodle soup more than any other kind because to him the meanings of this food are concern, affection, and maternal care.

2 A man may prefer meat grilled on an outdoor barbecue to meat prepared in any other manner because, years ago, he and his father cooked food in this way on camping trips. The meanings of grilled meat to this man include the father-son relationship and the masculinity of living away from civilization.

3 A woman's favorite kind of ice cream may be Neapolitan because that was the kind served at the first birthday party she remembers. To her, Neapolitan ice cream means gifts, affection, and being the center of attention for the whole day.

4 A college student may enjoy eating unusual, unfamiliar foods because she or he has always received praise and admiration for being willing to try anything new. Unusual foods help to identify this individual as adventurous, daring, unconventional, and more cosmopolitan than the person with a narrow and unchanging list of accepted foods.

5 Children beg their parents for coffee, tea, beer, and other "adult" beverages, even though they may grimace at the bitter taste. These drinks mean: grown-up, equal to parents, "big."

6 A person who often went hungry during childhood because of poverty may, as an adult, focus a disproportionate amount of value upon food. To this person, eating well may actually mean overeating. Food means: security, the prestige of wealth, the power to get all you want and more than you need.

Food aversions and dislikes

Sometimes, of course, a food itself or the way it is prepared may be the cause of its being disliked. Okra, liver, and sauerkraut, for example, are disliked by so many people that it is difficult to believe that unhappy personal or interpersonal experiences are often involved. More likely it is the texture of okra, the flavor of liver, and the odor and sourness of sauerkraut that prevent many people from liking these foods. However, a given individual may react negatively to a given food, a given meal, or even food in general because of associated meanings and past experiences, which may even have been forgotten.

1. A middle-aged woman may skip breakfast because, as a child, she had to prepare and eat her own breakfast alone while Mother occupied herself in caring for the new baby. The meanings of breakfast to her are: rejection, jealousy, loneliness.

2. A man may become angry and upset when his wife suggests that he carry his lunch to work in order to cut down on expenses. To him, carrying a lunch in a paper bag revives feelings of embarrassment and inferiority felt when he took a sack lunch to school instead of eating at the local snack shop with the more affluent, or more popular, students. A sack lunch means: inferiority, lack of success, "differentness."

3. An adult may detest cold breakfast cereal because, years ago, Mother prepared bacon and eggs for her husband's breakfast, but considered cold cereal "good enough for the kids." Cold cereal signals: second-class status, not worthy of people's best efforts.

Sometimes people develop negative feelings toward food and meals in general because the early home environment created an aura of unpleasantness around the very act of eating. Perhaps as children they were forced to eat certain things, not because the parents really believed that these foods were necessary for the child, but as a matter of rigid discipline ("No child of mine is going to tell me what he will or won't eat"). Other people cannot really enjoy food because of long-standing feelings of guilt ("What do you mean, you don't like carrots? Lots of little children in India would be glad to have those nice carrots!"). Still others associate meals with the tension and unhappiness resulting from their parents' use of the family dinner time to criticize manners, mete out punishments for the day's misbehavior, and complain about the hard day they had. Children may learn from such early experiences that eating is a chore to be gotten through as quickly as possible so that they can escape to a more pleasant activity.

A valuable activity for many people is to keep a written record of all the foods and beverages consumed, both in meals and as snacks, for two or more days. The foods which appear on the record may then be classed as follows:

1 Foods eaten because they are especially well liked.
2 Foods eaten because they were the only choices available because of economics, the decisions of the cook, the season of the year, or other reasons.
3 Foods eaten because of social factors, such as the overly sweet dessert you ate in order to avoid hurting the hostess's feelings.
4 Foods eaten for health reasons, real or assumed.

Foods which are common to most people's daily diets, but which do *not* appear on your record, may be categorized as follows:

1 Foods not eaten because of a physical intolerance, such as an allergy.
2 Foods not eaten because you dislike or have never tried them.
3 Foods not eaten because they were not available.
4 Foods not eaten because of social, educational, or cultural factors. These might include pork if you are an Orthodox Jew, meat of any kind if you are a vegetarian, expensive foods if you are on a strict budget, eggs if you have heard that they contain high levels of cholesterol, and many high-calorie foods if you are attempting to lose weight.

Many people, after analyzing a written record of food intake as described above, are surprised to discover that their eating behavior is very different than they would have assumed it to be. Even more surprises are in store for those who attempt to explain *why* they eat as they do. The basic factors that determine the kinds and amounts of food eaten will invariably be seen to include the following:

Hunger. This refers to the complex of unpleasant bodily feelings which drive people to seek food solely for the purpose of relieving those feelings.

Appetite. In contrast to hunger, appetite consists of the more or less pleasant sensations which accompany the desire for food or for certain kinds of food.

Satiety. Also called satisfaction, this refers to the feelings which cause people to stop eating when hunger and appetite are satisfied.

Anorexia. This is an abnormal lack of hunger or appetite, which is sometimes based on a biological factor but often is a result of emotional distress, when hunger and appetite would be more appropriate.

Sensory reactions. These are the responses of the individual to a food's taste, odor, appearance, texture, and even sound (as the breakfast cereal with "snap, crackle, pop" shows). The combination of taste and odor constitute flavor.

Availability of food. This refers to the amounts and kinds of food accessible to the person. It may be very restricted in certain situations, as in a hospital, a short-order type restaurant, or the home of a low-income family.

Ethnic group. Italian-Americans, for example, may feel that a good meal must include pasta; on the other hand, they may prefer Chinese food or "soul food" to pasta in order to emphasize the fact that they are *not* bound to their traditional ethnic patterns.
Religion. Although this is a less important factor in the United States than in some other areas of the world, certain food practices based on religious beliefs are of importance to various groups in this country; the best-known example is probably the Orthodox Jew's refusal to consume meat and dairy products in the same meal.
Socioeconomic status. Not only does this determine the amount of money currently available for purchasing food, but it may also have established food habits in the past as a result of socioeconomic factors existing during childhood.
Education. What people have learned, through formal education or otherwise, about food, weight control, malnutrition, and related subjects can determine whether they accept or reject certain eating practices. "Education" obtained from popular but inaccurate sources can have detrimental effects that are extremely resistant to change.
Motivation. Needs, desires, and similar impulses can act as incitements to actions related to eating behavior. The person who has tried to lose weight for years may finally be successful when motivated by a "diet or die" statement by a physician; the man who has always hated fried chicken from a concession stand may nevertheless be motivated to eat it if his wife insists that she needs an occasional night off from cooking.

An effort to explain your personal attitudes and practices regarding food can result in greater understanding of your own behavior as well as that of other people. Knowing certain basic concepts from some of the social sciences, which include psychology, sociology, anthropology, economics, political science, and history, can be very helpful in reaching this goal.

SUGGESTED READINGS

"Pickles and Humbug." *Journal of Irreproducible Results* 15 (1966):18.

Cardiovascular Center. *Bibliography of Nutritional Sources.* Omaha, Nebraska: University of Nebraska Medical Center, 1975.

Committee on Nutrition. "Factors Affecting Food Intake." *Pediatrics* 33 (1964): 135.

Darby, W. J. "The Unicorn and Other Lessons from History." *Nutrition Reviews* 32 (1974):57.

Harper, A. E. "Nutrition: Where Are We? Where Are We Going?" *American Journal of Clinical Nutrition* 22 (1969):87.

Henderson, L. M. "Programs to Combat Nutritional Quackery." *Journal of the American Dietetic Association* 64 (1974):372.

Index of Nutrition Education Materials. The Nutrition Foundation. Washington, D.C.: 1975.

Schanche, D. A. "Diet Books that Poison Your Mind . . . and Harm Your Body." *Today's Health* 52 (April 1974):56.

Villee, C. A. *Biology,* sixth edition. Philadelphia: Saunders, 1972. (Chapter 1).

Ziman, J. M. "Information, Communicaton, Knowledge." *Nature* 224 (1969): 318.

2

nutrition and the social sciences

The behavioral elements as well as the structural ones are vital aspects of our biologic heritage—a craving by each individual for response from his social environment is a craving as fundamental as that for food.

–L. Eisenberg, "The Social Development of Human Intelligence," *The Harvard Medical Alumni Bulletin* **43**:2–8, 1968.

Advances in the field of biological or physiological nutrition during recent decades have been rapid and spectacular. This was made possible largely by new methods developed through advances in other sciences such as physics and chemistry. The development of the electron microscope, for example, made possible the study of structures within living systems which cannot be seen with ordinary microscopes. The study of even smaller particles, such as genetic material and individual protein molecules, was possible only after certain modern methods of chemical analysis became available.

Perhaps because of the excitement generated by such new methods and discoveries, the emphasis in nutrition has, more and more, shifted away from the study of intact living things and toward the study of the minuscule parts of which living forms are composed. The effects of nutritional excesses and deficiencies on the size, number, form, and function of minute particles has become a major research emphasis. Although these studies have provided much valuable information on the underlying causes of the gross changes seen in malnutrition, one effect has been detrimental to the field of nutrition. By concentrating on the subcellular aspects of nutrition, people have tended to lose sight of the broad scope of the science, as illustrated in Figure 2–1.

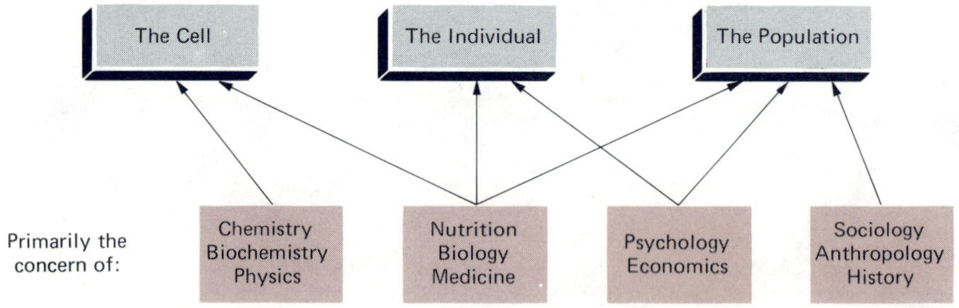

FIGURE 2–1. The scope of nutrition.

An individual or group cannot be understood on the basis of physical characteristics alone. A discussion of some of the principal ideas of the social sciences, which study behavior and the social components of the environment, is therefore essential.

PSYCHOLOGY AND NUTRITION

Psychology, the science of mental processes and behavior of individuals or of groups, seeks to understand and explain the way people act, function, or perform. *Behavior* may be defined as anything a person or other living thing does. This includes all of the movements a person makes, such as those involved in running, eating, breathing, or producing sounds such as speech or music. In addition, behavior can consist of looking, listening, thinking. These acts, although internal and hence less accessible to study than more obvious behavior, affect future behavior.

A major question asked by the psychologist is *why* a person acts in a particular way. A question in which nutritionists are particularly interested is, Why do people eat as they do? This question actually consists of two separate questions. The first is, To what goal is the act of eating directed, or What is the *result* of eating? One answer is that eating is necessary to sustain life itself, or that eating helps to insure survival.

The second question which may be what we mean when we wonder why people eat as they do involves not the effects of the behavior but the *causes.* Essentially, the causes of eating in a certain way consist of *internal* and *external stimuli,* without which the given eating pattern would not occur.

Conditioned and unconditioned responses

Often, psychologists must turn to animal experiments in order to control the conditions of their tests. The Russian physiologist, Pavlov, for instance, showed that dogs, which normally salivate at the sight of food, could be trained, or *conditioned,* to salivate upon hearing a bell which they had heard every time food was given them. Drooling at the sight of food is natural and instinctive; psychologists therefore say that it is *unconditioned.* Drooling at the sound of a bell is a conditioned response in that it requires learning. In short, a dog, or a human, can indicate readiness to eat because of internal signals such as hunger or because of external signals which have been learned. Any owner of a dog or cat can see this; the pet runs to the kitchen in response to the sound of a can opener.

In species with a very limited ability to learn, instinctive eating behavior is commonly as firmly ingrained as are form, color, and other physical traits. In humans, instinct is important in insuring *that* the person eats, but not in determining the *kinds* of foods which people eat. This is acquired mostly from the environment, and particularly from the people who make up the individual's social environment. The study of nutrition therefore leads to areas involving interactions between people.

SOCIOLOGY AND NUTRITION

Social behavior, the tendency of individuals to form organized groups and interact with each other, is not unique to humans. Bees, for example, are social insects with a caste system more rigid than the most extreme example in human society. Even among animals which tend to be solitary, social relationships may be evident under certain conditions, as when a male and female mate or when one or both parents care for the young.

Because social behavior is common to so many species, it is assumed to be of value in ensuring the survival of the species. Personal safety and efficiency of performing work through the division of labor are obvious advantages of being a member of a society. In addition, social behavior makes possible the social transmission of products of human work and thought, which is the *culture* of the society. However, it should be noted that social behavior in itself is not sufficient for the development of a culture. A flock of birds or a school of fish are social, but they lack the mental ability and language needed to develop the arts, beliefs, and other elements of a culture.

A very important point in relation to nutrition is the vast extent to which the social environment affects and modifies eating behavior. All human individuals have much the same physical needs for food. The manner in which these needs are met, however, varies not only from one society to another but also from one social group to another within each society.

A second important concept is that there is no one "best way" to eat, any more than there is a single best way to dress, build shelters, or dance. Many sincere attempts to improve the nutrition of people in other societies, including subgroups within our own society, have been weakened by a chauvinistic insistence that the nutritional practices of middle-class America are undoubtedly superior to any other. Social and cultural differences in eating behavior will be mentioned often in the following chapters. By no means will "different" necessarily mean "inferior." We are all bound to our own culture. It is important that this binding not be so firm that practices differing from ours are automatically labeled "illogical," "ignorant," or "wrong."

A third important idea is that the basic unit of human society is the family. It may be of the nuclear type, consisting of husband, wife, and children, or it may be of the extended type, in which grandparents, aunts, uncles, and others live in close association. Of all social units, the family is the single most significant determinant of eating behavior for most people. Eating habits, beliefs about food, religious taboos, and other sociocultural factors are all transmitted via the family to children while they are young enough to accept uncritically, and to imitate, the parents' ideas and behavior. Although other social units such as peer groups will later become important influences on eating behavior, for most of us the attitudes and behavior patterns or habits acquired early in life from the family remain very important reasons why we eat as we do.

ANTHROPOLOGY AND NUTRITION

The study of the development of human social and cultural characteristics is known as *social anthropology*. This field is often confused with the related field, archaeology, which is the study of material evidence remaining from human life and culture in past ages. Although the two areas frequently overlap, an important difference is that the anthropologist studies people living today as well as people from whom modern humans evolved.

When anthropologists study a society which died long ago, they must attempt to explain their findings by logic and speculation, and different explanations may be offered by different workers. Because there is no way to test these hypotheses by controlled experiment, many explanations must await new evidence before the issue can be resolved. An outstanding example is the case of the proposed relationships between food production and civilization. For years, the accepted sequence was that shown in Figure 2–2.

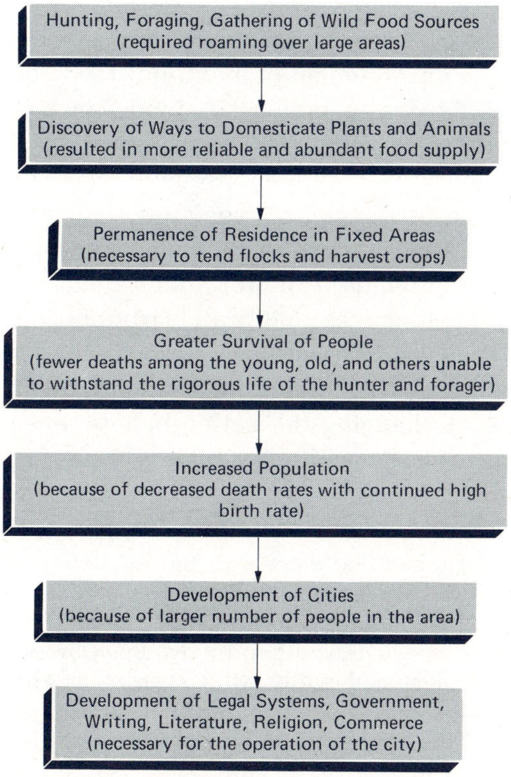

FIGURE 2–2. The proposed relationship between a "food production revolution" and the development of civilization.

Appealing as is the idea that a radical change in food production was at the very basis of the evolution of civilization, some evidence to the contrary has accumulated during the past quarter of a century. At one site in Syria, for example, established some 10,000 years ago and consisting of many levels of stone buildings, only wild plants and animals were used as food sources. The inhabitants of one of the cities at the ancient site of Jericho had the technology needed to build impressive walls for defense by the time they had begun to develop agriculture. However, in general a complex civilization requires agriculture, as modern agriculture depends upon the technology of civilization.

It is in the areas of the social and cultural development and behavior of people living today that the anthropologist's methods are most applicable to nutrition. Among Buddhists, for example, taking any form of animal life is abhorrent on the basis of the religious elements of their culture. Persuading Buddhists to eat meat or to use pesticides to prevent crop destruction by rodents, insects, and other pests clearly cannot be accomplished merely by pointing out the nutritional value of meat or the potential for increased food production through the use of pesticides. Suggesting alternate foods that are nutritionally equivalent to meat would be one way to solve the first problem. Developing pest-resistant food sources and devising ways to decrease the pest population through impairing their ability to reproduce, rather than killing them outright, are possible approaches to the second probolem.

A study of the development of a cultural taboo on a given food can sometimes suggest ways in which the food can be made acceptable. Because food habits are among the oldest and most firmly established aspects of many cultures, they are extremely resistant to change. There are hundreds of cases, among all societies, in which cultural beliefs forbid the consumption of certain foods, and the resulting eating patterns can become a problem if the forbidden foods are really important in human nutrition. Practices that are clearly detrimental, then, rather than those that seem illogical but are relatively innocuous, are the ones that should be studied with a view to changing them.

An example of changing the eating beliefs and practices of a society is the work done by multidisciplinary teams among Zulu tribesmen in the Union of South Africa. Each team consistcd of a physician, a nurse, and a health educator. The program proceeded as follows:

1 The teams determined that there was, indeed, extensive malnutrition among the people they served.

2 Diet surveys showed that the diet consisted mostly of corn supplemented by dried beans and a few other foods. Beer brewed from millet (sorghum) was consumed avidly. Milk, eggs, meat, and green vegetables were consumed in very small amounts by most of the people.

3 Examination of the environmental factors responsible for the existing diet revealed two main areas of factors:
a. The *physical* environment included impoverished soil and a lack of wild game, roots, berries, and greens which could have been used as food.

b. The *social and cultural* environment included the belief that the people's ancestors had been healthy on the same diet; the use of cooking practices which destroyed much of the nutritional value of the food; and certain emotional associations regarding milk and eggs.

4 Introduction of the missing foods was accomplished in the following manner:

a. Investigation of the past showed that the diets of the pastoral ancestors had been very different, including large amounts of milk, game, and wild plants. This was confirmed by the elders of the tribe, who added the prestige of age to the subject. This illustrates the importance of determining the leadership and decision-making patterns in a culture. In most American families, food decisions are made primarily by women; in many other cultures, a woman's opinion carries no authority and it is therefore necessary to deal with males or with older members of the group in order to bring about changes.

b. Seeds and instructions for gardening were supplied in order that domesticated greens could replace the formerly used wild ones. Within ten years, the percentage of families raising vegetable gardens increased from 3 percent to 80 percent, and cooking demonstrations helped the women to prepare these foods so that they tasted best and were of maximum nutritional value.

c. Eggs, in contrast to vegetables, were available but infrequently eaten because of definite emotional associations. Eating eggs was considered:

(1) uneconomical, because the egg, if not eaten, would become a chicken

(2) a sign of greed

(3) capable of arousing sexual desire in girls

Methods for increased egg production were introduced so that enough eggs for both eating and hatching were available. The nutritional value of eggs was stressed, and the people were assured that eating eggs was neither greedy nor a cause of passion. Because of the emotional views on the use of eggs, response was neither as rapid nor as extensive as in the case of green vegetables, but over a period of years egg consumption steadily increased.

d. Milk drinking was a much more complex situation. The amount available was small, averaging about 1 ounce for each person daily. In addition, women frequently could drink no milk whatsoever because of deep-seated beliefs. For example, it was believed that a woman exerted an evil influence on cattle if she drank milk during the menses or during pregnancy. Because the men of the household could never be sure that the women of the family were not menstruating or pregnant, they often routinely excluded milk from the diets of females after puberty. In addition, it was considered wrong for anyone, male or female, to drink milk produced by cows not owned by the head of the kin group, because cattle were regarded as the link between a man and his ancestors. When a woman married and went to live with her husband's family, she could not offend her husband's ancestors by drinking milk from his cows, and she lived too far from her own father's home to drink milk from his cows. Under these conditions, stressing the nutritional value and flavor of milk was useless. The solution lay in introducing milk which did not originate from cows belonging to any of the local people. Therefore, powdered milk obtained from distant places was imported. This was accepted so enthusiastically that the demand for milk became too great to be met by importing milk, and eventually some of the less conservative families agreed to

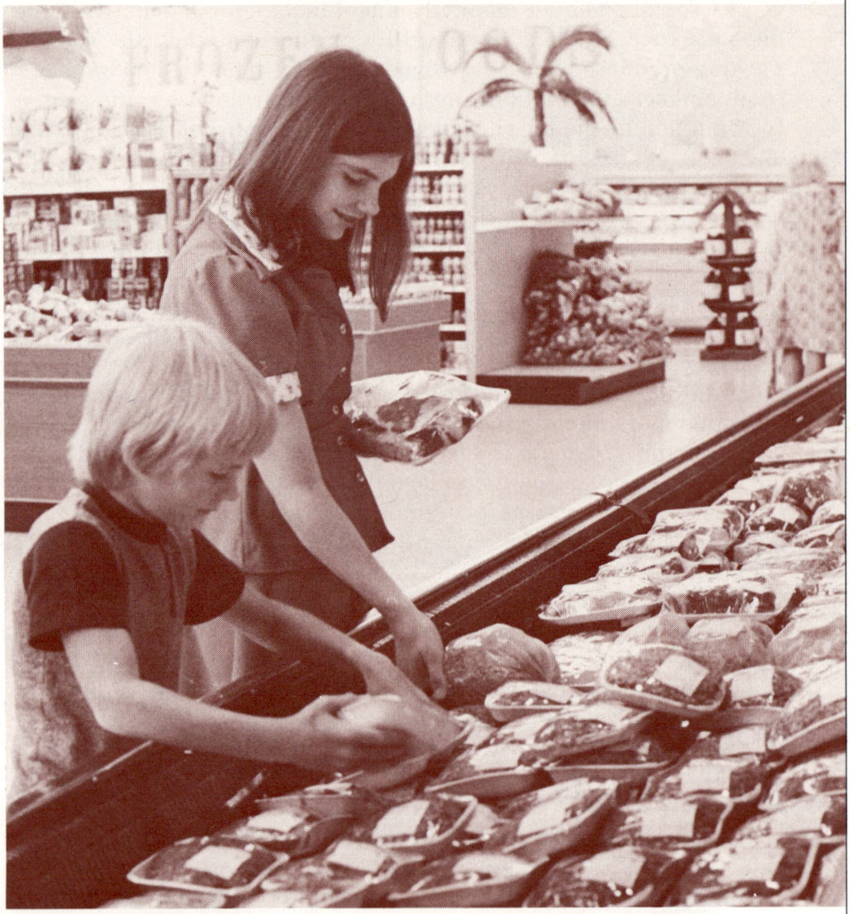

FIGURE 2–3

Even children can select a safe, nutritious food supply in our modern supermarkets.

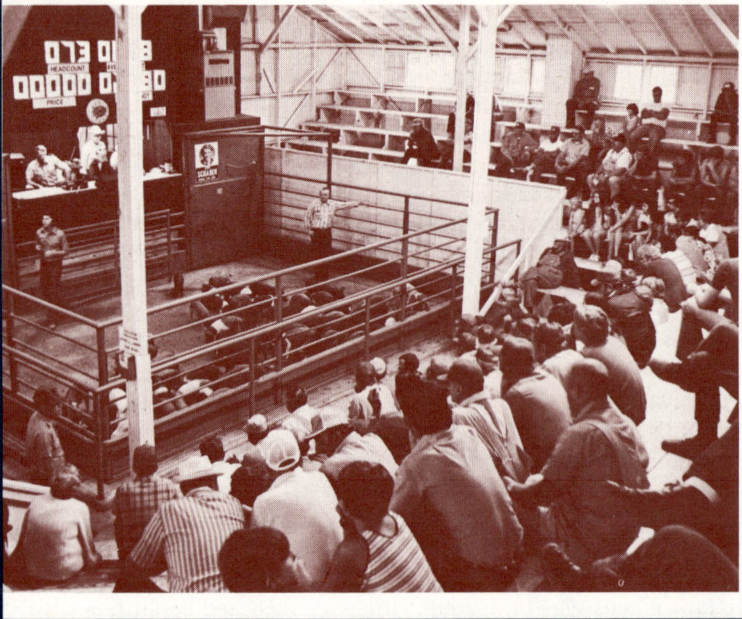

FIGURE 2–4

In some parts of the complex food market, such as this hog auction, the law of supply and demand is very evident; prospective buyers bid to get what they want at the lowest possible price.

allow women to drink milk from previously forbidden sources. During a period of 12 years, apparently as a result of increased ability of the better-nourished nursing mothers to produce milk for their infants, infant mortality decreased to one-third of its previous level, protein deficiency and a formerly common vitamin deficiency disease were virtually eradicated, and the growth rate of infants increased. Examples such as these illustrate that nutritional practices, although resistant to change, can be altered if the following conditions are met:

1 The investigator should have a firm knowledge of the people's beliefs and attitudes as well as of their eating behavior.

2 The functions performed by these beliefs, attitudes, and practices, or the way in which they fit into the total culture, must be evaluated.

3 Methods appropriate to the particular culture or subculture must be devised, because programs suitable for one group may be entirely inappropriate for another.

4 Possible repercussions of a successful program should be considered. For example, the acceptance of new ideas by the Zulu women in this study might have led to an eventual decrease of the status of males as decision makers, and acceptance of the fact that women can drink milk without fear of offending their husband's ancestors could weaken the religious worship of ancestors. Improving one aspect of a culture may have profound and sometimes detrimental effects on other cultural elements.

ECONOMICS AND NUTRITION

The production, distribution, and consumption of commodities are the subjects of the science of economics. Central to these subjects is some type of market system. Most Americans think only of a typical supermarket in relation to food, and casually accept the ease with which a shopper can obtain a safe, nutritious food supply (Figure 2–3). However, behind the food supermarket is a myriad of other markets: the auction at which animals are sold (Figure 2–4), the grain market which supplies the animals' feed, the seed market needed to grow the feed, the fuel and labor markets necessary to operate the agricultural equipment, and so on. A market, then, exists whenever people get together to exchange goods or services, and "the food market" actually consists of a complex web of interdependent markets.

Each time a person buys something or spends money for a service, this action causes a response in the market system. By buying, we indicate a demand, and this stimulates increased supply. Obviously, however, there are limitations to this. For example, during World War II the supply of sugar to civilians was restricted by the government's decision on rationing. A high demand did not, therefore, increase the civilians' supply as it ordinarily would. Also, in some cases the resources for meeting a demand are simply not available. If every individual in the world decided today that he or she wanted nothing less than a pound of high-quality steak at every dinner, this demand could not be met by the present supply of steak. Two alternatives would then be possible:

1 The demand might be met by greatly increasing the supply of steak. This would involve transferring resources such as land and labor, currently used for production of other goods, to the production of beef cattle.

2 The demand could be met for some people, but not for others, by changes in the price of steak. A similar example of this was seen in the case of supply, demand, and the price of liver some thirty or forty years ago. Before then, liver was almost unsalable because of the low demand for it, and because the supply was great relative to the demand, the price was virtually nil. Butchers gave liver away free to customers who fed it to their dogs and cats. During the 1920s, however, the value of liver as a specific treatment for a very serious, although rare, type of anemia was discovered. As a result, liver gained a reputation as a highly nutritious food which was generally valuable for health. Consequently, demand for liver increased very rapidly. As a practical matter, the supply could not very well be greatly increased; nobody raises whole animals simply to obtain the livers. Increased demand for liver therefore brought about a tremendous increase in the price. This served as an automatic control on distribution; only those who could afford the higher price could obtain liver. This also points out one of the weaknesses of the economic system; was it right that some of the people who actually needed liver for the treatment of anemia could not obtain it, because of its price?

This example illustrates a situation of increased demand for a *specific* food. A more serious problem is that of increased worldwide demand for food in general. This is of such magnitude economically and politically, as well as nutritionally, that it is not an exaggeration to place it among the most urgent problems of the modern world.

Malthus' theory of population and the theory of diminishing returns
One of the most famous ideas in economics was postulated not by an economist but by a clergyman. Thomas Malthus' *Essay on the Principle of Population,* published in 1798, advanced the hypothesis that population, unless checked by limits of the food supply, would increase geometrically: 1, 2, 4, 8, 16, 32 . . . Furthermore, food production inevitably would lag behind population growth, because of the law of diminishing returns. This law may be illustrated as follows:

If one man labors alone on a farm, he may produce 1000 bushels of corn in a year. If he hires a man to help him, the two together may produce 2200 bushels, or more than twice the output of one man, because of the greater efficiency possible from division of labor. However, if a third man is hired, production may be increased very slightly, say, to only 2700 bushels. This averages out to 900 bushels per man per year, or less than the production of each man working alone. The successively diminishing returns (or outputs) gained by adding more of some input such as labor is inevitable because of the limited ability of a given amount of land to produce food beyond a certain point.

Figure 2–5 shows how much population has increased in parts of the

world during the years 1948 to 1969, and how food production has increased in the same time. It is obvious that food *per person* has declined despite intensive attempts to increase it. Available food per person can be increased in only two ways: the total amount of food available must be increased, or the number of people available to consume it must be decreased.

Humanitarian concerns force us to attempt to alleviate the extreme hunger and malnutrition which exist throughout much of the world. In addition, a situation in which two-thirds of the world's people are hungry is dangerous, politically and economically, for the other one-third. Temporarily, improvement can result from increasing the food supply. Exporting food from the developed to the developing countries, and improving the yield and distribution of foods within the developing countries themselves, have been successful to some degree. However, the resources of the earth are finite and the ability of the earth to produce food is therefore limited, even if every available bit of land and water were used with maximum efficiency for food production. For this reason, attempts to increase the numerator in the ratio, Amount of Food/Number of People, must eventually be replaced by programs designed to decrease the denominator through population control.

Factors determining population growth

A population size is determined by the balance between the number of births and the number of deaths in the population. Since the latter part of the nineteenth century, family *fertility,* the actual number of children born per family, has declined in most Western societies. Death rates, however, have declined even more rapidly, largely as the result of medical advances and the higher living standards following the Industrial Revolution. The result has been a net growth of population despite decreased birth rates.

The picture is different throughout the large part of the world known as the *developing* or *underdeveloped* nations. In these areas, which include large parts of Asia, Africa, and Central and South America, family fertility is very close to family *fecundity,* or biological reproductive ability. Death rates here have declined, although the change has been much less dramatic than in the developed, industrialized nations. The net effect of decreased death rates without correspondingly decreased birth rates has been a rate of population growth so rapid that the term "population explosion" is appropriate.

Projections for the future range from the most dismal view, that starvation on a worldwide scale is inevitable within the next decade or so, to optimistic predictions that birth rates will fall in the developing countries before the already acute food supply situation further deteriorates. Economists as well as specialists in many other disciplines have vital roles to perform in the solution of this complex problem.

SUGGESTED READINGS

Berg, A. *The Nutrition Factor: Its Role in National Development.* Washington, D.C.: The Brookings Institution, 1973.

Bolton, J. M. "Food Taboos Among the Orang Asli in West Malaysia: A Potential Nutritional Hazard." *American Journal of Clinical Nutrition* 25 (1972):789.

Brown, L. R. "Population and Affluence: Growing Pressures on World Food Resources." *Population Bulletin* 29 (1973):No. 2.

Cassel, J. "Social and Cultural Implications of Food and Food Habits." *American Journal of Public Health* 47 (1957):732.

FIGURE 2–5. The amount of food available per person can decrease despite increased total food production if population growth is rapid. (From "World Agriculture, the Last Quarter Century," Food and Agriculture Organization of the United Nations, Rome, 1970).

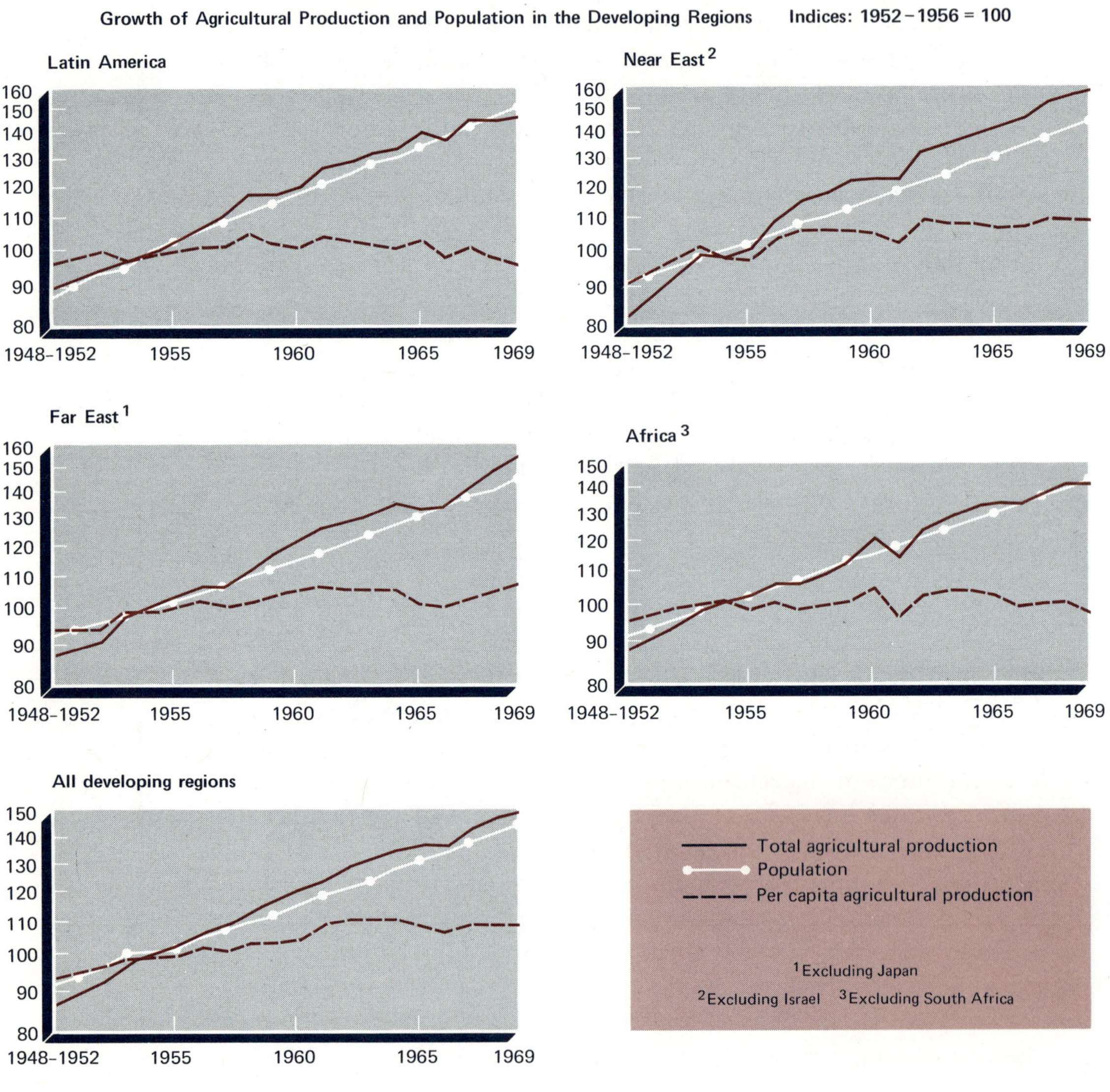

Cesal, L., L. Blakeslee, and E. O. Heady. "The World Food Situation." *World Review of Nutrition and Dietetics* 7 (1967):1.
Dupont, J., ed. *Dimensions of Nutrition*. Boulder, Colorado: Colorado Associated University Press, 1970.
Dwyer, J. T. and J. Mayer. "Beyond Economics and Nutrition: The Complex Basis of Food Policy." *Science* 188 (1975):566.
Gifft, H. H., M. B. Washbon, and G. G. Harrison. *Nutrition, Behavior and Change*. Englewood Cliffs, N. J.: Prentice-Hall, 1972.
Herman, M. W. "Excess Weight and Sociocultural Characteristics." *Journal of the American Dietetic Association* 63 (1973):161.
Human Fertility and National Development. United Nations, New York, 1971.
Jelliffe, D. B. "Parallel Food Classification in Developing and Industrialized Countries." *American Journal of Clinical Nutrition* 20 (1967):279.
Population. International Planned Parenthood Federation. London, 1973.
Sharman, A. "Nutrition and Social Planning." *Journal of Developmental Studies* 6 (1970):77.
Wilson, C. S. "Food Habits: A Selected Annotated Bibliography." *Journal of Nutrition Education* 5 (1973):Supplement 1.
Yudkin, J. "Psychological and Social Aspects of Dietary Habits." *Nutrition in Pre-school and School Age*. G. Blix, ed. Stockholm: Almquist & Wiksell, 1969.

3

nutrition and the natural sciences

The emphasis thus far has been upon the study of social and psychological factors that determine food choices which get nutrients into the body. Important as these are, an understanding of the roles played by nutrients after they are in the body depends upon knowing something of basic chemistry and physics. Occasionally people find it difficult to believe that knowledge of these sciences, which together constitute the physical sciences, is absolutely essential for understanding nutrition fully. However, it is important to remember that there are only two basic components of the entire universe, *matter* and *energy*, and that chemistry and physics are the study of these two components respectively. Therefore nutrition, like any other subject, can be understood most fully by knowing some of the basic concepts of these two most fundamental sciences and of the third natural science, biology.

SOME RELATIONSHIPS OF NUTRITION TO CHEMISTRY

Life is chemical. All living creatures, from the one-celled microscopic plant or animal to the large and complicated human, whale, or tree, act as harmonious systems of chemical reactions. Nutrients derived from foods are chemicals which must enter into the reactions of living things in order to supply materials for growth, repair, and renewal; to provide energy; and to regulate the organism's function.

Chemistry is the study of *matter*. Matter is anything which has mass (that is, which has weight when subjected to the force of gravity) and which occupies space. Matter can be divided and subdivided into categories, as shown in Figure 3–1.

Although *elements* are substances which cannot be converted into simpler substances by ordinary chemical means, as through the action of acids or other chemicals, atoms of certain elements can be split by extraordinary means, as in the atomic bomb. Living things, however, are incapable of splitting atoms in this manner.

By contrast, the millions of different *compounds* that exist can be broken down into simpler fragments, which are one or more of approximately one hundred kinds of atoms which combine to form compounds. A very familiar compound is water, H_2O. As seen from the formula, a molecule of water contains 2 atoms of hydrogen (H) and 1 atom of oxygen (O). Typically, each compound has its own set of properties, which may have no similarity to the properties of the elements of which the compound is made. For example, hydrogen (a gas) and oxygen (a gas) combine to form water (a liquid); carbon (a solid) and oxygen (a gas) combine to form carbon dioxide (a gas). Many of the compounds

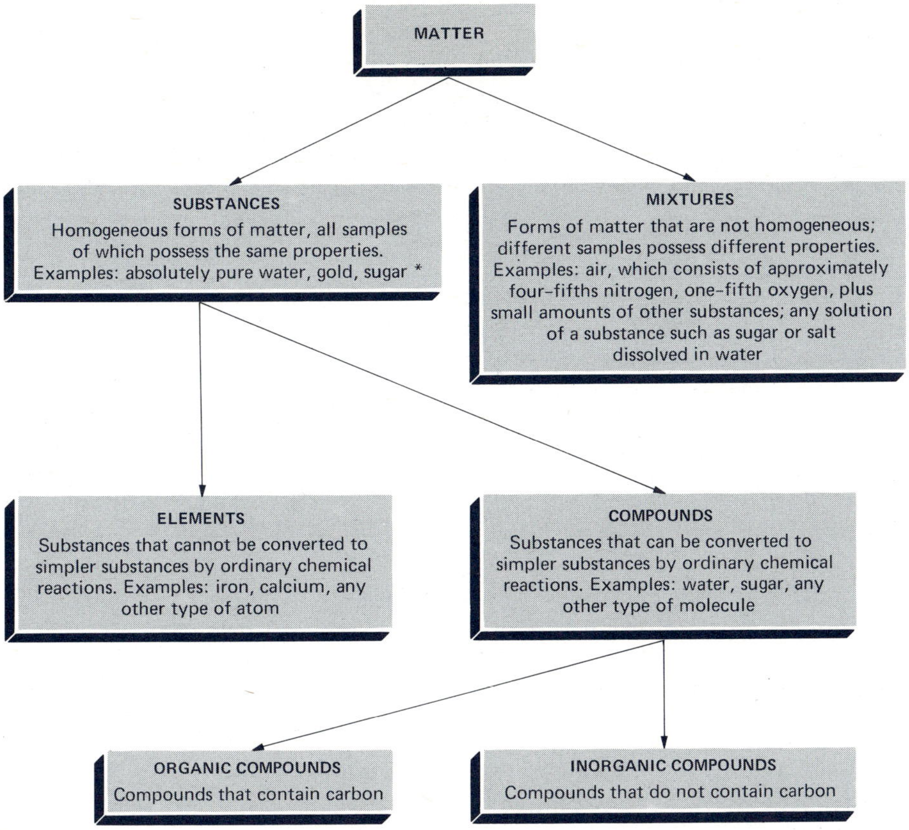

**Absolute* purity, in chemistry as in morality, is an ideal rather than a condition likely to be encountered in the real world.

FIGURE 3–1. The various forms of matter.

important in nutrition are extremely complex, consisting of thousands or millions of atoms held together by chemical bonds.

The two terms *organic* and *inorganic* are among those most commonly misunderstood by the public. To many, organic suggests life and vitality because it is believed to mean "from a living source, or organism," and inorganic implies inertness or lifelessness and is thought to mean *synthetic* or "from an inanimate source." This usage is quite understandable, because health food enthusiasts use the terms in this manner. However, it is entirely incorrect. Properly used, the term organic means that the compound contains the element carbon. Thus vitamin C, a carbon-containing compound, is organic and has exactly the same effects in the body whether it is obtained from an orange or produced synthetically in a chemistry laboratory. Similarly, water, which contains hydrogen and oxygen but no carbon, is inorganic whether it is in a lifeless raindrop or is part of a living plant or animal. Obviously, the terms *organic* and *inorganic* should have no value judgments attached to them. Water, an inorganic material, is absolutely essential to life, whereas botulism toxin, the most poisonous material known, is organic. It is therefore apparent that the "organic way" in nutrition is based on a confused definition of the term organic.

Mixtures are forms of matter that are not homogeneous, in that different samples taken from a mixture are found to possess different properties. An example of a mixture is granite, different particles of which can be seen to have different colors and hardness, and to melt at different temperatures. A solution of sugar in water appears to be homogeneous. However, if the water molecules are removed by evaporation, sugar molecules are left behind. The solution is therefore seen to be a mixture rather than a single substance.

Atomic building blocks

Although an atom cannot be broken down by ordinary means, it should not be thought of as a mere solid little sphere. Within the atom are fundamental smaller particles which are common to all atoms. The atoms of one element differ from those of other elements according to the number of the various particles found in the different atoms.

An atom contains a *nucleus* which is composed of two types of fundamental particles: the *neutron,* which has no electrical charge, and the *proton,* which has a positive charge. Circling the nucleus are tiny particles, *electrons,* which carry a negative electrical charge. The entire atom has a total, or net, charge of zero, because the number of negatively charged electrons is equal to the number of the positively charged protons.

Ions: charged atoms

If a person with a net financial worth of zero dollars somehow gets out of paying a debt (which represents negative financial worth), his *net* worth will increase. Conversely, a person with a bank balance of zero dollars can acquire a negative bank balance (or be overdrawn) by gaining additional debts which require writing more checks.

The rules governing atomic charges are the same. Atoms which have lost or gained one or more electrons are called *ions.* If an atom *loses* an electron (which has a negative charge) the atom as a whole becomes positively charged, and is called a *cation. Gain* of an electron produces a negatively charged atom known as an *anion.*

The concepts of charged atoms and gain and loss of electrons are important in two major areas of nutrition. First, one class of nutrients, the minerals, exist in foods and in the body as cations and anions rather than as uncharged atoms. Second, the release of energy from certain nutrients is possible only insofar as these nutrients can give up electrons, which are simultaneously gained by atoms in other molecules.

Chemical reactions or changes

Glucose, a particular type of sugar molecule, combines with many other glucose molecules to form the much larger starch molecule found in many foods.

Glucose burned in the presence of oxygen is converted to the smaller molecules, water and carbon dioxide.

In general, chemical changes transform one or more substances into one or more new and different substances. Of the many general types of chemical reactions, the ones most relevant to the study of nutrition are those in which the following occur:

1 Two substances, elements or compounds, *combine* to form one or more new substances. For example:

Many glucose molecules ⟶ One starch molecule

This type of reaction, a synthesis in which smaller units are built up into larger molecules, *requires* energy, just as does the building of a wood fence from individual boards.

2 One or more compounds break down to form smaller, simpler products, which may be either elements or compounds. For instance:

$C_6H_{12}O_6$	+	$6O_2$	⟶	$6CO_2$	+	$6H_2O$
glucose	plus	oxygen		carbon dioxide	plus	water
(1 molecule)		(6 molecules)		(6 molecules)		(6 molecules)

This second type of reaction, a degradation, commonly *releases* energy, just as energy is released as sound waves when a fence collapses into a disordered pile of boards.

It is readily apparent that, although the study of energy is more in the realm of physics than of chemistry, neither area can be understood without knowing something of the other.

BIOCHEMISTRY, ENZYMES, AND THE RATES OF REACTIONS

In biochemistry, which links the world of inanimate matter to the world of living things, the substances which are to be changed are called *substrates,* and the resulting substances are called *products.* In the breakdown of glucose, for example, glucose is a substrate, and carbon dioxide and water are products of the reaction.

Many vital reactions in living systems must occur at a very rapid rate in order to meet the demands of living things for the products of the reactions or for the energy released. In order to speed up reactions which would otherwise occur too slowly, living systems have developed special compounds called enzymes. These compounds act as catalysts; that is, they increase the *rate* of a reaction without being changed themselves. These relationships are depicted as follows:

$$\text{Substrate(s)} \xrightarrow{\text{enzyme}} \text{Product(s)}$$

Enzymes themselves are not required in the diet because the body can manufacture them, although of course the raw materials used must come from the diet. In the chemical reactions whereby nutrients perform their roles in a living system, enzymes produced from other nutrients are absolutely necessary.

RELATIONSHIPS OF PHYSICS TO THE STUDY OF NUTRITION

Originally, physics meant the study of all natural phenomena in the material world; thus, it included the areas now known as astronomy, biology, chemistry, and geology. Today physics is defined as the study of energy, but concepts in this field necessarily spill over into important areas in many other sciences.

Energy is the capacity to do work. Any time a change occurs in matter, work is being performed. The muscular efforts during exercise, the starting of a car, the moving of an object up a flight of stairs—all of these are forms of work and therefore require energy. Familiar forms of energy that we encounter every day are heat, light, and electricity. In nutrition, however, the form of energy which is of paramount interest is the form known as *chemical energy,* which is the energy stored in the chemical bonds which hold atoms together into molecules. When you burn a candle, the chemical energy of the wax or tallow is converted to other forms of energy, namely heat and light. Likewise, when cells "burn" certain nutrients, the chemical energy stored in the nutrient molecules is converted into forms of energy used by the cells for the work they must do to survive and function.

Conservation of energy

Energy changes in a chemical system are governed by precise laws called the laws of *thermodynamics.* Although *thermo* might suggest that only the form of energy known as heat is involved, thermodynamics encompasses changes in all forms of energy.

The first law of thermodynamics states that, although energy can be converted from one form to another, it cannot be created or destroyed; the total amount of energy present before the change is the same as at the end of the change. This is an extremely important concept in nutrition. Energy, measured in units known as calories, is used by living systems according to need. Any energy in excess of needs cannot simply be destroyed; it must be used, hence conserved, in some way. As almost everyone in our calorie-conscious society is aware, excess energy (calories) in the body is used principally to produce fat from excess nutrients. Conversely, the amount of fat in the body can decrease only if the intake of energy is decreased to a level below the amount needed.

Obtaining energy

The continuous, controlled utilization or consumption of energy is a requirement of life. All forms of life must therefore somehow obtain energy from the environment. Green plants are capable of trapping the energy of sunlight and using it to convert simple substances into the materials of which the plant is made. This energy-trapping process, known as *photosynthesis,* produces an estimated 500 billion tons of organic matter on earth each year. Plant-eating animals then obtain their energy from the plants. Other animals, including humans, obtain energy by eating the bodies of both plants and animals. Ancient peoples who worshipped the sun as the ultimate source of life were therefore not entirely wrong, for all of the energy used by living systems comes ultimately from the sun.

Release of chemical energy in living systems

If a food such as a peanut, a lump of sugar, or a piece of meat is burned, the materials in the food combine with oxygen and energy is released as heat and light. Obviously, the release of large amounts of heat and light in the body would be not only useless, but detrimental. Therefore, the energy released from food materials must in some way be made available in forms usable by the body. A special molecule, *adenosine triphosphate,* or ATP for short, enables living creatures to use the chemical energy in foods. ATP is formed by combining *adenosine diphosphate* (ADP) and a smaller phosphorous-containing part, designated P. When certain food components are broken down in the body, the energy released is used to link ADP and P together, thus forming ATP. When ATP in its turn is broken down, its chemical energy is released and thereby made available for energy-requiring reactions. Thus *ATP is the connecting link between energy-yielding and energy-requiring processes in life.* The amount of ATP produced daily in the body is astonishing; it is, in fact, roughly equal to the total weight of the body itself. Why, then, do we not become solid blocks of ATP by the end of the day? The answer is that, just as ATP is continuously produced, so it is continuously broken down in the body in order to release its trapped energy, as shown in Figure 3–2.

One of the leading uses of energy in a living system is to maintain the complex and highly orderly structure of the creature. Life does not occur if all the materials found in living things are simply mixed together in any old way; rather, the components must be arranged in specific patterns and combinations. A useful analogy is to compare a pile of bricks with an orderly arrangement of bricks in the form of a wall. The material in the pile of bricks is the same as the material in the wall. To create the wall from the bricks, however, it is necessary to supply energy and to do work. Not only must cells create order from chaos, but they must ever afterward continuously use energy to keep

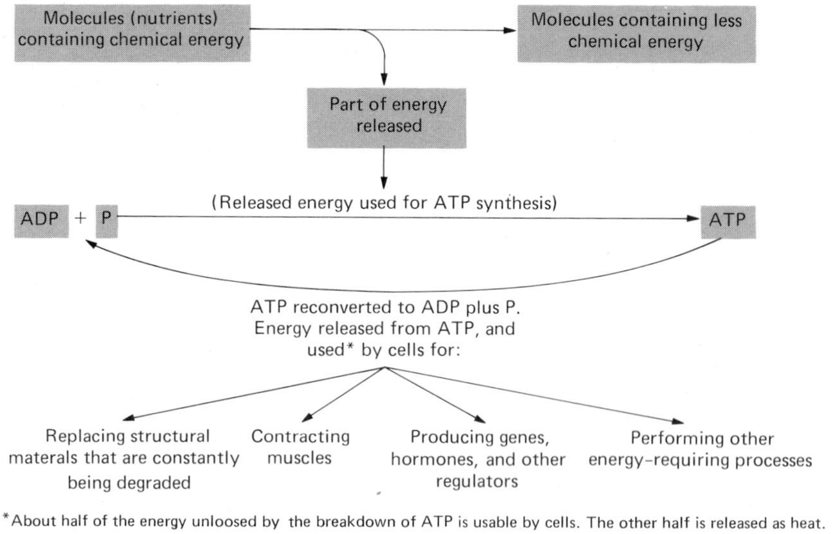

FIGURE 3–2. Life demands the continuous production and the continuous breakdown of ATP.

the orderly pattern from regressing to a random, disordered state. A living system which becomes random and disordered does not long remain alive.

Energy is also required for the movement of the body or parts of the body, and ATP must be broken down to release the energy required by the muscle which contracts to produce the movement. Everyone is aware that energy is required for familiar forms of muscular work such as walking, running, and playing (really "working at") games such as golf or tennis. Less commonly recognized is the need for energy to move the internal muscles, such as the heart muscles, the muscles that move the lungs in the act of breathing, and the organs that allow us to extract what we can use from food by the act of digestion itself.

Many other activities of living things also require energy; the light of the firefly's tail and the shock of the electric eel, for example, represent the conversion of the chemical energy of ATP to light and electrical energy. All of this energy was derived in turn from certain components of the animal's diet.

RELATIONSHIPS OF NUTRITION TO BIOLOGY

Biology is the science of life and life processes, including the study of structure, function, growth, and evolution of living things as well as the relationships of living things to their environments. Some of the important areas of biology are shown in Figure 3–3.

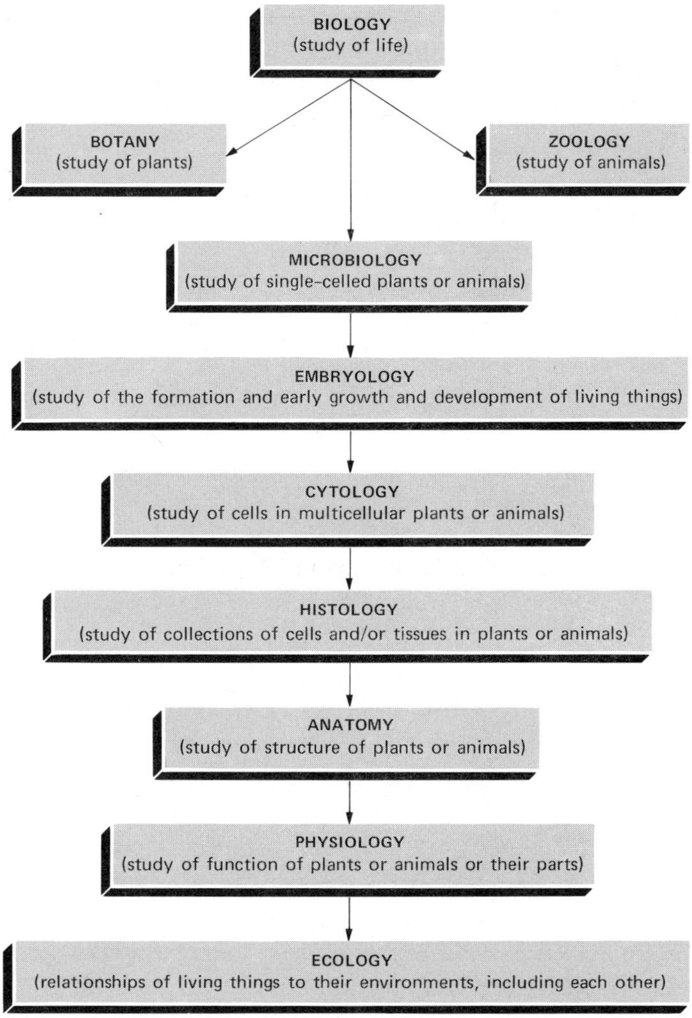

FIGURE 3–3. Biology—the science of life—actually includes many areas, each a science in itself.

Any living thing can be called an *organism*. Organisms may consist of a single cell or of trillions of cells. Because the cell is the basic unit of life, the smallest portion that has all the characteristics of life, a description of a hypothetical "typical cell" is in order.

The material of which cells are composed is called *protoplasm*. This should not be confused with the somewhat similar term *protein*. Proteins are simply large organic molecules, and each protein is therefore an individual substance. Protoplasm contains proteins, to be sure, but it also contains water (the principal constituent of living things), inorganic minerals, sugars, fats, vitamins, and a myriad of other substances. Protoplasm is, then, an incredibly complex mixture. Within this mixture, certain components form highly organized subcellular structures, some of the most important of which are shown in Figure 3–4.

The *cell membranes,* including the outer covering of the cell, appear microscopically to consist of three layers. They are often thought of as extremely thin bread and butter sandwiches, the "slices of bread" being layers of protein and the "butter" consisting of special fatlike materials called *phospholipids.* However, this is inaccurate, as cell membrances actually consist of complexes of proteins and phospholipids linked together by chemical bonds. The membrane that delineates the cell as a separate being is not merely a covering which keeps the cell contents from spilling out. It is also important in controlling materials within the cell, because all materials, including nutrients, entering the cell must cross this barrier, as must all waste materials leaving the cell.

Within the cell, usually near the center, is a small structure called the *nucleus.* This contains rod-shaped bodies called *chromosomes,* which in turn contain still smaller units known as *genes.* The genes are the units of heredity, controlling the inherited traits of the organism; chemically they consist of molecules of a special compound known as *deoxyribonucleic acid,* or DNA.

Cytoplasm is the term used for all the cellular material outside the nucleus. In this semifluid material is a highly complex system of tubes, spaces, and other organized structures. Much of the cytoplasm is filled with a maze of membrane-enclosed spaces known collectively as the *endoplasmic reticulum,* some sections of which are indicated in the diagram. Two types of endoplasmic reticulum exist, both of which may be present in the same cell. The rough, or granular, endoplasmic reticulum appears granular because numerous small particles called *ribosomes* are bound to it. Cell proteins are produced on these particles. The smooth, or granular, endoplasmic reticulum consists of membranes without any such particles attached.

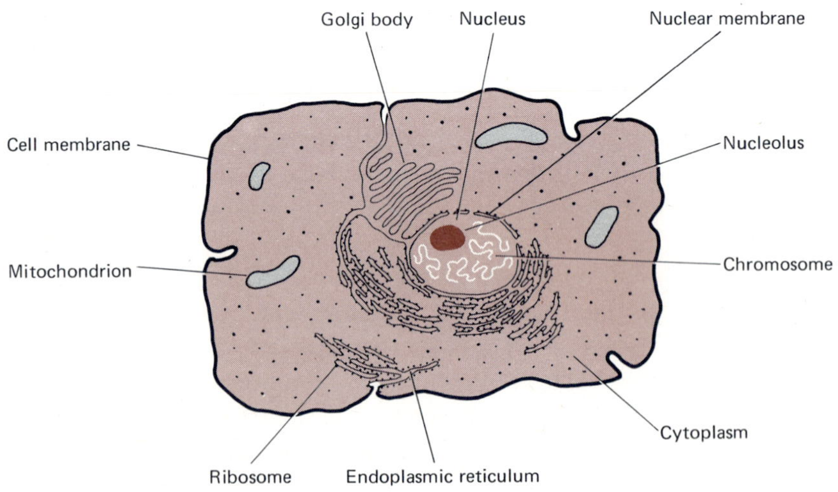

FIGURE 3–4. The main features of a hypothetical "typical cell."

Mitochondria, the sausage-shaped structures shown in Figure 3–4, are the powerhouses of the cell. It is inside the mitochondria that most of certain food components are broken down, thereby releasing energy to be trapped in the form of ATP, and subsequently used.

In addition to the structures discussed here, cells may contain other specialized structures with specific functions. Some of these are found in some cells but not in others. For example, *chloroplasts,* which contain the green pigment *chlorophyll,* are found in cells of green plants but not in cells of animals or of colorless plants such as bacteria or mushrooms. It must be recognized, therefore, that the "typical cell" does not really exist. It is, however, a useful abstraction for discussing the important features that most cells have in common with each other.

Cell specialization and differentiation

The cells in the body of a multicellular organism are not all alike; various cell types within the organism are differentiated or specialized to perform certain functions. The advantage of this specialization is that each cell type is superbly adapted to do one or a few things very well, rather than being like a jack-of-all trades—doing many things less well. For example, a mature red blood cell is marvelously adapted to carrying oxygen to other cells in the body, but completely lacking in the ability to reproduce itself by dividing; muscle cells are specialists at contracting, thereby allowing the organism to move; nerve cells, or *neurons,* are experts at conducting electrochemical nerve impulses. The *disadvantage* of specialization is that the various cell types have become completely dependent upon each other, so that injury or disease of a vital organ such as the heart, lung, or brain can bring about the death of all the cells of the organism as well as that of the injured organ itself.

Tissues and organs

When a group of similarly specialized cells function together to perform certain duties, the collection of cells is known as a *tissue.* Not all biologists agree on the number of types of tissue there are. A common classification of animal tissues consists of the following six types:

1 **Epithelial.** This type of tissue, which consists of closely packed cells arranged in layers or sheets, forms the covering of internal surfaces and internal organs as well as the outer surface of the animal. Examples are the surface of the skin, the lining of the digestive tract, and the lining of the lungs.

2 **Connective.** Connective tissue, as the name implies, forms the supporting and connecting structures of the body. Cells of this tissue produce and secrete nonliving material, called the *matrix*; it is this matrix, rather than the cells themselves, that characteristically performs the actual functions of supporting and connecting. Examples of connective tissue include the tissues of bones, tendons, ligaments, and *adipose* (fat) tissue.

TABLE 3–1

Human organ systems and nutrition

System and major functions	Major components	Examples of relationships to nutrition
1. **Circulatory** Transports materials to all parts of body.	Heart, blood vessels, blood, lymph vessels and lymph, tissue fluid, cerebrospinal fluid.	Transports nutrients, the oxygen needed for the use of nutrients as fuel, and hormones which regulate nutrient utilization.
2. **Digestive** Cleaves large molecules into smaller molecules.	Mouth, tongue, teeth, salivary glands, pharynx, esophagus, stomach, small and large intestines, liver, gallbladder, pancreas.	Splits large nutrient molecules into molecules small enough to pass from the digestive tract into the rest of the body.
3. **Endocrine** Produces chemical messengers (hormones) which integrate activities of different body parts.	Pituitary, thyroid, parathyroids, certain digestive organs, adrenals, gonads (testes in male, ovaries in female).	Regulates the utilization of virtually every nutrient in the body.
4. **Excretory** Eliminates waste products.	Kidneys, digestive tract (colon), lungs, skin.	Eliminates useless and/or toxic materials formed from nutrients in the body or ingested incidentally in foods.
5. **Integument** Covers and protects the body.	Skin and its derivatives: hair, nails, oil glands, sweat glands.	Produces vitamin D (skin); excretes significant amounts of certain nutrients, such as water and minerals in sweat.
6. **Muscular** Allows movement of whole body and of body parts.	Skeletal muscles, heart (cardiac) muscle, smooth muscle of internal organs.	Allows people to move about in search of food; moves food through digestive tract; pumps blood, thereby allowing nutrients and oxygen to be carried throughout body; increases need for calories during conscious muscular activity (exercise).
7. **Nervous** Coordinates activities of other systems by conducting impulses throughout the body.	Brain, spinal cord, nerves.	Coordinates behavior involved in obtaining food, eating, digestion, and other phases of nutrition.
8. **Reproductive** Allows perpetuation of the species.	Testes, connecting ducts, and penis in male; ovaries, fallopian tubes, uterus,	In females, increases nutritional requirements in general because of the needs of the fetus during

System and major functions	Major components	Examples of relationships to nutrition
	and vagina in female.	gestation; increases iron needs because of iron lost through menstruation. In males, sex hormones produced by testes stimulate growth, thereby increasing nutritional requirements.
9. Respiratory Allows oxygen to enter the body and carbon dioxide to leave.	Nostrils, pharynx, trachea, bronchi, lungs.	Provides oxygen required for combustion of energy-yielding nutrients; eliminates carbon dioxide produced as a result of nutrient combustion.
10. Sensory Receives stimuli from the external environment as well as from internal organs.	Eyes; ears; taste buds in tongue; tactile sensors in skin; olfactory receptors in nasal cavity; sensors in muscles, joints, and internal organs which sense muscle tension, hunger, thirst, and other internal sensations.	Allows people to detect, eat, and enjoy food; causes them to seek food and water to relieve hunger and thirst.
11. Skeletal Supports the body; along with muscular system, allows movement of body.	Bones; ligaments attaching bones to other bones; tendons attaching bones to muscles.	Allows people to move about to seek food and to escape predators which seek them as food; demands large amounts of certain nutrients, such as calcium, to support growth and maintenance of bones.

3 **Muscle.** Muscular tissue performs mechanical work by contracting; the muscle cells shorten and thicken, thereby pulling the bone or other body part to which the muscle is attached. Without muscle tissue, the animal could not move about in its environment in order to seek food, find a mate, or avoid danger, nor could it perform the less obvious internal movements, such as the beating of the heart, the contraction of muscles involved in breathing, or the churning of the stomach and intestine during digestion.

4 **Nerve.** Nervous tissue, containing specialized cells called neurons, functions to regulate and integrate the activities of distant body parts through the conduction of nerve impulses along thin fibers that extend out from the main part of the neuron. Some of these fibers may be a yard or more in length in the arm or leg of a human.

5 **Reproductive.** Reproductive tissue consists of cells whose only function is to produce a new generation. The female reproductive cell, the ovum or egg, is the largest single cell in the human body; the male reproductive cell, or sperm cell, is the smallest. Having little cytoplasm and a

"tail" with which they move themselves toward the egg, sperm cells are wonderfully adapted to their sole function of fertilizing an egg which may then develop into a new individual. For any other purpose, however, they are useless.

6 **Blood.** Blood is sometimes classified as a special type of connective tissue. However, blood has such unique roles in the body, serving to transport nutrients, oxygen, wastes, and other materials, that classifying it as a separate tissue is justified. Blood is also unique in that it is the only fluid tissue, consisting of red and white cells and other entities suspended in the liquid, plasma.

Organs and organ systems

In complex multicellular organisms such as humans, different types of tissues are arranged into more complex structures known as *organs*. Familiar examples of organs are the heart, lungs, stomach, kidneys, brain, thyroid gland, ovary, and skin. When a number of different organs function together to carry out one of the essential life functions, the collection of organs is called an *organ system*. The organ systems found in humans and other higher animals are shown in Table 3–1. It is evident that all organ systems are related to nutrition. This does not, of course, mean that being nourished is the only, or even the principal, basis of having developed each of the systems. One could just as well write Table 3–1 in terms of the relationship of each organ system to sexual activity, for example, Then, the function of the circulatory system in transporting materials needed for reproduction would be emphasized, as would the importance of the digestive system in assimilating food to support courtship, sexual intercourse, and reproduction. Because this is a book on nutrition rather than on sex, the stress has been placed upon the relationships of each system to nutrition; this in no way implies that all the parts of the body exist solely to nourish the body. The question, "Do we eat to live, or do we live to eat?" is no less than a form of the question, "What is the meaning or purpose of life?" And this is not a properly scientific question.

SUGGESTED READINGS

Fruton, J. S. *Molecules and Life. Historical Essays on the Interplay of Chemistry and Biology*. New York: Wiley, 1972.

Goldsby, R. A. *Cells and Energy*. New York: Macmillan, 1967.

Lapp, R. E. and the Editors of Time-Life Books. *Matter*. New York: Time-Life, 1974.

McGilvery, R. W. *Biochemical Concepts*. Philadelphia: Saunders, 1975.

Thomas, L. *The Lives of a Cell*. New York: Viking, 1974.

Villee, C. A. *Biology*, sixth edition. Philadelphia: Saunders, 1972.

4

foods and nutrients: comparisons and contrasts

The words *food* and *nutrient* are commonly, although incorrectly, used as if they were synonyms: "essential foods such as vitamins," "breads and other starches," "proteins such as meats and eggs." It is important that foods and nutrients be distinguished clearly from each other with respect to what they are as well as to what they do. Otherwise, much of the material in the following chapters may be misinterpreted.

FOOD AND CULTURE

Literally hundreds of different items are accepted as foods in one or more parts of the world. All of them are derived from once-living plants or animals, and are generally safe for all normal humans. But what is considered *suitable* as food in one culture may be totally unacceptable in another. For example, how many of you would eat the following?

Raw fish. Considered excellent in many parts of the Far East.
Camel. Delicious to the nomads of Near Eastern countries.
Locust. Considered a delicacy in certain Near East desert areas.
Blood mixed with milk. A staple food to the people of the Masai tribe of Africa.
Duck and chick eggs containing well-developed embryos. Highly prized in the Philippines.
Guinea pigs. Roasted and eaten in parts of South America.
Octopus. Valued as fine food in Mediterranean countries, many Pacific islands, Asia, Central and South America, and the Caribbean.

In addition to differences between cultures, there is considerable variation in what is considered suitable by various subgroups within a culture. The *average* American has eating beliefs and practices different from the following, which characterize certain groups within the United States:

Pork. Forbidden to Orthodox Jews and Moslems.
Meat of any kind. Forbidden to Seventh Day Adventists, rejected by various other groups for reasons ranging from health beliefs to ethical objections to killing animals.
Meat which has not been drained of blood as thoroughly as possible. Forbidden to Orthodox Jews, frowned upon by Jehovah's Witnesses.
Combinations of meat and dairy products. Forbidden to Orthodox Jews.
Goat's milk. Preferred to cow's milk by many Americans of Italian and Greek descent.
Rice. Used as a staple food daily by many of Oriental and Puerto Rican origin.
Unleavened bread. Required of Orthodox Jews during the Passover.
"Greens" such as collards and turnip tops, cooked with salt pork for an extended period of time. Enjoyed by Southerners more than by people of other areas in the United States.
Olive oil. Definitely preferred to other cooking fats by Italian-Americans and those of Near Eastern origin, such as Syrian, Greek, and Armenian.

Soy sauce. Used as a seasoning in almost every main dish by traditional Chinese-Americans.
Red chili powder. Considered an indispensible seasoning by many Mexican-Americans.
Alcoholic beverages. Absolutely prohibited by some religions, allowed with reservation by others, casually accepted as a part of daily meals by some ethnic groups.
Food in general. Forbidden at certain times by groups in which fasting is a religious obligation.

Changes in ethnic food habits

Distinctive food habits of a group help to promote feelings of solidarity and group loyalty. Nevertheless, many well-defined ethnic differences are becoming less marked than previously in the United States. One reason is that most present-day Americans are generations removed from the ancestors who came from countries with distinctive food habits. Also, social and educational forces such as advertising and school lunch programs have done much to level the eating practices of the majority of Americans to the same standard of quality (some would say "mediocrity"). As a result, foods once familiar to only one or a few ethnic groups have become accepted by others outside the group; for example, tacos, eaten mostly in the Southwest and especially by Mexican-Americans twenty-five years ago, are acceptable to people of all groups throughout the United States today.

Another factor in the fading of many ethnic eating habits is the desire of members of minority groups to become fully assimilated into the mainstream of American society. People can more easily become typical members of a society if their eating patterns do not vary greatly from the accepted norm. Also, particularly among younger people, there is a tendency to reject food habits dictated by religion and marking one as "different" in this respect.

Finally, the tendency to think or at least to speak of certain foods as typical of a given group has decreased as people have become more sensitive to the issue of civil rights. In the past, food habits, real or imagined, have sometimes been used in a very unfeeling manner to stereotype racial and ethnic groups. The old-fashioned cartoon of the black boy grinning over his slice of watermelon, the picture of the Irishman eating and getting roaring drunk at a wake, the image of the Greek or Italian reeking of garlic and strong cheese are repugnant to those who see such stereotyping as incompatible with the concept of universal human dignity.

Conversely, in some cases group pride has brought about a modern resurgence of interest in traditional eating patterns, such as the recently revived interest in traditional foods of Black Americans. Why, after all, should greens such as collards, or chitterlings ("chitlins," the small intestines of pigs) be avoided or eaten in shameful secret by racially proud blacks? Black is beautiful; therefore soul food is acceptable.

Individual differences in food acceptance

Although it is common to assume that all members of a group adhere to their group's "typical" pattern, there actually may be much diversification between members of a given subculture. An interesting activity is to rate a number of foods as "enjoyable," "acceptable but not enjoyable," or "unacceptable," and then to compare your own responses with those of others in your general social group. The following list of foods may serve to suggest others which could be rated in this manner:

- pork
- horsemeat
- goat meat
- liver
- kidneys
- sweetbreads (pancreas or thymus of animals)
- brains
- chicken eggs
- fish eggs (caviar)
- testes (also called "mountain oysters")
- ovaries
- cow's milk
- sheep's milk
- American cheese
- blue cheese (blue because it contains a particular type of mold)
- eggplant
- okra
- spinach
- zucchini
- ordinary white bread
- garlic bread
- sourdough bread

One item—ovaries—could legitimately bring forth the complaint, "trick question," for the ripened ovaries of seed-bearing plants are fruits. Nevertheless, varying numbers of individuals will reject every other item on the list precisely because they *can* identify the item—and they identify it as something they don't like.

NUTRIENTS: THE COMMON DENOMINATORS

In contrast to foods, relatively few items are classed as nutrients for humans. Also in contrast to foods, nutrients are commonly derived from nonliving as well as living sources; minerals, for example, may be extracted directly from the soil, and most of the water ingested by organisms comes from sources such as wells and rivers rather than from the bodies of plants and animals.

There are no cultural differences for nutrients as there are for foods; a substance that is a nutrient for the average middle-class American is also a nutrient for the average poor American and for the average member of a small religious sect. There *are* certain racial differences, but these are biologically inherited rather than culturally transmitted. A race is, after all, simply a group of people which differs from another group with respect to certain inherited genetic characteristics. An example of a nutritionally significant racial difference is the higher frequency of intolerance to milk in nonwhites compared to whites. Properly speaking, the reaction is not to the food as a whole but to one specific nutrient in milk: *lactose*, or "milk sugar." Compared to whites, members of other races are more likely to lack the ability to digest this sugar. Because undigested lactose remains in the intestinal tract rather than being assimilated into the body, it can cause severe intestinal distress.

Two points, however, should be noted. First, the majority of nonwhites, like the majority of whites, *can* digest lactose. Second, the similarities in nutrient needs and utilization are far more numerous than the differences between various races. In general, therefore, it can be stated that the substances used as nutrients are much the same for all cultures, subcultures, and individuals within the human species.

The six nutrient classes—or is it seven?

All nutrients can be placed in one of the following classes:

Carbohydrates	Proteins	Vitamins
Fats	Minerals	Water

In addition, *alcohol,* which in several respects is unlike any of the above six classes, is unquestionably a nutrient and should therefore perhaps be considered a seventh nutrient class in itself. Alcohol, however, is generally not discussed as a nutrient, perhaps because it is consumed primarily as a drug rather than for any nutritional value. Also, there is a tendency to dismiss alcohol as a significant part of the diet, especially the diets of college students, who constitute the largest group of readers of nutrition textbooks. The fact is, of course, that alcohol is used to some degree by the majority of adults, and to excess by a disturbingly large number; ignoring it by omitting it from the list of nutrients is hardly likely to change these realities.

Essential and nonessential nutrients

The term *essential* is used differently in nutrition than in general conversation. An essential nutrient is *one which the organism cannot synthesize (produce) in amounts sufficient to meet its needs.* The following points deserve emphasis:

1 "Essential" does not merely mean "important." Glucose, the principal sugar found in the bloodstream, is extremely *important* to the functioning of the brain; however, it is not an *essential* nutrient because the body can, if necessary, synthesize it in sufficient amounts from other dietary materials.

2 Any nutrient which is necessary for life, and which cannot be synthesized in sufficient amounts in the organism, must be obtained from the environment and is therefore by definition *essential.* Except for unusual cases, such as injection of a nutrient directly into the blood or other tissues, nutrients are obtained from the environment by ingestion of food and water.

3 The *amount* synthesized is an important part of the definition of an essential nutrient. Water, for example, is produced when certain nutrients are broken down in cells. However, the amount produced in this way is far too small to sustain life in most species, and water is therefore an essential nutrient.

4 Some nutrients cannot be synthesized in any amount whatever by cells. For example, minerals, which are elements, cannot be produced

from other materials; turning lead into gold, the medieval alchemist's dream, is impossible by any chemical means. Therefore, any mineral needed for life is an essential nutrient because the body cannot produce it, either from another mineral or from any other substance.

5 A *nonessential* nutrient is one which *can* be synthesized in amounts sufficient to satisfy the organism's needs. Nonessential does not in any way imply lack of importance; in a wide variety of living systems, many vitally important biochemicals are nonessential because the organism's cells can produce adequate amounts of them. However, one species' essential nutrient may be nonessential to other species. For example, plants can produce vitamins and other organic compounds which are dietary essentials for humans and other animals, as humans can produce certain materials which must be obtained from the environment by other forms of life.

Each of the six major nutrient classes will be discussed in some detail in later chapters. For the time being, the important point is that certain specific *nutrients* within these classes are needed in the diet. By contrast, no single specific *food* is essential. Vitamin C, for example, is needed in the diet by all humans; if the supply is inadequate, disease occurs and eventually the person dies. However, there are no such requirements for specific *foods* as vitamin C sources. Vitamin C from green peppers or broccoli, or, for that matter, from vitamin C tablets, is fully as effective as vitamin C from oranges. Thus many foods can be substituted for any one given food, whereas no nutrient can take the place of another essential nutrient.

THE FUNCTIONS OF FOODS AND OF NUTRIENTS

The functions of foods, that is, the things they do for us, have been discussed previously. To reiterate, foods have three general functions:

1 **Biological function.** Foods supply nutrients needed to sustain the organism's life.
2 **Psychological function.** Foods meet needs related to the mind, the emotions, and individual behavior.
3 **Social function.** Foods fulfill certain needs of interacting groups.

A single given food may perform two or even all three of these functions. Something as simple as a cup of black coffee has biological value (in providing the essential nutrient, water); psychological value (by containing the stimulant caffeine and by signaling "Wake up!" when the first cup is drunk in the morning); and social value (at events such as coffee breaks and coffee klatches). To take another example, steak fulfills no more biological function than stewing beef, but has much more value for many people because of its ability to meet psychological and social needs.

What is the minimum number of foods which, in combination, could fairly well satisfy the nutrient needs of an average person? This question is rather commonly asked. One such combination would be a steady diet of the following:

milk: 1 quart or more daily
enriched or whole grain bread: 1 to 2 pounds daily
tomatoes (canned or fresh): 1 pound daily

However, for how long would most people be willing to restrict themselves to this biologically adequate diet? Unmet social and psychological needs and the resulting dissatisfaction would drive almost anyone to seek other foods to meet these needs—perhaps even at the cost of lower nutrient intakes.

Nutrients, in contrast to foods, do not serve primarily social and psychological functions. Instead they have three general functions, all related to biological needs:

1. **Building and maintaining the structure of the organism.**
2. **Serving as energy sources.**
3. **Regulating biological processes.**

The role of nutrients in building and maintenance of organisms

All forms of life that can be studied scientifically have a physical structure. (If any such entities as living disembodied spirits exist, the study of these is in the field of theology rather than in the natural sciences.) Nutrients are the materials necessary for building and maintaining physical structure, including the solid materials and fluids surrounding the cells as well as the cells themselves.

Traditionally, water, proteins, and minerals are listed as the most important building materials because together these three nutrient classes make up a very large part of the body's total lean (or fat-free) mass, as shown in Table 4–1.

Although carbohydrates and vitamins together constitute less than one one-hundredth of the weight of the body, these nutrients are nevertheless extremely important parts of body structure. Certain carbohydrates are integral parts of hormones and other important molecules, and the significance of vitamins in body structure is illustrated dramatically by the decreased growth which occurs in many vitamin deficiencies. Thus, although vitamins and carbohydrates are not *quantitatively* great parts of biological structure, they are extremely important parts nevertheless.

Fat was once considered merely an inert storehouse of excess energy, to be drawn on in time of need. Today we know that fat tissue is a vital, active part of the body. In addition, certain specialized fatty substances have important roles as parts of cells and organs; the phospholipids, for example, are part of the membrances of cells. It is therefore inaccurate to look upon fats as expendable body components as compared to the materials that constitute lean body tissues.

Finally, the old concept of body structure should be revised. Structure was once believed to be a relatively permanent arrangement, like that of a formal living room, whereas materials such as carbohydrates and fats were considered analogous to the fuels expended to heat the room. Today we know that the situation is much more complicated. It

TABLE 4–1
Composition of the human body

Approximate percent of:	**Normal adult male**	**Normal adult female**
Water	60.0	60.0
Protein	15.0	15.0
Minerals	5.0	5.0
Fats	15.0	20.0 or more
Carbohydrates	0.5	0.5
Vitamins	Very small part of 1 percent	Very small part of 1 percent

The above figures do not add up to 100 percent because they are very rough estimates, presented for the purpose of making certain points. Note that men and women are similar in body composition except for the difference in fat content.

is as if the very walls and furniture of the room itself are continuously being broken down, some to be consumed as fuel and some to be recycled for building new walls and furniture. At the same time, the materials formerly thought of as mere fuels are now known to be used to some extent as building materials for the room and furnishings. The modern concept of this continuous, dynamic process of change, called *turnover* of body constituents, makes the former classification obsolete. All six nutrient classes, and not just water, proteins, and minerals, play major roles in the growth and maintenance of living systems.

The function of nutrients as energy sources

Because the nutrients which human cells break down in order to obtain energy are carbohydrates, fats, and proteins, plus alcohol, these substances are called *energy nutrients.*

Note the word *human* in the previous sentence, for different species are capable of using other nutrients as energy sources. Certain bacteria, for example, can obtain energy from organic compounds useless to higher species such as humans; reports of "making food from oil" refer to studies on the feasibility of growing edible microorganisms on petroleum, or crude oil. These microorganisms can use petroleum as an energy source, as an automobile can—and as a human obviously cannot. Microorganisms in the intestines of termites produce enzymes that digest the compound, cellulose, in wood. Human cells cannot, of course, use wood as an energy source; desperate attempts of people to survive famine by making bread from sawdust invariably led to death by starvation. Properly speaking, the cells of termites cannot digest cellulose either. It is only through the intervention of the microbes in the termite's digestive tract that termites live by eating wood.

The energy nutrients used by humans have the following characteristics:

1. They are all organic compounds which cells can break down to simpler compounds.
2. As a result of their breakdown, energy is released; the number of units of energy resulting from the breakdown of a given amount varies from nutrient to nutrient, however.
3. *Energy nutrients* do *not* include vitamins, minerals, or water. There is a good deal of misunderstanding on this point, partly because the term *energy* is commonly misused. Energy is *not* a feeling of vigor, enthusiasm, or determination; it is the physical capacity to do work. Very often, however, this is obscured, as in the following examples:

Vitamin-fortified foods such as breakfast cereals have been advertised as "high energy" foods.

Vitamin supplements such as pills and tonics, with or without added iron, are touted as "providing energy." One brand used the slogan "tired blood" to suggest the "lack of energy" which supposedly existed unless the supplement were taken.

People often feel as if they "lack energy" when they are hot, tired, and thirsty; they "regain their energy" after a drink of cold water.

The relationship of minerals, vitamins, and water to energy, when the term is used correctly, are all indirect. It will be recalled that any biochemical reaction can be represented as follows:

$$\text{Substrate(s)} \xrightarrow{\text{(enzyme)}} \text{Product(s)}$$

In energy-releasing reactions the *substrates* are energy nutrients. Vitamins and minerals are frequently necessary parts of the structures of enzymes, which catalyze biochemical reactions, and water molecules may enter into reactions as well as being the liquid in which biochemical reactions occur. The term "energy nutrient," however, should be reserved exclusively for those nutrients that serve as substrates in biochemical reactions whereby energy can be released, and the only nutrients in human diets that meet this criterion are carbohydrates, fats, and proteins, as well as alcohol.

The functions of nutrients in regulating biological processes

Because life can continue only within a certain narrow range of conditions, everything that goes on in a living system must be regulated, or controlled. If an organism becomes too hot, too cold, too acid, too non-acid (also called *alkaline* or *basic*), too abundant with respect to toxic materials or too lacking in needed substances, the organism will die. The process of regulating the conditions inside the organism, thereby maintaining a relatively constant internal environment, is called *homeostasis,* a word that means literally "staying the same or similar." However, as the old French saying puts it, "The more things change, the more they remain the same." The constant internal conditions actually constitute a state of dynamic equilibrium achieved through continual changes dictated by the organism's needs. Too hot? Sweat, and lose body heat through the evaporation of the water in sweat. Too cold? Increase the rate of energy nutrient breakdown, thereby releasing energy as heat; or shiver, thus releasing energy as heat as well as for the uncontrolled muscle contractions known as shivering. Too high a level of sugar (glucose) in the blood? Release more insulin, which lowers blood glucose. Too much of some toxic material in the body? Excrete it, or produce larger amounts of an enzyme that converts the toxin to an innocuous substance. In short, great deviations from ideal conditions must be avoided by making continual adjustments.

The mechanisms for controlling the internal environment include certain nutrients in the same form in which they occur in the diet, as well as many substances that are *not* properly called nutrients. Genes and hormones, for example, need not be ingested because the body is capable of producing them. However, the materials from which they are produced must all be provided from the animal's diet. In summary, then, regulation of biological functions by nutrients occurs in the following two general ways:

FIGURE 4–1. The composition of some common foods. The vitamin content is too small to be shown on the graph.

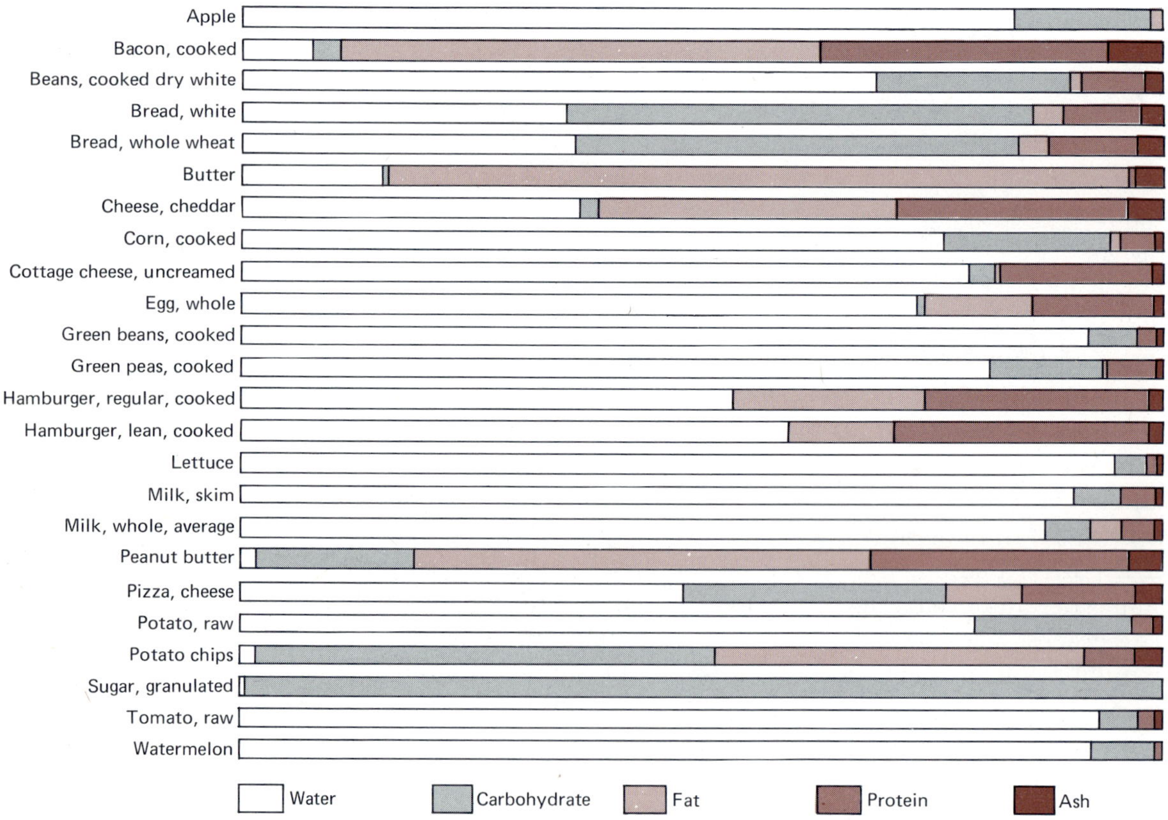

Nutrients per se function as regulators, in the original forms in which they are found in the diet.
Nutrients provide raw materials for synthesizing regulators which originate within the organism itself.

THE COMPOSITION OF FOODS: THE CHEMICALS WE EAT

Although it is not correct to refer to meats as "proteins" or breads as "starches," it *is* correct to classify foods in terms of the relative amounts of various nutrients in them. Figure 4–1 shows the composition of a number of common foods in terms of the percentage of water, proteins, fats, carbohydrates, and minerals which they contain. The vitamin contents of foods, like the vitamin content of the body, are far too small to be shown on any reasonable-sized graph. The following points can readily be seen from the chart:

1. Foods as they are obtained from nature are not pure substances (elements or compounds) by any means. They are wild mixtures of all the nutrient classes, and often contain nonnutrient materials as well.

2. By contrast, foods that are very highly processed, such as table sugar, vegetable oils, or plain unflavored gelatin, may consist of virtually 100 percent carbohydrate, fat, or protein.

3. Intermediate between unprocessed foods and very highly refined foods are such processed items as flour, corn meal, and cheese. The nutrient content of these foods is different than the composition of the whole wheat, corn, and milk from which they were made, but this does not necessarily imply that their nutritional value has been significantly decreased.

4. The most abundant component of most foods is water. A "solid" food such as watermelon may actually contain a higher percent of water than a liquid food such as milk; a raw potato, which appears to be very solid compared to a raw egg, in fact contains a slightly higher percent of water than does the egg.

5. The most abundant *solid* component of a food may be carbohydrate, fat, or protein.

6. Except for very highly processed foods such as sugar, oils, and corn starch, all foods contain protein; this is to be expected in view of the origin of foods from living things, all of which contain proteins. Not all foods, however, contain *enough* protein or the right *kinds* of proteins to make them valuable as dietary protein sources.

7. A food may be classified as "high protein" even though it contains less protein than fat or carbohydrate. For example, nuts contain more fat than protein, and dried mature beans and peas contain more carbohydrate than protein. However, in categorizing a food as high in protein, the important consideration is whether the food is a *nutritionally significant* protein source, because it is much easier to obtain sufficient fat or carbohydrate than sufficient protein.

8. Foods of animal origin tend to be rich in protein and fat and in general contain very little carbohydrate. Exceptions are milk (which contains slightly more milk sugar than either fat or protein), and fatty foods such as lard, bacon, and salt pork, which contain little or no protein. Liver is the one meat which may contain up to 5 percent of carbohydrate because carbohydrate is stored in rather high concentration in the animal's liver.

9. Foods of plant origin are, in general, much higher in carbohydrate content than in fat or protein content. Exceptions include nuts, olives, and avocados which are rich in fat, and mushrooms which contain about equal proportions of carbohydrate and protein.

10. Fruits and vegetables are generally high in water content. The carbohydrates present may be sugars or starches (which supply energy) or cellulose (which is not an energy source for humans). The energy (calorie) values of various fruits and vegetables will therefore depend upon the type as well as the amount of carbohydrates present.

11. The mineral or *ash* content of foods (so-called because it remains as incombustible ash after a sample of food is burned completely) is generally small. This is partly because the tissues with the highest concentrations of minerals in an animal's body are the teeth and bones, which of course are not ordinarily used as food. The mineral content of many foods has been increased considerably over "natural" levels by the use of sodium chloride (common salt) as an additive. Even so, ash usually accounts for no more than a few percent of the total weight of foods.

12. Even unusually rich sources of vitamins contain too little of these to represent on a graph. A 4 ounce serving of orange juice, for example, contains approximately 0.002 ounce of vitamin C, or 0.05 percent of the total weight of the juice. People who know that vitamin C is another name for ascorbic acid sometimes assume that it is this vitamin which gives citrus fruits their acid flavor. Actually, the acidity of citrus fruits is caused by substances such as citric acid, and not by a vitamin. With few exceptions, vitamins in foods are present in amounts far too small to affect taste, odor, appearance, or other *organoleptic* qualities.

SUGGESTED READINGS

Benarde, M. A. *The Chemicals We Eat*. New York: American Heritage Publishing, 1971.

"Diet as a Regulator of Metabolism." *Dairy Council Digest* 42 (1971):28.

Food and Nutrition Board, National Research Council–National Academy of Sciences. *Recommended Dietary Allowances,* eighth edition. Washington, D.C., 1974.

Hegarty, P. V. J. "Some Biological Considerations in the Nutritional Evaluation of Foods." *Food Technology* 29 (1975):52.

"Treating Alcoholism: The Illness, The Symptoms, The Treatment." National Institute on Alcohol Abuse and Alcoholism, Rockville, Maryland, 1975.

5

the nutrients: some basics

In contrast to foods, which are complex mixtures, nutrients are pure substances. Nutrients can therefore be classed largely on the basis of their chemical and biochemical characteristics, as shown in Table 5–1.

Because members within each nutrient class may differ greatly from each other, an introduction to the chemistry and biology of important representatives of each class is in order. People commonly find it somewhat more difficult to become familiar with the chemical struc-

TABLE 5–1
Classification of nutrients as biochemicals

Class	Element or compound	Organic or inorganic	Energy nutrient
Carbohydrates	Compounds	Organic	Yes
Fats	Compounds	Organic	Yes
Proteins	Compounds	Organic	Yes
Minerals	Elements	Inorganic	No
Vitamins	Compounds	Organic	No
Water	Compound	Inorganic	No

FIGURE 5–1. Carbohydrates significant in nutrition.

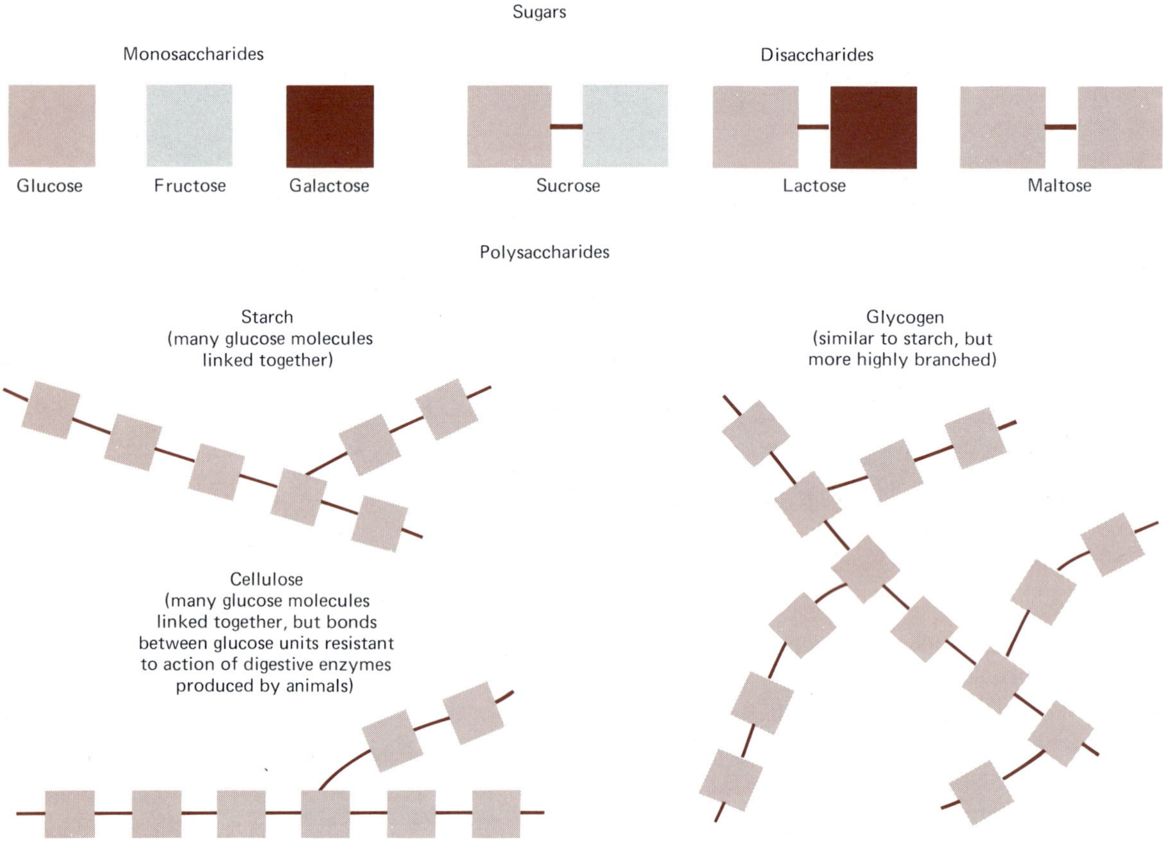

tures of the nutrients than to learn about their purely physiological aspects. However, structure and function are so intimately related that the time required to learn the general features of nutrient structure is well spent. The chemistry can be ignored only at the cost of later difficulty in understanding the functions of nutrients.

CARBOHYDRATES

A number of nutritionally important carbohydrate molecules are represented in Figure 5–1. All contain atoms of carbon, hydrogen, and oxygen, with hydrogen and oxygen present in the same proportion (two to one) as in water, H_2O; hence the name carbohydrate (hydrate = water).

Monosaccharides, or simple sugars, are carbohydrates that contain 4, 5, 6, or slightly more carbon atoms. Most of the nutritionally important simple sugars contain 6 carbons and are therefore called *hexoses.* The ones with which we will be most concerned are the following:

Glucose. This is the principal form of carbohydrate in the blood of humans and other animals. In foods, it occurs as such in a relatively small number of items, including honey and certain fruits; other items, ranging from intravenous feedings to candies, have glucose as an important ingredient. It is often listed on the label under its alternate name, *dextrose.* In addition to occurring in nature as the free, uncombined molecule, glucose is part of the structure of most larger carbohydrates. If this enormous amount of combined glucose is considered, as well as that which occurs in free form, glucose is the most abundant organic molecule in foods, and indeed in the world.

Fructose. Also called *levulose,* this is found mostly linked chemically to glucose to form sucrose, or common table sugar. The sweetest of all sugars, fructose in the uncombined form gives honey its extremely sweet taste and imparts a distinct sweetness to many fruits in which it is found in small amounts.

Galactose. This is almost invariably found linked to glucose to form lactose, or milk sugar, although extremely small amounts of galactose are also found in the uncombined form.

Disaccharides are molecules formed by the linking together of two monosaccharides. During digestion, the bond between the two simple sugars is broken, and the resulting free monosaccharides are absorbed into the organism's bloodstream. The disaccharides found most commonly in foods are the following:

Sucrose. Common table sugar, sucrose is formed by chemical combination of glucose and fructose, and is found in many fruits and vegetables. Sucrose obtained from sugar beets or other plants is identical to sucrose from sugar cane, because it is chemical structure, and not origin, which determines a molecule's characteristics.

Lactose. This is milk sugar, which consists of glucose and galactose linked together, and is found in milk; all mammals secrete milk containing lactose and no other sugars. Physicians, nutritionists, and geneticists are particularly interested in studying this disaccharide because of two distinct types of inherited diseases. In one type, the individual is unable to digest lactose, that is, to split the chemical bond which holds the two monosaccharide units together. In the second type, the person can digest lactose but cannot subsequently utilize the galactose subunit normally.

Maltose. This consists of two glucose molecules linked together, and is found most commonly in sprouting grains, such as those used in the production of beer and distilled liquors. Otherwise, it is an uncommon component of foods.

These carbohydrates, monosaccharides and disaccharides, all have the following characteristics in common:

1. In contrast to the large polysaccharides (to be discussed next), they are sugars, having a sweet taste. The degree of sweetness varies from one sugar to another; lactose, for example, is much less sweet than is an equal amount of sucrose.

2. They are identified as sugars by the characteristic *ose* ending of their names.

Polysaccharides are large carbohydrates consisting of hundreds or thousands of glucose molecules linked together. For this reason, they are called *polymers* of glucose (poly = many, mer = part). When polysaccharides are digested, the individual simple sugars are liberated, as beads are when the string of a necklace is cut.

Starch. This is found only in plants, where it functions as a reserve form of energy. During digestion, it is cleaved first to dextrins, which are smaller molecules than starch but still far larger than sugars; further digestion produces maltose, and finally glucose.

Glycogen. Also called *animal starch,* this is the storage form of carbohydrate in animals. The maximum amount of glycogen that can be stored in the human body is approximately one pound, about one-fifth of which is found in the liver alone. The remainder is distributed throughout other body parts, especially the muscles.

Cellulose. Like starch, this is found in plants and not in animals. Unlike starch, however, it functions as an integral part of the plant's cell walls, rather than as an energy reserve. Because the bonds between adjacent glucose units in the cellulose molecule are different from the bonds in glycogen and starch, cellulose is resistant to the digestive enzymes which break the bonds of other polysaccharides. Consequently, cellulose cannot be utilized as an energy source by humans. Nevertheless, it has important functions in nutrition. First, it provides roughage, also called fiber or bulk, which stimulates contraction of muscles in the intestinal walls. This helps to move food material along the digestive tract. Second, it absorbs water, just as a paper towel (which is largely cellulose) absorbs spilled liquid; this helps to keep the material in the intestines soft and moist. Third, cellulose can be an *indirect* source of energy for animals which cannot digest it. Bacteria digest cellulose inside the rumen, or specialized stomach, of cud-chewing animals such as cattle, sheep, and goats. These animals can then produce milk and flesh by utilizing the glucose and products of glucose breakdown yielded from cellulose by the bacteria. Therefore, people consuming meat or milk from these animals are obtaining nutrients derived originally from cellulose in the plants the animals grazed upon.

FATS AND OILS

Fats and oils differ from carbohydrates in several important respects. First, they are insoluble in water, but are soluble in organic solvents such as ether and carbon tetrachloride, which is the reason people use these solvents for removing grease spots from clothing. Second, they have a much higher ratio of hydrogen to oxygen than carbohydrates or proteins have; as will be shown later, this is why fats and oils furnish far more energy than do equal weights of other energy nutrients. Third, they may be either solids (in which case they are called *fats*) or liquids (which are called *oils*). Finally, they are made up of two types of distinctly different basic units, *fatty acids* and *glycerol*. Because typical fats or oils consist of three fatty acids linked to a glycerol molecule, they are called *triglycerides* (Figure 5–2). The consistent fea-

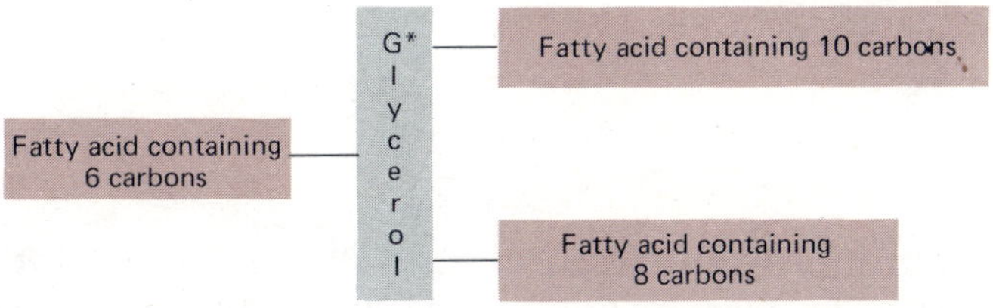

*Glycerol is a 3-carbon compound. To each of the 3 carbons is attached a fatty acid, which may have as few as 4 or as many as 20 or more carbons atoms. Thus the structure of one triglyceride may vary greatly from that of others, depending upon the particular fatty acids linked to the glycerol molecule.

FIGURE 5–2. A typical fat or oil is a triglyceride; 3 fatty acids are chemically linked to glycerol.

ture of structure in a fat or oil is the glycerol part of the molecule. By contrast, the fatty acid units may vary with respect to the number of carbons in the chain, the type of chemical bond between adjacent carbons, and the ability of the organism to synthesize one or another specific fatty acid.

A word which is sometimes used as a synonym for fat, though not quite accurately, is the term *lipid*. Lipids, however, include *all* substances which dissolve in organic solvents. Materials of little or no nutritional importance, such as waxes and certain hormones, are lipids, as are some vitamins. Therefore, in nutrition the term *fat* or *oil* is preferable to the broader term *lipid*.

Fats are generally given much less credit for their value in the diet than they actually deserve. As will be seen later, fats perform several important functions other than merely providing calories.

PROTEINS

Proteins are very large molecules or polymers made up of *amino acids* linked together. The structures of a few of the approximately 20 amino acids found as subunits of proteins are shown in Figure 5–3.

Like carbohydrates and fats, proteins contain carbon, hydrogen,

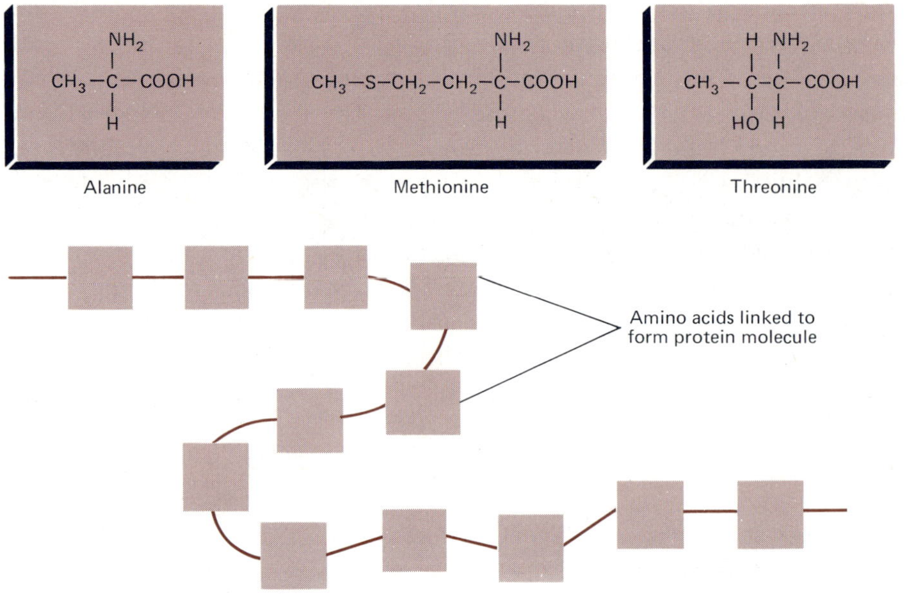

FIGURE 5–3. The structures of 3 of the 20 or so different amino acids. Hundreds, or perhaps many thousands, of amino acids are chemically linked together in a single protein molecule.

and oxygen. However, all proteins contain the element *nitrogen* as well, and some, although not all, also contain sulfur and other elements.

No single specific protein is essential in the diet; people could remain healthy throughout life without ever once ingesting a molecule of *hemoglobin, collagen,* or any other given protein. What *are* essential in the human diet are 8 specific amino acids. The others can be produced in sufficient amounts by the cells themselves and are therefore nonessential.

Many people apparently do not realize that a deficiency of one or more essential amino acids is possible despite a high total protein intake. Thus the diet of a strict vegetarian, which may contain an adequate amount of total protein, may nevertheless lack adequate amounts of one or more essential amino acids. This is because the quality as well as quantity of dietary protein is crucial, and the quality of proteins depends upon the particular amino acids that make up the protein molecules.

Interest in this class of nutrients is currently high because protein deficiency is a severe problem in many of the less developed areas of the world. The reasons can be divided into two great classes: those related to the physico-chemical-biological environment, which limit availability, and those of the sociocultural environment, which limit acceptance.

Physical, chemical, and biological factors in protein availability

Simple nitrogen sources in the soil are absorbed by plants and used for synthesis of amino acids, and subsequently of plant proteins. Relatively few of the amino acids produced by plants are the kinds which are essential for animals such as humans. After all, from the point of view of the plant, its goal is its own survival rather than the nourishing of animals which devour it. Thus plant proteins, which have evolved in such a way that they consist largely of nonessential amino acids, function very satisfactorily as parts of plant cells.

A transfer of nitrogen-containing compounds occurs when plant proteins are eaten by an animal. Many animals are very efficient at concentrating the essential amino acids. This they do by using most of them for synthesis of their own body proteins, which contain a higher proportion of essential amino acids than do plant proteins. The large amounts of extra nonessential amino acids are mostly burned as energy sources.

Another transfer occurs when humans ingest animal proteins in flesh, eggs, or milk. In utilizing the amino acids from an animal, human cells do not need to interconvert most of them to other amino acids or to burn them for energy, for many of the amino acids present in animal proteins are precisely those needed by human cells. Thus, although the utilization of amino acids of animal proteins for synthesis of human cell proteins is not 100 per cent efficient, far fewer amino acids are "wasted" for other purposes than if only plant proteins had been eaten.

Because some nitrogen compounds are lost at each transfer, the various stages are best represented not as a chain but as a pyramid (Figure 5–4). A relatively small mass of humans is supported by a large

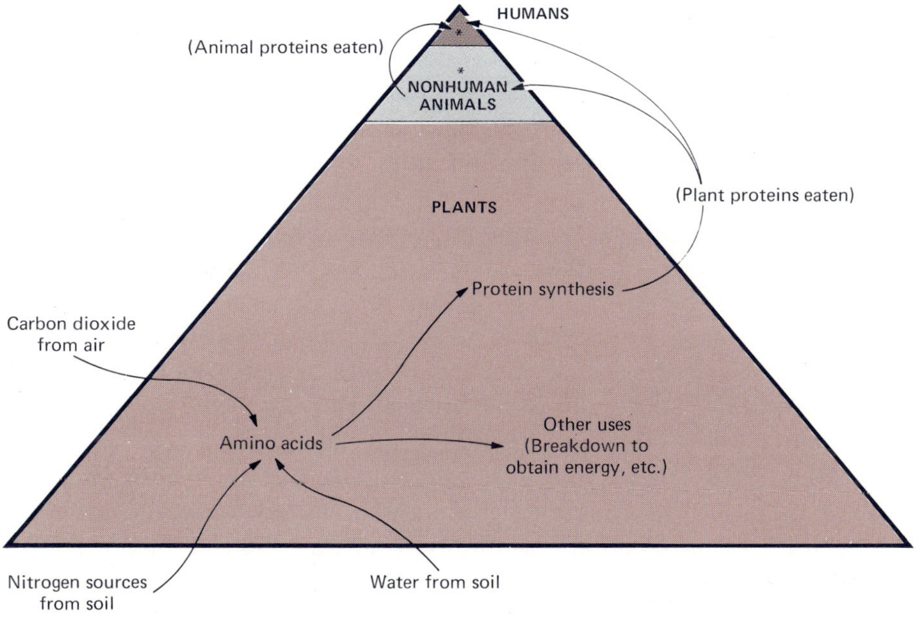

*Of the proteins ingested by humans and other animals, roughly one-tenth are retained in the body through use of amino acids to synthesize proteins for growth. The other nine-tenths are used for other purposes, such as breakdown to yield energy, replacement of previous cell components, or production of nonprotein compounds.

FIGURE 5–4. The protein pyramid.

mass of animals, which in turn is supported by an enormous mass of plant life. Therefore, one important reason for protein deficiency is that, where land and food are scarce and populations are dense, people cannot afford the luxury of wasting part of the available protein by feeding plants to animals, but must eat the plants directly instead. Lack of one or more amino acids, as well as inadequate total protein quantity, then becomes more probable than if reasonable amounts of animal proteins are eaten.

Sociocultural factors in protein intake

In many societies, custom dictates that males, especially adult males, get most of the high-quality protein sources and that young children and pregnant women are restricted in this respect. Thus, although making more, and better quality, proteins available to the world's people is necessary, it may not be sufficient for solving the problem of protein deficiency. The altering of customs and habits that dictate intake may prove to be even more difficult than solving the technical problems of availability.

MINERALS

Unlike the nutrient classes discussed previously, minerals are *inorganic* substances. Unlike *all* other nutrient classes, the minerals useful as nutrients are *electrically charged* particles. For example, sodium chloride (common salt) does not consist of electrically neutral sodium and chlorine atoms. In fact, these neutral elements themselves are highly poisonous; chlorine, for example, is the very irritating gas easily detected by sniffing chlorine laundry bleaches. However, when such substances lose or gain electrical charges, thereby becoming *ions,* they become remarkably gentler and, indeed, in that form are necessary parts of protoplasm.

Minerals function in two general roles. The first is as *structural* material. Iron is part of the structure of the oxygen-carrying protein, hemoglobin, in the red blood cells; calcium, phosphorus (or, more accurately, the phosphate ion), and other minerals constitute a significant part of the mass of teeth and bones; and sodium, potassium, phosphate, sulfate, chloride, and many other minerals are important constituents of the fluids both inside and outside all the body cells.

The second general role of minerals is their function in *regulating* numerous biological functions. Calcium in minute concentrations is necessary for normal blood clotting; magnesium stimulates the activity of many enzymes; and a number of minerals control the contraction of muscle cells and the transmission of impulses by nerve cells.

Because minerals are water-soluble substances that occur naturally in soils, even very pure water contains at least minute amounts of many minerals. This helps to insure that minerals needed in very small amounts will generally be obtained in adequate amounts. Indeed, in the case of a few minerals, the chief problem for some individuals is that the intake is too high rather than too low. Problems of excesses as well as deficiencies will be discussed in later sections in connection with the individual minerals.

Because no living system is able to produce a given element from any other material, *all* of the many members of the nutrient class of minerals are essential nutrients. However, different species have qualitatively different mineral requirements. A striking example is seen in the case of *iodine;* plants have no need for this mineral, nor do many species of animals. The reason is that iodine has only one known biological function: it constitutes part of the structure of *thyroid hormones* and is therefore essential for any species that has a thyroid gland, but useless for all other organisms. The mineral *boron* is apparently not needed by any species of animal, but lack of it causes barrenness (lack of seed production) in seed-bearing plants. *Fluoride,* in minute amounts, protects against dental decay in humans and other animals, but seems to have no value whatever to plants.

In addition to differences in the kinds of minerals needed, there are many species differences in the uses to which these minerals are put. Two outstanding examples are *iron* and *magnesium,* both of which are required by plants and animals alike. Iron is part of the hemoglobin molecule, which plants of course do not produce, and magnesium forms part of the plant pigment chlorophyll, which is not produced by animal cells.

One current fad is for so-called "organic minerals," an expression that is chemically absurd. Minerals do not contain carbon, and therefore are all inorganic substances. From the point of view of the seller of such products, "organic minerals" are those derived from once-living sources, such as iron extracted from liver, or calcium obtained from bones or even eggshells and oyster shells. Somehow the cells of the person taking such products are supposed to recognize them as superior because of their "vital, living" origin, although precisely how a cell is to distinguish between an iron ion from liver and an iron ion derived directly from the earth is never explained. Presumably an ion is believed to become suddenly "alive" when it becomes part of an animal's liver. Actually, of course, no unit smaller than a cell can properly be called "living." A mineral ion may be absorbed from the soil, become part of the cell of a plant, be eaten by an animal, enter a human's body, and finally return to the soil after the human dies. It does not achieve "life" when it becomes part of an organism, any more than it "dies" when it returns to the soil. All it has done is repeatedly change its address.

A rather sad commentary on the economic pressures that operate on usually reputable firms is seen in the case of one large department store chain. It now offers, in addition to its regular line, "organic" mineral supplements that consist of minerals linked chemically to carbon-containing substances. Technically, these are "organic mineral compounds" because of the presence of the carbon-containing part. Nutritionally, they are identical to the same materials from any other sources. Ethically, one can question whether it is right to exploit for profit the public's lack of nutritional information.

VITAMINS

Like the energy nutrients, vitamins are organic compounds. But unlike energy nutrients, vitamins are needed only in very minute amounts, and they are not broken down to provide energy. Vitamins as such, as well as compounds formed in the cells from ingested vitamins, function as *coenzymes* or *cofactors* (Figure 5–5), forming necessary parts of enzymes that catalyze reactions in living systems.

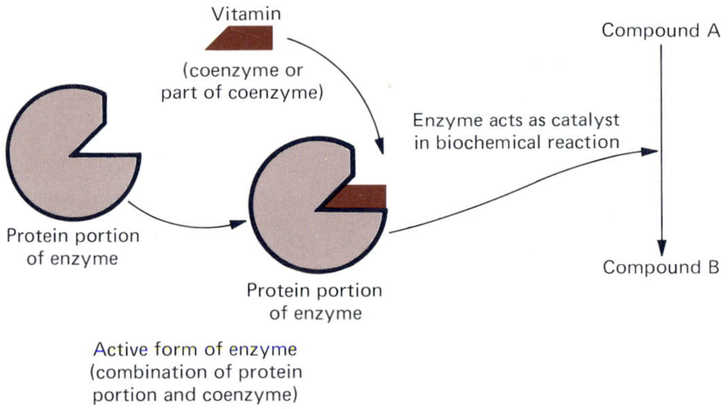

FIGURE 5–5. The function of a vitamin as a coenzyme.

The enormous importance of vitamins to biological functions is dramatically illustrated by the severe and sometimes fatal diseases that occur as a result of prolonged lack of even one vitamin. Unfortunately, the result too often is that people think of vitamins as "miracle drugs" that can be used to prevent and cure any and all diseases. Of all the nutrient products promoted as cure-alls by faddists, the majority are vitamins. Of all the money wasted on unnecessary nutrient-containing pills, capsules, and liquids, most is spent on vitamins. It appears therefore that of all nutrient classes, this is the one most often exploited for profit.

One reason for the public's gullibility on this subject is that certain terms are commonly misunderstood. The terms *water-soluble* and *fat-soluble,* for example, simply mean that certain vitamins have been found to dissolve in water whereas others dissolve in organic solvents such as ether. It does *not* mean that fat-soluble vitamins are found only in high-fat foods. Yet one supposed nutrition expert solemnly stated in one of her books that pregnant women can "rarely get sufficient amounts (of the fat-soluble vitamin A) from foods" because of the need to avoid large amounts of cream and butter in order to control weight. This indicates a very poor understanding of food sources of vitamins, because low-fat foods such as carrots, spinach, and yellow squash are rich in vitamin A value. Some people, nevertheless, assume that they will be lacking in fat-soluble vitamins if they avoid eating large amounts of fat, and are easily persuaded that supplements containing fat-soluble vitamins are necessary if they decrease their fat intake even slightly. Actually, fat-soluble vitamins are found in many low-fat foods, and some high-fat foods are devoid of them.

A second point of confusion is that a compound that is a vitamin for one species may be of no value to another. A visit to any "health food" store will demonstrate this. Vitamin supplements sold in such establishments often contain substances such as *inositol* and *lipoic acid,* which are not essential for humans although they are vitamins for certain other organisms. The reason is that human cells have the ability to synthesize these from other dietary compounds, whereas certain other species, during evolutionary development, have lost the ability to produce them.

A third problem is the by now familiar topic of "organic versus inorganic" nutrients. All vitamins are, chemically speaking, organic compounds. A molecule of thiamin, niacin, or any other vitamin will have the same structure, and therefore the same activity and function, whether it was synthesized in a chemical laboratory or in an animal or plant cell. As is the case with any other nutrients, cells cannot distinguish between a synthetic molecule and a "natural" one of the same structure.

A final reason for the vast amount of misunderstanding on the subject of vitamins is the large number of books and magazine articles based on the opinions of self-appointed nutrition experts. In the past few years, the public has been informed that one vitamin will prevent heart attacks, another will cure the common cold, while still others are effective in the treatment of mental illness. Although nutritionists concede that they do not yet have all the answers regarding nutrition and disease, they insist that many of the claims made for vitamins do not stand up under the scrutiny of careful investigation. Where controversy exists, it should be clearly stated. However, when cautious statements are made, they are often overwhelmed by the stridency of those with products, books, or ideas to sell.

WATER

If the nutrient classes had been discussed in order of either importance or amount needed, water would have come first, for if any nutrient

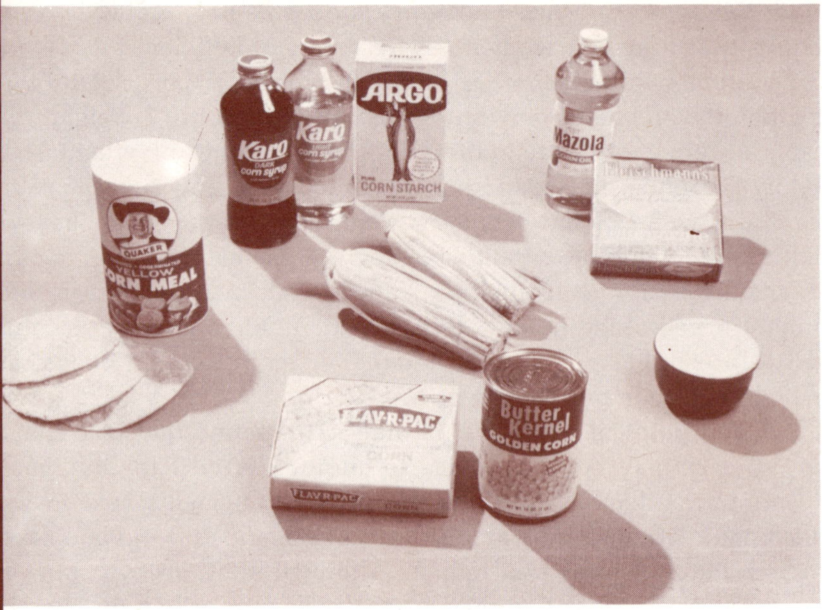

FIGURE 5–6
Processed foods of varying nutritive value compared to fresh corn.

TABLE 5–2
Sources of water

Sources	**Typical daily amounts for adults**
External	
Liquids	1000 milliliters (approximately 1.1 quarts)
Water in solid foods	500–1000 milliliters
Internal	
Water of oxidation	250–400 milliliters
Total	1750–2400 milliliters

Note: Intake of liquids (coffee, tea, milk, soft drinks, and other beverages, as well as plain water) can vary greatly. Water from solid foods generally varies less. Internally produced water varies least.

can be called the *most* essential one, it is water. During complete deprivation of all nutrients, people can lose virtually all of their body fat and carbohydrate reserves, and up to one-half of the body's protein. Loss of only one-fifth of the body's water, however, is usually fatal, and a loss of this magnitude can occur within only a few days.

One function of water is its role as structural material, because almost two-thirds of most cells consist of water. In addition, water performs a variety of regulatory roles: excretion of wastes by the kidneys requires the excretion of an obligatory minimum of water; control of body temperature is accomplished in large part through the evaporation of water in sweat; special watery solutions lubricate joints and spaces between organs. These are only a few examples of the many regulatory roles that can be listed for water.

The minimum amount of water needed, even under ideal conditions, is enormous compared to any other nutrient. The average person, given enough nonspecific calorie sources to prevent starvation, could survive indefinitely on daily intakes of a small fraction of an ounce of each of the other nutrients, such as essential amino acids, vitamins, and minerals, whereas the absolute minimum amount of water required daily by the adult human is over 2 *pounds*.

However, not all of the water ingested need be in the form of water itself, or even of liquids in general (Table 5–2). Solid foods also provide some water; for example, 1 pound of a fruit and vegetable may supply almost that much water. In addition, there is a third source of water, that which is formed within cells themselves. When energy nutrients are broken down, hydrogen is removed from them and combined with oxygen from the air. The resulting water, however, amounts to only about 1 cup per day in the average adult human—far too little to replace the amount lost daily.

FOOD PROCESSING AND NUTRIENTS

We can now take a second look at a previously stated fact: Processing can change the nutrient content of foods. Figure 5–6 illustrates what can happen to corn as it undergoes various types of processing. Drying of whole corn to remove much of the water has relatively little effect on the content of other nutrients, except, of course, that as the percent of water *decreases*, the percent of other constituents *increases*. Very extensive processing, such as separating a single component from others, results in a food such as starch or corn oil, which consist of virtually 100 percent of a single nutrient. One of these pure components may then be processed even further to yield still other products, as in the case of producing syrup from cornstarch.

Significant versus insignificant alterations as the result of food processing

One point to be emphasized is that *some* of the nutrient changes that occur as a result of processing are nutritionally important, whereas others are of so little practical importance that they can safely be ignored. For example, removal of the germ (or embryo) from whole grain corn removes much of the mineral iron and of the vitamins thiamin, riboflavin, and niacin. Because grains are significant sources of these nutrients, enrichment is commonly practiced to restore their levels to the original whole grain values, or even to levels higher than nature originally provided. On the other hand, the loss of fiber, fat, vitamin E, calcium, phosphorus, a small amount of protein, and certain other nutrients when corn is degerminated is not important, because grains are not major sources of these in Western diets. For this reason, no attempt is made to replace these nutrients through enrichment. The characterization of processed foods as "lifeless," "devitalized," and "inferior to natural foods," common to many groups of food faddists, indicates that they do not understand the difference between a nutritionally important change because of processing, and a trivial one.

SUGGESTED READINGS

Handbook on Human Nutritional Requirements. United Nations: FAO/WHO, Rome, 1974.

Food and Nutrition Board, National Research Council–National Academy of Sciences. "General Policies in Regard to Improvement of Nutritive Values of Foods." Washington, D.C., 1973.

Food and Nutrition Board, National Research Council–National Academy of Sciences. *Recommended Dietary Allowances,* eighth edition. Washington, D.C., 1974.

White, A., P. Handler, and E. L. Smith. *Principles of Biochemistry,* fifth edition. New York: McGraw-Hill, 1973.

6

nutrition and health: the individual

A very large number of people, perhaps the majority, have one or more health practices or ideas that could be considered examples of food faddism or nutrition misinformation. Many of these popular fashions in nutrition are relatively harmless. The person who takes a vitamin pill to "fight off the infection" at the first sign of a cold, or the cook who sprinkles wheat germ over every main dish, are hardly a threat to the public's health.

In the case of the big business known as the "health food movement," however, faddism and misinformation are more serious matters. Health food stores sell more than food and nutrient supplements; they also supply the vast amount of misinformation necessary to create and sustain interest in their products. When the books, magazines, and brochures distributed by professional food faddists are examined, amazing "facts" are disclosed:

A "normal, natural, ecobiological" way of eating is claimed to be capable of arresting, if not actually curing, any disease within ten days. The Macrobiotic diet, consisting almost entirely of brown rice, supposedly cures diseases ranging from baldness and sterility to cancer. Enormous doses of vitamin C are purportedly both safe and effective in treating all types of infection, including pneumonia, encephalitis, polio, measles, and chicken pox. "Well-known authorities" (who, if named at all, may be found to have no authority or competence in nutrition) declare that diseases such as cystic fibrosis, leukemia, and muscular dystrophy are caused by nutritional deficiencies. Lack of B vitamins is said to be a major cause of alcoholism, drug addiction, schizophrenia, and hyperactivity in children; and organic foods supplemented with the correct proportions of vitamins and minerals are claimed to cause sexual difficulties to disappear, enabling one to have sex every day, at least until the age of eighty.

Claims such as these, which are representative of many more examples that could be given, can be summarized as follows:

> **You are what you eat. Therefore, if your health—physical or mental—is not perfect, it must be because of faulty diet, since all diseases can be prevented or cured by proper nutrition.**

To analyze and evaluate such claims, certain questions must be answered:

What are health and disease?

What factors are important in determining health?

Why are statements such as the foregoing so readily accepted by many people?

What are the possible consequences of acting upon such beliefs?

HEALTH AND DISEASE—WHAT ARE THEY?

Susan, a successful research scientist, works a ten-hour day and still has vitality to spare for an active social life. She dismisses as unimportant her recurring headaches and episodes of depression, which require frequent treatment with drugs. On a job application, she would undoubtedly list her health status as "excellent."

Dan owns his own business, enjoys an income far above average, and proudly states, "I've never been sick a day in my life." His business associates see him as a gregarious, extroverted person; only his family knows that he spends many of his evenings staring at the television screen, drinking one bourbon and water after another.

Are these people as healthy as they think they are? According to the World Health Organization (WHO) of the United Nations, they are not, for this group has defined health as "the state of complete physical, mental, and social well-being." Accordingly, a person in superb physical condition could still be unhealthy because of lack of emotional or social well-being, as another could be socially and psychologically healthy and yet have some physical defect that prevents attainment of total health. Flawless health is therefore an ideal rather than a state likely to be enjoyed throughout life by any given individual.

The World Health Organization definition further states that health is "not merely the absence of disease or infirmity." A disease is any abnormality of structure or function of an organism. Because *normal* generally means usual, typical, average, or common, people can certainly be normal even though not in a continuous state of "complete physical, mental, and social well-being."

As shown in Figure 6–1, nutrition is *one* important factor in health, but it is by no means the only one. Both internal and external factors contribute to health and disease. These interact with each other, and there is much controversy as to their relative importance. The "nature versus nurture" question regarding mental health is an outstanding example; many believe that environmental or external factors primarily control psychological health, yet others insist that inherited or internal factors are equally, or even more, important. Although the question of physical health is at least somewhat less difficult to study, even here various factors are sometimes so intertwined that their relative importance remains largely unknown.

INTRINSIC (INTERNAL) FACTORS IN HEALTH

The internal factors important in determining health include the *genes* and the *hormones*. They are classed as intrinsic factors because they are produced inside the organism, rather than being obtained per se

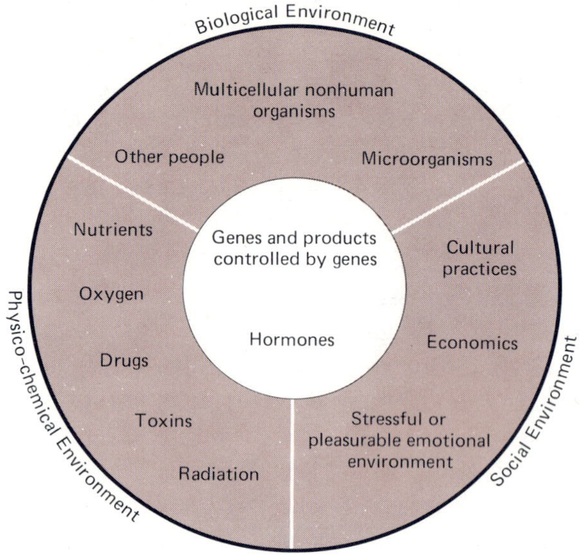

FIGURE 6–1. Intrinsic and extrinsic factors in health.

from the environment, although the raw materials required for their production must come from outside the organism.

GENES: THE BLUEPRINTS FOR PROTEIN STRUCTURE

The process of building complex orderly cells from randomly arranged substances requires more than just energy and raw materials; in addition, exactly as in the construction of a building, some sort of detailed plan or program is required. A construction company uses the information in a set of blueprints. A cell uses the information in its genetic material to build its own cellular structure according to specifications.

Fundamentally, what a cell is and does depends largely on what its internally produced proteins allow it to be and do. Therefore, cells with given characteristics result from using the genetic material *deoxyribonucleic acid,* or DNA, to regulate the kinds and amounts of proteins in the cells.

Functions of DNA

For a basic understanding of the functions of genes, it is necessary to know of the three main functions which genes (DNA molecules) perform.

First, all genes serve as *patterns,* or *templates,* upon which identical genes are produced. This is a prerequisite for growth or for replacement of dead cells, because all the genes must be duplicated (or *replicated*) before a cell can divide. Division forms two "daughter" cells, which contain DNA identical in kind and amount to that in the original cell.

Second, the so-called "classical" or "structural" genes dictate the *structure* of proteins by determining the kinds and sequences of amino acids which link together to form protein molecules.

Third, special DNA molecules, known as *operator* and *regulator* genes, control the *amounts* of proteins produced. This they do by acting as switches to turn on and off the structural genes that dictate protein structure.

Because DNA resides in the nucleus, whereas protein synthesis occurs on the ribosomes, how is the information coded in DNA carried from the nucleus to the ribosomes, where it is used? This is accomplished by molecules of a material similar to DNA, which is *ribonucleic acid,* or *RNA.* Actually, there are three types of RNA molecules. *Messenger* RNA, as the name implies, carries the "message" coded in DNA from the nucleus to the ribosomes. *Transfer* RNA links to amino acids and transports them to the ribosomes. *Ribosomal* RNA remains in the ribosomes, forming an integral part of their structure.

The control of protein structure by DNA can therefore be represented as follows:

DNA ⟶ RNA ⟶ Protein structure

This is analogous to the use of other types of plans, as in the following

Master blueprint ⟶ Working copies of blueprint ⟶ Structure of a building

It should not be thought that DNA is converted to RNA, or RNA to protein, any more than it could be assumed that a blueprint or a working copy of it becomes an actual part of the finished building. The DNA acts as a pattern or *template* upon wihch a closely similar RNA molecule is synthesized, a process known as *transcription* because the coded information of DNA is transcribed into RNA. The RNA molecules then move to the ribosomes, where they dictate the amino acid sequences of protein molecules. This process is called *translation* because the information originally obtained from the structure of genetic material is translated into the entirely different structure of a protein molecule.

The "one gene—one enzyme" hypothesis is an expression of the fact that each specific protein molecule has a particular structure dictated by the structure of a given gene. Because all enzymes are proteins, a defect in a gene can result in a defective enzyme. As a result, a change in the rate of a given biochemical reaction catalyzed by the enzyme, or even the complete loss of a biochemical reaction, can occur. Changes in gene structure, or *mutations,* can in this manner cause a profound alteration in one or more of the biochemical reactions that collectively determine the organism's health.

Genetic aspects of nutrition

Of the many fascinating aspects of the relationships of genes to health, the following are of particular interest to nutrition.

First, genes are very important in determining nutrient needs and intakes in many species. The total amount of food and the kinds of food needed and obtained may be determined almost exclusively by the size, instinctive behavior, and other inherited characteristics of the organism. The lion may lie down with the lamb, but not for long; it is not in the nature of lions—which are inherently incapable of surviving on a vegetarian diet—to browse peacefully beside lambs. Humans, however, have great variation in food choices compatible with survival and health. Unlike most other animals, humans are not exclusively *carnivorous* (flesh-eating) or *herbivorous* (plant-eating). Rather, they are *omnivorous,* genetically able to eat virtually all foods of either plant or animal origin. Because of the wide range in their food choices, whether people "lie down with the lamb" or turn it into chops is largely determined by the culture of the society into which they were born.

Second, the *specific* nutrients that are essential for various animals are determined by genes. Consider the hypothetical case of nutrients produced, as follows, in cells:

$$\text{Compound A} \xrightarrow[\text{(enzyme 1)}]{} \text{Compound B} \xrightarrow[\text{(enzyme 2)}]{} \text{Compound C}$$

As long as the genes controlling both enzyme 1 and enzyme 2 are normal, B and C can be produced by the cells and are therefore, by definition, nonessential nutrients.

If, however, a structural change known as a mutation occurs in the gene controlling Enzyme 1, this enzyme may no longer be produced. Now Compound A cannot be converted to B and subsequently to C; therefore these formerly nonessential nutrients become essential dietary components. In fact, studies of lower organisms, in which nutrient needs were changed by damaging genes with x-rays, provided much of the information that led to the "one gene—one enzyme" hypothesis.

A third and very important point is that no form of malnutrition can cause a gene mutation. One well-known faddist has stated that inborn diseases caused by gene mutations are on the increase, apparently as a result of inadequate prenatal diets. This is absurd. Genetic diseases *appear* to have increased greatly in recent decades because physicians are better able to diagnose them today than in the past. Although mutations can occur as the result of environmental agents such as x-rays and other high-energy radiation, or simply because cells for unknown reasons sometimes produce abnormal DNA, no nutrient excess or deficiency has ever been shown to cause mutation of any gene in any species.

However, certain nutrient deficiencies and excesses *can* cause congenital malformations in a variety of animals, although the importance of this to human health is largely unknown. Cleft palate, heart defects, and club foot, which are examples of congenital malformations, are commonly confused with gene mutations. However, the *phenotype* of an organism (the outward expression of its genes) should not be confused with the *genotype* (the actual structure of the genes). For example, a person with the genotype for normal height may, as the result of disease, develop the same phenotype as one who is genetically dwarfed. A congenital malformation (or anomaly or defect) is simply a structural or functional abnormality that is *present at birth;* it may or may not be caused by an abnormal genotype.

How malnutrition can result in congenital malformations that mimic genetically caused defects is shown in Figure 6–2. It can be seen

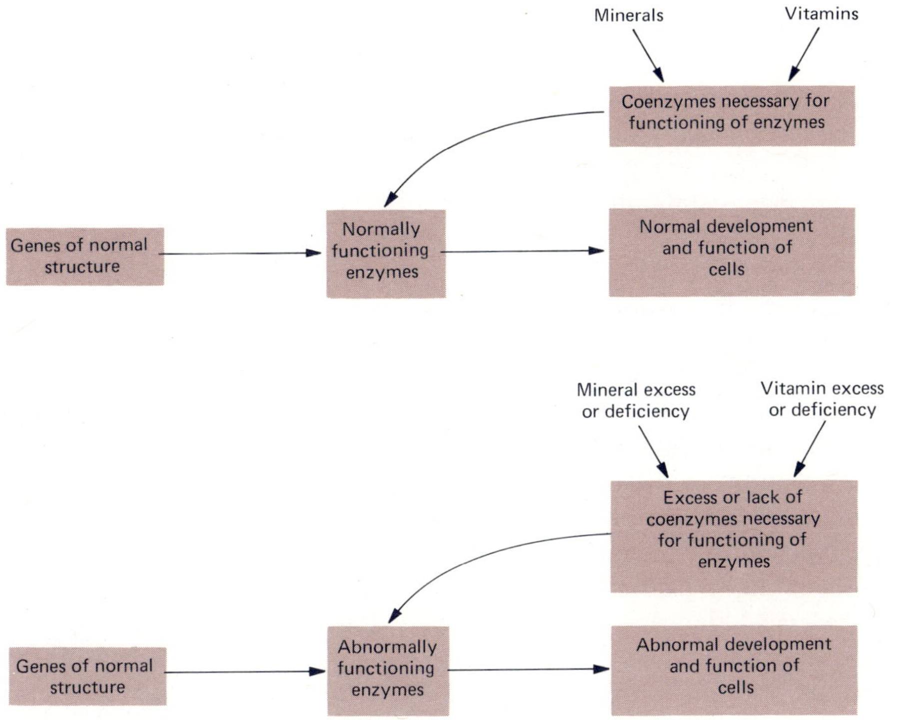

FIGURE 6–2. How malnutrition can produce malformations resembling those caused by gene mutations.

that normal development depends not only upon normal genes, but also upon normal amounts of *coenzymes* needed for many enzymes to function. Consequently, abnormal levels of vitamins or minerals can lead to abnormal levels of coenzymes within the cells, which can in turn lead to abnormal development that may resemble genetic defects.

Most of the evidence that malnutrition causes congenital abnormalities has been obtained from studies of animals such as rats and pigs. These results cannot necessarily be applied to humans, and there is no conclusive evidence that malnutrition is a major cause of the congenital defects commonly seen in humans.

It should be emphasized that large *excesses* as well as deficiencies of certain nutrients have been shown to cause congenital defects in animals. Food faddists who recommend enormous doses of nutrients for pregnant women "in order to insure normal development in the growing fetus" are apparently unaware of this.

It may be asked, "What difference does it make to the person born with a serious defect whether or not it was caused by abnormal genes?" The answer is that, although it may make no difference to the individual, it is vitally important to the species. A genetic mutation can be passed on to a person's children and children's children; a congenital malformation in a genetically normal person cannot.

DNA and RNA in the diet

The materials cells use to produce DNA and RNA are easily obtained even from relatively poor diets. These molecules, collectively called *nucleic acids,* are polymers of *nucleotides,* each of which consists of a nitrogen-containing part, a 5-carbon sugar, and a phosphate group. The nitrogen-containing parts, called *purines* and *pyrimidines,* are all readily synthesized in human cells; the 5-carbon sugars, *ribose* in RNA and *deoxyribose* in DNA, are also easily produced in abundance. Only the phosphate portion is an essential nutrient, and phosphate is one of the most easily obtained minerals.

Although vitamins are not actual parts of DNA molecules, certain of them are cofactors in DNA synthesis. If they are lacking, the *amount* of DNA produced will be decreased, which will interfere with the multiplication of cells. However, the DNA produced will be normal in *structure* regardless of the kind or severity of malnutrition.

Nucleic acid supplements are therefore a complete waste of money, although many health food stores offer DNA and RNA, obtained from sources such as yeast and beef liver, in the form of pills and capsules. The sales pitch is as follows: "Nucleic acids are involved in cell division and reproduction." (True.) "Cell division and reproduction decline with aging." (Also true.) "Therefore nucleic acid supplements will rejuvenate you, protect your heart, and retard the aging process." (Absolutely false.) Because nucleic acids are digested to simple subunits in the intestine, any absorbed products are no longer intact DNA or RNA, and hence are unable to function as units of heredity. As Ronald Deutsch lightheartedly states it:

> **Some promoters claim that we can use ingested RNA and DNA to replace that already in our cells, or to add more instructions for making more proteins. This, if true, would be a disturbing idea. For consider: we know that each bit of RNA and DNA carries instructions for making the organism in whose cells it was born. Some of the RNA and DNA being promoted as a reprieve from aging are from yeast. Others are from the meats of animals. So if the promoters are right, the author is concerned about the possibility of people rising to much greater size if left in a warm place overnight . . . (or) that those receiving animal**

DNA may begin to grow wool, hooves, or horns—and perhaps be inclined to moo in public places.

–Ronald M. Deutsch. "The Family Guide to Better Food and Better Health," Des Moines, Iowa: Meridith Press, 1971, p. 56.

Products of nucleic acid activity, such as specific enzymes, are likewise of no value in the diet. Certain food faddists object strongly to processes such as the refining of wheat and even to the canning, freezing, and cooking of food because "vital enzyme activity" is lost as a result of these processes. In point of fact, one of the very reasons for these processes is to halt the activity of enzymes that would otherwise cause food quality to deteriorate. At any rate, enzymes, like other proteins, are digested in the intestine and only the amino acid subunits are absorbed and utilized by the body. Enzymes in foods therefore cannot function as biological catalysts inside human cells, any more than can the enzymes in the pills and capsules sold in health food stores, despite the advertising of these as "vital," "energy-releasing," "fat-blasting," or "natural digestants."

Genetic abnormalities necessitating dietary modifications

Inherited diseases can be divided into three large groups: those caused by a single defective or mutant gene, those related to a number of genes, and those associated with an abnormality of one or more entire chromosomes.

Single-gene defects: inborn errors of metabolism

Over one hundred genetic diseases caused by a defect in a single gene have been identified in humans. Of these, a relatively small number can be treated by a special diet. One that has been studied very extensively is *phenylketonuria,* or PKU. Fortunately a rare disease, occurring in about one out of 20,000 births, it leads to permanent mental retardation if untreated. The condition can be diagrammed as shown in Figure 6–3.

If gene number 1 is defective, enzyme number 1 will be inoperative. Therefore, the amino acid *phenylalanine* will be forced to take a "detour," a reaction catalyzed by enzyme number 2 and little used in

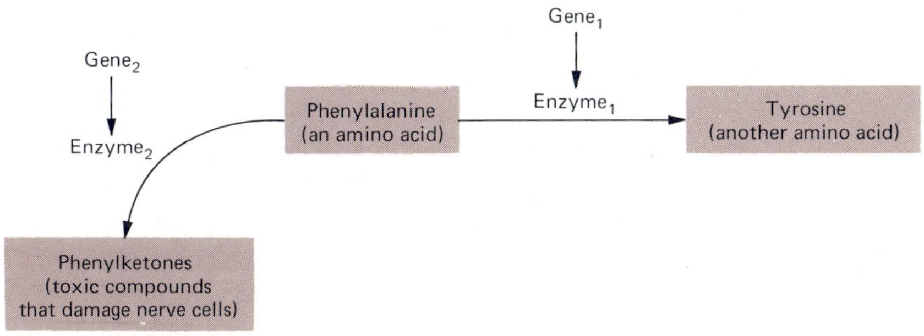

FIGURE 6–3. The biochemical basis of the disease phenylketonuria.

the normal person's cells. Enormous amounts of the toxic *phenylketones* will be produced, until these actually appear in the urine, where they can be detected by chemical tests.

Dietary treatment, using a special artificial formula which is low in phenylalanine, can prevent the formation of excess phenylketones and hence the retardation which otherwise occurs. This fact has led to a good deal of misunderstanding. First, the diet does not "cure" the disease; the defective gene remains and can be passed on to the offspring. Second, PKU is not a nutritional disease; it is a *genetic* disease in which the symptoms are merely controlled by diet. Third, the diet used in PKU will not produce superintelligence in normal children; although it prevents mental retardation in the child with PKU, it is so lacking in phenylalanine that its effects in normal children would be nothing short of disastrous.

Although other inborn errors with nutritional implications will be discussed later, it is important to keep in mind that, although *some* inborn errors can be treated with diet, others must be treated with drugs or by other means, and the majority cannot be treated by any means at present.

Multigenetic diseases

Most traits are polygenic or *multigenetic;* in contrast to monogenic traits such as eye color and the various inborn errors, they depend on multiple genes which may be located on many different chromosomes. Thus these traits can vary in many possible ways rather than in an "all or none" manner.

Of the diseases that are at present believed to be related to multiple abnormal genes, one with the greatest implications for nutrition is *diabetes mellitus.* This disease is characterized by excessively high blood glucose levels resulting from abnormally decreased secretion of the hormone, insulin. Although some cases of the disease can be controlled largely or entirely by diet, others must be treated by daily injections of insulin. Taking insulin by mouth would be useless, because insulin is a protein; it would be digested and only the amino acid subunits would be absorbed. Certain *oral hypoglycemic agents,* taken by mouth, stimulate the pancreas to secrete larger amounts of insulin, but not all diabetics respond to such agents.

Many other diseases, including arthritis, cancer, diseases of the heart and blood vessels, and even obesity have been postulated to be at least partly caused by multiple gene defects because they tend to occur more commonly in some families than in others. However, familial occurrence does not necessarily implicate the genes, because environmental factors, which are commonly similar for the various members of a family, could equally be responsible.

Chromosome abnormalities

In some individuals there is a gross alteration in the number or structure of the rod-shaped structures found in the nucleus and known as *chromosomes.* A typical human cell contains 23 pairs of chromosomes. Many genes are found on each chromosome, and these genes therefore also occur in pairs. Thus "the gene for eye color" actually means the *pair* of genes which together determine eye color.

Of the 23 chromosome pairs in human cells, the members of 22 pairs, called *autosomes,* are alike in males and females. The 23rd pair is known as the *sex chromosomes;* the larger of the 2 sex chromosomes is called an *X chromosome* and the smaller a *Y chromosome.* Normal female humans have 2 X chromosomes, whereas normal males have 1 X and 1 Y chromosome. It is for this reason that certain inherited diseases such as hemophilia are "sex linked," carried by females but suffered only by males. If a female has a defective gene on one X chromosome, its effect can be counterbalanced by a normal member of that gene pair on the other X chromosome. However, a male who inherits the defect will lack a second X chromosome carrying a normal gene to cancel out the effect of the mutant gene. Therefore, he will suffer the disease, although the mother from whom he inherited the defective gene did not. From this point of view, a male can perhaps be considered an incomplete female.

Abnormalities of the sex chromosomes sometimes occur, as in the disease known as Turner's syndrome, characterized by 1 X chromosome and no Y chromosome. Such people are dwarfed, sterile, and often mentally retarded females in appearance. In other diseases, an extra X or Y chromosome may be present; for example, a person with Klein-felter's syndrome has one Y and two X chromosomes, and is an abnormal male, usually sterile and commonly with multiple abnormalities in mental and physical development. People with 1 X and 2 Y chromosomes received a great deal of attention within recent years because of reports that prison populations had unusually large numbers of these individuals. A film was even produced, complete with lurid advertising ("The Y Chromosome! One makes a man—two make a monster!"). However, more recent studies have failed to confirm the spectacular earlier reports.

Abnormal numbers of autosomes generally have much more severe effects on health than abnormal numbers of sex chromosomes. Lack of one member of an autosome pair is almost invariably lethal, causing the embryo to cease development soon after conception. Although possession of three autosomes instead of the normal pair is compatible with life, it can cause profound developmental anomalies. For example, *Down's syndrome,* once called "mongolism" because of the supposed mongoloid appearance, is caused by an extra autosome. Many other even more rare autosomal diseases are associated with extreme malformations of the heart, brain, and other organs.

It has been estimated that 10 percent of all fertilized ova, 40 percent of all spontaneous abortions, and 1 percent of all live births in humans are associated with gross chromosome abnormalities, the causes of which are largely unknown. Various chemicals have been reported to cause abnormal numbers of chromosomes or breakage of chromosomes; *lysergic acid diethylamide* (LSD) and the artificial sweetening agents known as *cyclamates* have both been suspected of causing chromosome breaks. However, recent studies suggest that the conclusions were hasty.

Parents of children born retarded or deformed as a result of a chromosome disease are often preyed upon by charlatans offering various treatments, including dietary cures, none of which are of any benefit whatever. The only nutritional implications of these diseases are that the afflicted individuals often present special feeding problems and needs. They may never be able to feed themselves, or they may choke because of a convulsion during feeding. Drugs to control behavior such as hyperactivity, and surgery to correct malformations such as cleft palate and defects of the heart and other organs, are the only treatments presently available to make life happier for many of these people and their families.

Genetics in psychological and social health

The idea that inborn body chemistry determines human feelings and temperament goes far back in time. Medieval physiologists supposed that the body had four "humors" or fluids: blood, phlegm, black bile, and yellow bile. Ideal proportions of the four were believed necessary for good health, and too much of one or another "humor" was thought to cause characteristic changes in disposition. An excess of blood made one "sanguine"—passionate and fond of "mirth and music, wine and women." Excess phlegm gave rise to a "phlegmatic" personality, sluggish and calm. Overabundance of "black bile" led to "melancholy," or a state of depression, and extreme amounts of yellow bile characterized the "choleric" person, ill-tempered and violent.

Although the idea of "humors" has long been discarded, modern controversy now centers on whether genes can determine mental and social traits. People may speak of the "born criminal" or the person who is "an alcoholic like his father before him," overlooking the vast difficulty of separating the effects of heredity from those of the unfavorable environment into which children of criminals and alcoholics are often born. A recent furor was raised when racial differences were reported as being the reason for higher or lower scores on aptitude and intelligence tests. Some investigators claimed that these findings proved that the average genetic potential of whites was greater than that of blacks. Certainly it is possible that racial differences exist with respect to intelligence, as they do with respect to skin color, hair texture, and other characteristics. However, given the poorer environment in which most American black children are raised and educated, it would be naïve to suggest that test score differences prove anything about inherent ability. Until all children are given environments which permit optimal development, social and psychological as well as physical, conclusions regarding the relative importance of heredity and environment are premature.

HORMONES

The study of hormones is known as *endocrinology.* These intrinsic factors in health are secreted by the *endocrine* or *ductless glands.* These are glands that secrete into the bloodstream, in contrast to the exocrine glands—such as the mammary glands, sweat glands, and salivary glands—which secrete to body surfaces via tubes or ducts.

Like the nervous system, the endocrine system is specialized for regulation and integration of the functioning of other parts of the body. However, the endocrine system has slower, more sustained effects mediated via the chemicals called hormones, in contrast to the nervous system which responds rapidly via electrical impulses as well as by certain chemical mediators.

Although a hormone is itself not an enzyme, it may modify the rate of synthesis of an enzyme by acting upon genes, or it may alter the activity of already existing enzyme molecules, or it may regulate the rate at which a substrate (such as glucose) enters cells. In each case the cell type or molecule affected by the hormone is called its *target.* Some hormones have very specific targets, even including other glands within the endocrine system. These are called *trophic* hormones. Other hormones have a broad spectrum of targets, affecting virtually every part of the body, and hence many aspects of biological function.

Hormones, which are themselves regulators, are in turn regulated. This is accomplished in three general ways: Hormones may be secreted in response to other hormones, to nutrients, or to nerve activity. For example, the thyroid-stimulating hormone stimulates secretion of the hormone, *thyroxine;* increased blood glucose stimulates *insulin* secretion; and stimulation by nerves increases the release of *adrenaline.*

The principal features of the endocrine system are shown in Figure 6–4 and in Table 6–1. It is apparent that some endocrine organs are members of other organ systems as well; the intestine and pancreas, for example, are parts of the digestive system, and the gonads and placenta are parts of the reproductive system.

The information presented in Table 6–1 is worth particular study and review, because understanding how nutrients are utilized in the body is possible only if hormone activities are known. Hormones are often unfairly blamed for overweight ("It's my glands") and are used in questionable forms of medical treatment, including some for obesity. A knowledge of basic endocrinology is therefore very helpful in dispelling certain fallacies in nutrition.

Table 6–1 does not include all of the compounds that function as hormones even in humans. In addition, there are plant hormones that

TABLE 6–1
Hormones and nutrition

Endocrine gland	Major hormones	Examples of functions; diseases of excess or lack of hormones
Pituitary gland		
a. Posterior	Oxytocin	Stimulates contraction of smooth muscles in uterus and breast.
	Antidiuretic hormone (ADH), (vasopressin)	Increases water reabsorption in kidneys. Deficiency: diabetes insipidus.
b. Anterior	Growth hormone ("somatotrophin")	Stimulates utilization of amino acids, minerals, and other nutrients; a major determinant of stature. Deficiency: hypopituitary dwarfism. Excess: giantism in the child; acromegaly in the adult.
	Trophic hormones Adrenocorticotrophic hormone (ACTH)	Stimulate other endocrine glands to secrete; the adrenal cortex, thyroid gland, and gonads are regulated by these five trophic hormones.
	Thyroid stimulating hormone (TSH) Gonadotrophins: FSH (follicle stimulating hormone) LH (luteinizing (hormone) LTH (luteotrophic hormone or prolactin)	
Thyroid gland	Thyroxine	Regulates metabolic rate (the rate at which energy nutrients are utilized for vital life functions, exclusive of voluntary muscular activity). Important determinant of mental development as well as skeletal and tooth development. Deficiency: cretinism in the infant or child; simple goiter, myxedema in the adult. Excess: "toxic goiter."
Parathyroid gland	Parathyroid hormone	Regulates the level of calcium in the blood plasma.
Adrenal glands		
a. Medulla	Epinephrine (adrenaline)	Stimulates an enzyme involved in converting glycogen to glucose ("fight or flight" reaction) which helps prepare the organism to survive emergencies.
b. Cortex	Aldosterone (a "mineralocorticoid")	Increases reabsorption of sodium in kidney. Deficiency: Addison's disease.

Endocrine gland	Major hormones	Examples of functions; diseases of excess or lack of hormones
	Cortisol, cortisone, and corticosterone ("glucocorticoids")	Increase conversion of amino acids to glucose. Excess: Cushing's syndrome.
	Testosterone (an androgen, or male sex hormone)	See functions of sex hormones under the heading "Gonads."
	Estrogens and progesterone (female sex hormones)	
Intestine	Pancreozymin	Stimulates pancreas to synthesize digestive juice enzymes.
	Secretin	Stimulates pancreas to secrete digestive juice into intestine.
	Cholecystokinin	Stimulates gallbladder to eject bile into intestine.
Pancreas	Insulin	Decreases blood glucose by facilitating passage of glucose from blood into cells. Deficiency: diabetes mellitus.
	Glucagon	Increases blood glucose by stimulating conversion of glycogen to glucose. (Action similar to that of epinephrine, but slower and longer-lasting.)
Gonads Ovary (the female gonad)	Estrogens	Promote growth and development of uterus and vagina and development of female characteristics (breasts, wide pelvis, etc.). May inhibit linear bone growth; promotes fat deposition in typical female pattern.
	Progesterone	Important in maintaining pregnancy. Regulates growth and development of uterine lining (endometrium).
Testis (the male gonad)	Testosterone and other androgens	Promote growth and development of sex organs and development of male characteristics (wide shoulders, deep voice, body hair, beard, etc.). Stimulate linear growth; promote muscle growth. Stimulate development of bones to mature form in which growth is complete.
Placenta	Chorionic gonadotrophin (early in pregnancy)	Stimulates synthesis of sex hormones by ovaries.
	Estrogens and progesterone (later in pregnancy)	Prepare breasts for lactation; maintain pregnancy.

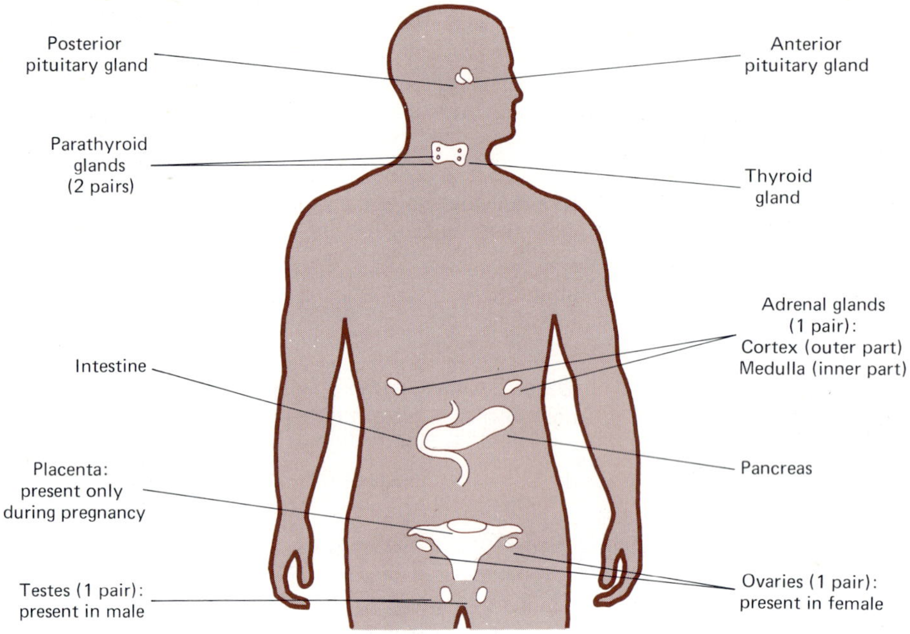

FIGURE 6–4. The location of the principal endocrine glands. A helpful memory device is to think of the thyroid and parathyroid glands as a bow tie with 4 polka dots. The glands located lower form a pattern that resembles a face, if you use enough imagination.

control the growth and development of plants, and insect hormones that regulate molting and metamorphosis. Many insects also produce so-called "social hormones" or *pheromones,* which serve as chemical means of communication. In fact, control of some species of insect pests through using pheromones as sex attractants is being studied intensively; luring an insect to its death by use of a sex attractant has obvious environmental advantages over spraying insecticides over an entire area. Also, the use of hormones which cause certain species of insects to fail to change into adults at the proper time can control their numbers by interrupting their normal life cycle.

Although Table 6–1 does not show all of the known endocrine diseases, those most relevant to nutrition are included. Addison's disease, for example, demands a very high sodium intake which can be provided by large amounts of salt; Cushing's syndrome requires an unusually high protein intake to offset the effects of excessive amino acid breakdown; and diabetes insipidus results in a need for enormous fluid intakes to replace the copious urinary losses of water. However, it is important to recognize that treatment of most endocrine diseases requires hormone therapy as well as nutritional changes.

Although individual hormones will be mentioned later in relation to various aspects of nutrition, this introduction should help to place them in perspective and to highlight their importance to nutrition and health.

SUGGESTED READINGS

Ballin, J. C. and P. L. White. "Fallacy and Hazard: Human Chorionic Gonadotropin/500-Calorie Diet and Weight Reduction." *Journal of the American Medical Association* 230 (1974):693.

Brown, J. "Nutrition-Endocrine Relationships." *Medical Clinics of North America* 48 (1964):1241.

Burns, G. W. *The Science of Genetics*, second edition. New York: Macmillan, 1972.

Frye, B. E. *Hormonal Control in Vertebrates*. New York: Macmillan, 1967.

Garn, S. M. and C. G. Rohmann. "Interaction of Nutrition and Genetics in the Timing of Growth and Development." *Pediatric Clinics of North America* 13 (1966):353.

Hamwi, G. J. and M. Tzagournis. "Nutrition and Diseases of the Endocrine Glands." *American Journal of Clinical Nutrition* 23 (1970):311.

Hirschhorn, K. "Human Genetics." *Journal of the American Medical Association* 224 (1973):597.

Kretchmer, N. and R. E. Greenberg. "Some Physiologic and Biochemical Determinants of Development." *Advances in Pediatrics* 14 (1966):201.

Meltzer, Y. L. *Hormonal and Attractant Pesticide Technology*. Park Ridge, N.J.: Noyes Data Corporation, 1971.

Scarr-Salapatek, S. "Race, Social Class, and IQ." *Science* 174 (1971):1285.

Slater, E. and V. Cowie. *The Genetics of Mental Disorders*. New York: Oxford University Press, 1971.

Turner, C. D. and J. T. Bagnara. *General Endocrinology*, fifth edition. Philadelphia: Saunders, 1971.

7

nutrition and health: environmental influences

The environmental, or extrinsic, factors in your health can be considered in three great classes:

1 **Biological.** The living things in your environment, including people other than yourself, as well as all kinds and sizes of plants and animals.
2 **Physical and chemical.** The forms of energy (such as sunlight, heat, x-rays), and the inanimate matter (such as nutrients, oxygen, drugs, toxins) which act upon you.
3 **Social.** The organized group in which you live, with its characteristic habits, traditions, and institutions.

The intrinsic factors in health do not always fit neatly into separate categories; diabetes mellitus, for example, is a genetic as well as a hormonal disease. When we consider the *extrinsic* factors, it is even more difficult, and in some cases impossible, to place each separate facet into one and only one class.

THE BIOLOGICAL ENVIRONMENT AND HEALTH

Others of your own species, plants and animals of considerable size but of different species, and microscopic plants and animals are biological factors in health. For each of these categories, a few examples can illustrate their impact on human health and on nutrition.

Other people

Malthus long ago stated that the human birth rate produced rapid increases in numbers which are checked only by the limits of the food supply. This implies that members of a given species *compete* with each other for resources such as food.

Charles Darwin, in the nineteenth century, applied Malthus' principle to biology. The *theory of evolution,* one of the great unifying ideas of the biological sciences, was the result. The theory is based on three observations:

First, organisms *vary,* so that the members of a given species are not all exactly alike. Although Darwin had no way of knowing it, we recognize today that these inherited variations are caused by gene mutations.

Second, many more organisms are born than can possibly survive on the available resources such as food and space.

Third, despite the high birth rates seen in each species, the number of surviving individuals does not ordinarily increase rapidly.

It follows from these facts that there is a *struggle for existence.* This may be open conflict, as when two animals fight for possession of a single food source or mate. In many cases, however, the struggle is silent and nonviolent; Darwin used the example of two plants struggling to survive drought by putting out more and more roots to obtain water.

A second conclusion is that, in the struggle for existence, the organisms that survive are those most "fitted" for survival. In many cases, however, fitness and hence the probability of survival are enhanced by cooperation as well as by competition between members of a species. A group of hunters, for example, has a greater chance of killing prey than has any single member of the group; at the same time, the crowding within the group may elicit aggressiveness within the group, which would not be possible with isolated individuals.

Human development, including an unknown number of social and psychological elements of modern humans as well as their physical characteristics, is therefore the culmination of our ancestors' interactions with each other as well as with other aspects of their environment. Although biological evolution is still occurring, another important influence on human well-being is in the social development of the species. Cooperation in protecting the environment while providing the resources necessary for optimal health throughout the world has replaced biological change as the most important determinant of human survival. However, the capacity or fitness to think and plan toward these goals is the end result of past eons of biological evolution.

Animals and plants other than microorganisms

Except for human flesh, eaten in a few societies, and certain microbes such as yeast, which some people eat as a food in itself, all foods eaten by people are derived from living or once-living nonhuman organisms of fairly large size—although modern urban dwellers, far removed from the sites of food production, may overlook this obvious fact.

A variety of birds, mammals, and other animals decrease the populations of organisms that are potentially harmful to humans. Cats kill rats; the insect known as the praying mantis kills many other insects which would otherwise have adverse effects on human welfare. Conversely, many organisms kill other organisms which humans find useful, and humans must therefore often compromise in deciding whether a given organism is "good" or "bad." The cat that kills rats may also eat birds which would have destroyed harmful insects. The web of life is so complex that no organism can be categorized as valuable or detrimental without qualification.

In addition to contributing to physical health, many plants and animals are important to psychological health by providing emotional satisfaction. Pets, house plants, flower gardens, the animals and plants of wilderness areas, indeed green plants in general, virtually synonymous with the renewal of life in the spring, all lift the human

FIGURE 7–1

Pest control through pitting one organism against another. A potato field is sprayed with a solution containing the spores of a fungus. This microorganism causes disease that kills the aphids feeding on the potato plants. (USDA photo.)

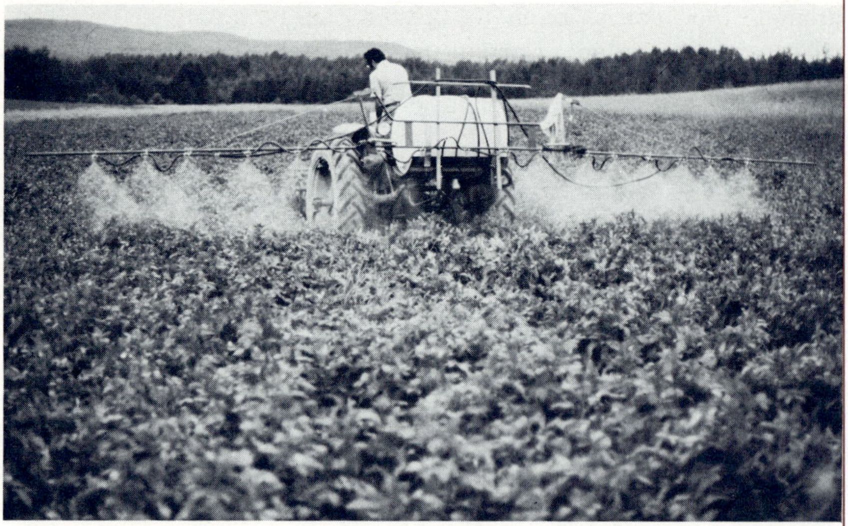

spirit. How bleak the world would be if overcrowding forced us to regard these as unnecessary competitors for space, or as mere additional food sources.

Many nonhuman organisms, however, have negative effects on human health, and these are classified as "pests." Thus a "pesticide" (pest-killer) may be an insecticide, a rodenticide, or a herbicide that kills "undesirable" plants known as weeds. Of course, a dandelion plant would consider a gardener or a rose bush a pest; and rats would benefit if they could use a pesticide known as a "homicide." From a human's point of view, though, pests are those organisms with interests inimical to those of people (Figure 7–1).

Pests affect human health in many ways; they may decrease the available amount of food directly, by consuming plants and animals intended for use by humans, or indirectly, by transmitting diseases that cause crops or domestic animals to sicken or die. Pests can also spoil food by blemishing it, as the worm in the apple does, or by making it unclean, as rat feces and insect parts do in stored grain. In these examples, pests are in competition with humans for available food sources.

In addition to affecting food supply, certain pests transmit infectious diseases to humans. The Great Plague of London, which in the seventeenth century killed over 30,000 people in a single month, was actually caused by a species of bacteria. It was spread, however, by fleas which bit infected rats and then bit humans. In fact, the decline in plague in Europe after the early part of the eighteenth century has been traced, not to a change in the bacterium, but to the disappearance of the black rats which transmitted the bacteria; brown rats coming to Western Europe from Russia competed so successfully with the black rats that they eventually replaced them completely. Fortunately, brown rats are sewer dwellers and avoid the houses of humans, and the fleas on these rats therefore had little opportunity to bite humans.

When the insecticide DDT was introduced in the 1940s, the incidence of malaria decreased dramatically because the pesticide killed the mosquitoes which transmit this disease to humans. Simultaneously, there was a marked increase in crop yields, 100 percent or more in some areas, because of the control of plant-eating insects by DDT. Those who insist that the use of such chemicals inevitably results in disaster to the environment should be informed that disastrous results to human health would surely result from a complete ban on pesticides.

Microorganisms

Microorganisms, too small to be visible without the aid of a microscope, include many varieties of organisms. Although yeasts and molds are also significant, the two most important groups in relation to human health are the *bacteria,* which are one-celled plants, and the *protozoa,* which are one-celled animals. Viruses, which consist of enormous molecules of nucleic acid linked to proteins, are often considered in this category; however, because they do not consist of cells, they are actually on the border between living and nonliving things.

The beneficial effects of microorganisms on human health are enormous. For example, microorganisms in the digestive tracts of animals perform functions that produce usable materials for the animal, such as the digestion of cellulose in the rumens of animals such as cattle, sheep, and goats. Chickens and rats can remain healthy on food devoid of vitamin B_{12} if they are allowed to eat their own feces, because the bacteria in their intestines produced the vitamin B_{12}. At least one nutrient, vitamin K, is absorbed in significant amounts by humans in whose intestines the vitamin is produced by bacteria.

A very important group of soil organisms, known as *nitrogen-fixing bacteria,* act as tiny fertilizer factories. Although green plants cannot use atmospheric nitrogen directly, these bacteria in the soil convert it to nitrogen-containing compounds which can then be absorbed by the plants' roots.

Saprophytic, or "corpse-eating," bacteria perform an indispensable role in decomposing dead organisms. Many of the components of your own body were in past eons parts of long-dead trees, dinosaurs, and other forms of life. Were it not for saprophytic bacteria, much of the raw materials necessary for life would have remained locked forever in the dead bodies of plants and animals instead of being recycled to simpler materials, which were then incorporated into other living things.

As is true in the case of larger organisms, microorganisms may act to the detriment as well as the benefit of human health. Those that cause infectious diseases are called *pathogenic;* if the disease is readily communicated, or spread, to other individuals, it is called a *contagious* disease. By causing disease in humans, pathogens affect human health directly; by causing disease in domesticated plants and animals, they can affect health indirectly but profoundly by decreasing food supplies.

Since ancient times, it has been recognized that malnutrition and infection frequently occur together, although both were believed to be divine punishment for sins. It was not until the Middle Ages that the first tentative notions of contagion appeared; diseases which were epidemic, appearing in large numbers of people in the same area, were thought to result from "poisonous fumes" or "bad air" (from which the word "malaria" comes).

More recently, a direct relationship between "famine" and "pestilence," or, more precisely, between malnutrition and infection, has been the subject of intensive study. This relationship represents an extremely important example of an interaction between nutrients and another class of extrinsic factors.

Synergism of malnutrition and infection

If two factors act independently, the combined effect of them together is the simple sum of the two separately. For example, a certain degree and kind of disease may cause death in 2 percent of the affected individuals, and a given degree of another type of disease may kill 5 percent of the victims. If the two act independently, the death rate of people who are simultaneously affected by both would be approximately 7 percent, or the sum of the two separate effects.

By contrast, in a *synergistic* relationship two factors working together produce an effect greater than the sum of the two separate effects. For example, red measles, also called *hard* or *ten day* measles, is ordinarily not a fatal disease in children; in the United States, only one case out of 10,000 cases of measles ends in death. In some of the developing countries, however, death rates from measles may be two hundred to four hundred times this high. Controlled studies, using high-protein foods to improve the nutritional status of children, have shown that these high death rates can be lowered to the same level as in the United States. This is because the majority of deaths seen in cases of measles in malnourished children are not solely the result of measles nor solely the result of malnutrition. Rather, they result from the synergism of these two; therefore the death rate in protein-deficient children with measles is far greater than the simple sum of the death rate from measles alone plus the death rate from protein deficiency alone.

Some of the reasons that malnutrition and infection act synergistically (shown in Figure 7–2) are seen to be biological. For example, antibodies, the specific proteins produced by the body in response to invasion, combat infection and can cause the person to be immune (nonsusceptible) to a later attack of the same infectious agent. *Phagocytes,* a type of white blood cell, engulf microorganisms and destroy

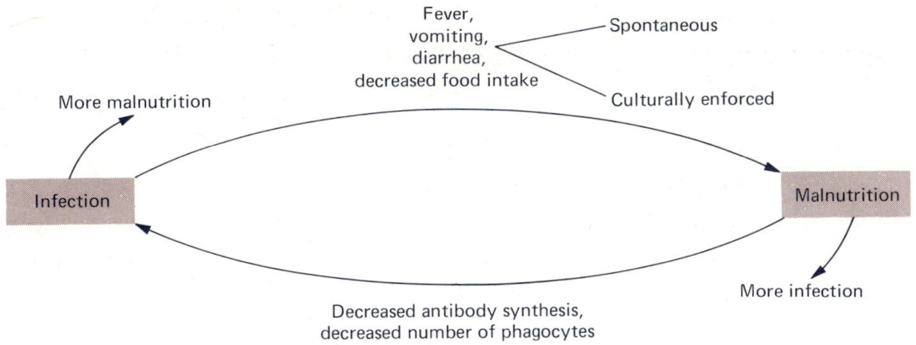

FIGURE 7–2. The synergism of malnutrition and infection.

them. Production of both antibody molecules and phagocytes is decreased by severe degrees of certain nutritional deficiencies.

Just as malnutrition decreases resistance to infection, infection can increase the degree of malnutrition. Appetite may decrease; vomiting and diarrhea cause nutrients to be lost from the digestive system before they can be absorbed into the body; fever increases the rate of energy-nutrient breakdown because chemical reactions generally occur more rapidly at higher temperatures.

Moreover, in addition to these biological factors, cultural practices may work to produce malnutrition in infected children. In Western countries, there is a saying: "Starve a cold and feed a fever." (It is difficult to know how such a practice could be applied to the person with a cold *and* a fever.) Other societies may have even more stringent and untenable customs regarding diet during illness. It may be firmly believed, for example, that a sick child should have no food at all, or only very thin broths or gruels. The effects of a prolonged period of such treatment, detrimental even to a healthy child, can be disastrous to an already sick one who is suffering from both infection and malnutrition.

Medical care, public health practices, and nutrition

Good nutrition, although important to health, cannot replace medical procedures necessary to the prevention and treatment of infectious diseases. For example, although adequate nutrition helps to insure that measles will not be fatal, innoculation is necessary to *prevent* measles and other infectious diseases. The bacterium, virus, or other infectious agent is attenuated, or subjected to processes which make it less dangerous; a measured dose of this material is then injected, and the person responds by producing antibodies which prevent future disease caused by the same agent.

Sanitation of food and water supplies, prompt treatment of disease, isolation of infected individuals, and control of disease-carrying pests are also important in protecting the health of the public. Despite the claims of certain fanatics, the majority of infectious diseases can neither be prevented nor treated by nutrition alone.

THE PHYSICAL ENVIRONMENT AND HEALTH

Because physical and chemical agents include all forms of radiation and of inanimate matter, the discussion of these is necessarily very selective.

Nutrients

These are the chemical agents with which the rest of this book will be primarily concerned. Therefore, they are merely being mentioned, rather than discussed, at this point.

Oxygen

This atmospheric gas, necessary for the utilization of energy nutrients by animal cells, has been produced mostly through the process of photosynthesis by green plants. This illustrates interrelationships between various extrinsic factors; green plants, the organisms which originally produce energy nutrients, are also the source of the oxygen needed for nutrient utilization by animals.

Despite the importance of oxygen to life, excessively great concentrations can be detrimental, as in the cases of blindness caused in many premature babies by exposure to artifically high oxygen concentrations. Although many of these babies would have died without oxygen administration, the amount given was, unfortunately, sometimes great enough to cause severe eye damage.

Radiation

Life could not exist at all without various types of radiation. The energy of sunlight, or *solar* radiation, is used by green plants for the process of photosynthesis, by which nutrients are produced. In the case of one specific nutrient, vitamin D, sunlight allows animals to produce the nutrient in their own skins, thereby making it unnecessary to have it in their diets if exposure to sunlight is adequate.

However, some forms of radiation are injurious to health. Certain radioactive chemicals, which emit radiation of various forms, can cause cancer. Years ago, factory workers who painted luminous numbers on watch dials with radium were exposed to excessive amounts of this material; as a result, many later died of cancer.

Exposure to X-rays can cause gene mutations in some cases, or cause malformation in fetuses if the pregnant female is exposed excessively. Even sunlight can be damaging, as anyone who has suffered a painful sunburn knows. Less well known is the fact that the incidence of skin cancer is increased in people who are excessively exposed to sunlight; light-skinned people are more susceptible to this form of cancer than are dark-skinned people.

Drugs

Broadly speaking, drugs are chemicals which are used to treat diseases; use for other purposes, such as to avoid reality, is generally termed drug *abuse*. A major problem in relation to drugs is that they are commonly potent materials that may have serious side effects. The tranqualizer, Thalidomide, which seemed, when first used in Europe, to be a safe, effective drug, was later shown to be the cause of tragic malformations in human fetuses. Americans were protected only by the refusal of the U.S. Food and Drug Administration to allow the drug to be sold in this country until it had been more thoroughly tested than it had been in Europe.

A second problem with drugs is that most of them have been developed very recently. Of the myriad of drugs used today, only a few were in use one hundred years ago, and the majority have been available for less than twenty-five years. For this reason, the long-term effects of many drugs are not yet known, and some may prove to have side effects more serious than the conditions which they are intended to treat.

A third problem is that it is very difficult to define terms such as *drug* and *abuse*. If the term *drug* is confined solely to those chemicals used to prevent and treat disease, an oral contraceptive could not be called a drug, unless pregnancy is defined as a disease. Although alcohol is a drug, alcoholism is generally considered distinct from drug addiction. Some drugs are taken solely to depress the appetite, or otherwise act as an emotional crutch. Is this use or abuse of a drug?

Nutrients are considered drugs when they are supplied in the form of products such as pills, capsules, or liquids. However, the only diseases that nutrients can treat successfully are nutritional deficiency diseases. Thus iron is effective in the treatment of iron deficiency anemia, just as ascorbic acid is effective against scurvy, the disease caused by a lack of vitamin C. However, nutrients are *not* effective as drugs in cases of diseases with causes other than malnutrition, and this includes the majority of diseases.

Toxins

Sola dosis facit venenum—"only the dose makes the poison"—said the sixteenth-century alchemist Paracelsus, meaning that the danger of any substance is related to the amount taken, as well as to the inherent toxicity of the material.

Because many materials are dangerous only in extremely high doses, they are commonly called *nontoxic*, but it should be recognized that no substance can really be considered "safe in unlimited amounts." Any substance, including oxygen, ordinarily safe drugs, or even essential nutrients, can be toxic if taken in large enough amounts. Certain vitamins, iron, table salt, and many other substances have caused death by poisoning in people who ingested them in very large amounts.

It is unfortunate that many people fail to realize that something which is "natural" can be highly toxic, although many *synthetic* compounds are relatively nontoxic. Botulism toxin, the toxin produced in contaminated foods by the bacterium *Clostridium botulinum,* is an example of a natural yet highly poisonous compound, as are snake and insect venoms. Moreover, many foods contain natural toxins. If a plant or animal part contains a high concentration of a toxin, one of three things can be done. People can avoid using these as foods at all; they can process them to remove or inactivate the toxic material; or they can use them in very small amounts. An example of the first possibility is avoiding the use of rhubarb leaves as food in order to avoid a large dose of oxalic acid, a poison sometimes used as a rust remover. An example of the second method is the heating of soybeans to inactivate a growth-inhibiting factor in the raw beans. The third alternative is seen in using only sparing amounts of nutmeg, because it contains the hallucination-producing compound *myristicin.* However, most foods contain only very small amounts of toxins. Materials with high concentrations of toxins have generally been rejected as food because people found, through the hard school of human experience, that they were unsuitable.

THE SOCIAL ENVIRONMENT AND HEALTH

Without question, the social environment profoundly affects social and psychological health. However, because the standards of behavioral

FIGURE 7–3. Emotional deprivation as an indirect cause of growth retardation.

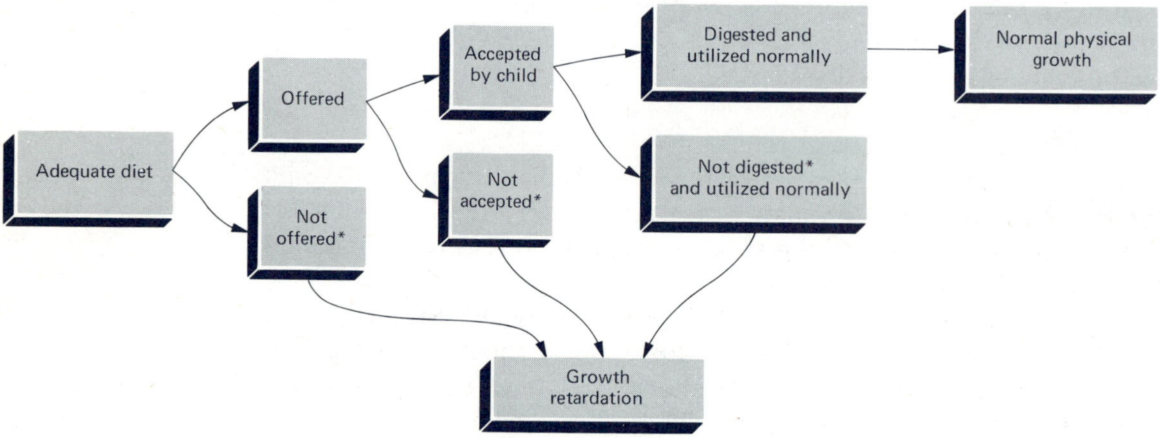

normalcy vary from one culture to another, the kind of behavior fostered by one social environment may actually be considered abnormal in another.

A good deal of confusion exists with respect to the effects of the social environment on physical health. Certainly the health of the body can be affected by the mind, which in turn is influenced by the social environment. For example, emotions can increase the release of hormones which alter the function of the heart and other organs, and certain diseases, such as stomach ulcers and allergies, are believed to be at least partly *psychosomatic* in that they may be caused by an interplay between the mind (*psyche*) and body (*soma*).

However, in some cases the social factors offered as reasons for impaired physical health may be at most only indirectly responsible. An example may illustrate this point:

Among children of the same age, there is considerable variation in size; some will be below average in height and weight, as some will be above average. Those in the lowest 3 percent for both height and weight are classed as cases of *failure to thrive*. In the majority of such children, a physical factor of some kind can be identified as the cause of the growth failure; these defects include severe allergies, inability to digest and absorb nutrients normally, and similar well-defined physical conditions.

Sometimes, however, examination of a child fails to disclose any definite medical basis for the growth failure, and it is often noted that the condition is particularly common in emotionally deprived children. Many are in institutions, and others are neglected or actually mistreated in their own homes. Because of the frequent association of emotional deprivation and growth failure, such children are sometimes said to be suffering from *deprivational dwarfism,* or growth impairment assumed to be caused entirely by lack of a normal social and emotional environment.

However, the question of exactly how emotions are related to growth retardation must ultimately be answered in physical and chemical terms (Figure 7–3). A well-fed and physically normal child cannot fail to grow, for the materials supplied in the diet cannot simply disappear into thin air. One possible explanation is that children offered an adequate diet may nevertheless refuse to eat, or may vomit or experience diarrhea as a result of emotional stress. In thse cases, the resulting lack of nutrients is a logical cause of the growth failure, and the emotional environment is therefore only indirectly responsible. Parents who deprive a child emotionally may also withhold adequate food, perhaps unconsciously. In one controlled study, children given an adequate diet showed striking gains in height and weight when they were fed adequately, even though the emotional environment was as unfavorable as previously. There seems, therefore, to be no basis for the commonly held belief that lack of love can, in itself, impair physical growth in children. However, the effects of emotional deprivation on social and psychological health can of course be very unfavorable.

SUSCEPTIBILITY TO HEALTH-RELATED NUTRITION MISINFORMATION

Although it is clear that nutrition is only one of many determinants of health and disease, claims that all diseases are caused by faulty diet persist, and are accepted by many. Those who accept such beliefs are sometimes dismissed as ignorant and gullible, perhaps even deserving of being misled because they are seeking impossibly quick simple solutions to complex problems; it may be difficult to imagine an intelligent person, reasonably familiar with the rational scientific attitudes of the twentieth century, accepting the bizarre and illusory promises of the modern version of the old-time medicine man.

Yet the number and variety of people who are or have been followers of various fad diets and forms of nutrition quackery are too large to be explained on the basis of a lack of information alone. Deep-seated hopes and fears, rather than rational considerations, can lead to acceptance of ideas and promises which, if examined critically and unemotionally, would be found to be unbased in fact.

Eating is a form of behavior that is charged with emotional connotations from the time of birth. To the infant, food is equated with security; it protects against the internal pain of hunger and acts as a buffer against inner senses of helplessness and vulnerability. As the child grows older, the early impressions are reinforced by parental admonitions: "Eat your vegetables; they'll make you healthy"; "Don't eat that; it can make you sick." Traces of childish beliefs in the power of food to relieve pain and to protect against harm may persist to a greater or lesser degree long afterward. People who retain these mystical ideas about food to an unusually large degree may be excessively vulnerable to suggestions that food can somehow allay all fears and fulfill all hopes. Because even the most emotionally mature person retains at least vestiges of primitive forms of unrealistic thinking, perhaps all people are potential believers of misinformation regarding the powers of foods, or of specific nutrients found in foods.

Desire for immortality, youth, and health

One of the strongest human desires is the wish to live forever, or, failing this, at least to achieve the longest possible life span. Furthermore, people hope to live in an eternal state of youth, or at least to retain the vitality and outward attractiveness of youth; to avoid the sickness and physical pain of disease; and to escape the deterioration associated with the aging process. Above all, they wish to avoid death, which is the inevitable and final consequence of aging.

In some people, fear of disease and deterioration is greatly exaggerated. Every magazine article, newspaper item, or television program on health and disease evokes the suspicion that this latest dread disease is even now claiming another victim. People who react in this manner are known as hypochondriacs, and are often a severe drain on the time and patience of many reputable physicians. After being assured repeatedly that there is no physical basis for their fears, they may encounter a food faddist or another charlatan who confirms their fears but offers a cure for their imaginary diseases.

Other people have very real reasons for fear of disease in themselves or in those close to them. In his book, *Death Be Not Proud,* John Gunther wrote poignantly of the family's desperate attempts to find a cure for the brain cancer which eventually killed their son at the age of sixteen. When neurologists and surgeons in a famed medical center could hold out no further hope, this intelligent, well-educated family turned at last to health food remedies in the conviction that no effort to save their son could be rejected without at least a trial. Of the decision to try a dietary treatment which had been attacked by the American Medical Association, Gunther writes:

> **We had tried orthodoxy, both static and advanced, and so now we would give heterodoxy a chance. If only we could stave Death off a little longer! And—once more—there was absolutely nothing to lose.**

And when his son died in spite of every treatment tried, he wrote:

> **All the doctors!—helpless flies now, climbing across the granite face of death.**

Desire for beauty and social acceptance

The longing for beauty and the love and acceptance that can come with it is a powerful consumer motivation that is fully exploited in the advertising of many products.

The nutrients that have been promoted for cosmetic purposes include some from almost every nutrient class. Gelatin has long been promoted as a treatment for "fragile, thin, breaking nails," and proteins of various types have been touted as shampoo ingredients which add "natural body" to hair. Of the vitamins, vitamin E is the latest one to enjoy a reputation as beneficial to skin and hair, and shows promise of replacing vitamin A, vitamin D, and *pantothenic acid,* which have been sold for this purpose in the past. According to current advertising, vitamin E used before tinting or bleaching hair will "protect against chemicals"; used as a deodorant, it provides "protection from offensive underarm perspiration odor"; and as a skin cream, it is reputed to remove blemishes, scars, and even the *straie* or "stretch marks" that sometimes appear during pregnancy. Calcium and magnesium, in the form of the mineral mixture, *dolomite,* are supposed to be effective cleansing agents in dentifrices, and certain fatlike materials such as lanolin and lecithins are advertised as effective in softening skin and hair.

In addition to specific nutrients to be applied externally or taken internally, certain foods are often advertised as beauty aids as well as health aids. Shining hair, a clear, unlined complexion, straight teeth free of cavities, perfect facial bones, and ideal body proportions are all promised to those who follow suggested regimens based on health foods, with or without supplemental nutrients in pills or capsules. That all of these physical characteristics are affected by heredity as well as by many external factors is of course ignored.

Longing for purity and freedom from modern technology

Among those who have become disenchanted with our highly technological society and with the seeming lack of emphasis on ethical values, the appeal to purity is very strong. Some find sinister connotations in the very words *chemical* and *industrial.* Organized medicine, with its armaments of drugs, surgical instruments, and other equipment, is viewed with suspicion. Because modern agriculture uses chemical fertilizers in place of manure or compost, and depends upon "poisonous chemicals" to control insect pests, it is denigrated as "agribusiness" which is "raping the environment." The farmer of the past, romanticized almost beyond recognition, is seen as having been "in tune with nature," able to produce bountiful yields with nothing more than a team of horses and a presumably unlimited supply of their manure.

To such people, security and health are equated with purity and with that which is natural. A pure environment, including pure and natural foods, may therefore be seen as a means of attaining physical and spiritual purity, and of counteracting internal feelings of corruption or uncleanness. Processed foods, foods raised with commercial fertilizers or pesticides, food additives, and a host of other entities are rejected as artificial and hence corrupt. Paradoxically, some who react in this way are nevertheless not adverse to the use of chemicals as "mind-expanding" drugs.

Distrust of the "establishment"

Rejection of conventional practices regarding food, health, and medical care may be motivated by beliefs that all of these are under the control of powerful groups against whom the individual is helpless. Physicians are seen as members of "medical trusts" who fear that they would be put out of business by products such as health foods. Food industries, it is claimed, deliberately remove nutritional value from food and add dangerous chemicals in order to make larger profits at the expense of the consumer's health. Some even suspect that the health of the American public is being systematically undermined in order to enable a foreign government to take over the nation. And, of course, the Educational Establishment is suspected of supporting the nefarious activities of other segments of the Establishment because of control by "refined food and drug" industries which threaten to withhold research funds from professors who refuse to cooperate.

CHARACTERISTICS OF PROFESSIONAL FOOD FADDISTS

Like any other group, professional food faddists come in a wide variety of forms. Many, despite their glib use of scientific-sounding jargon, have had little or no education in nutrition or medicine, although a small minority are legally entitled to the use of titles such as M.S., D.Sc., and Ph.D. Both men and women have gained, through food faddism, publicity and financial gain rarely achieved by those who accomplish legitimate work in nutrition. Because food faddists vary so much in their opinions, approaches, and methods and frequently disagree vehemently among themselves, it is impossible to list characteristics which are true of all. However, most of the following will be found to apply generally.

Knowledgeability of value of merchandising methods

Door-to-door peddling as practiced by medical charlatans of the past has largely been replaced by wide use of advertising via radio, television, magazines, newspapers, and mailorder campaigns. Vast audiences are thus reached, with the result that food faddism and nutrition misinformation constitute a multibillion-dollar business. The money-back guarantees commonly offered are of small risk to the seller because few disappointed customers bother to demand their money back.

The technique known as the "testimonial" is very common in the advertising of faddists' products; these are particularly effective if they come from well-known people in professions such as the performing arts and sports. The aura surrounding famous personalities may lead their followers to accept opinions regarding diet and health without questioning whether nutritional expertise necessarily follows from the ability to hit either a high note or a baseball. The "breakfast of champions" slogan has undoubtedly sold many a box of a certain cereal.

Claims of persecution

Charges that the faddist's statements are not accepted by nutritional and medical science elicit the indignant reply that "medical trusts and cartels" and "ivory tower professors" are trying to silence the faddist because they see him as a powerful rival who can cure diseases which are beyond the understanding of science. The "truth" about health foods and dietary supplements would make present knowledge obsolete, states the quack, and the "medical and scientific establishment" would, literally, rather see sick people die than allow this to happen.

Drug and food industries, also, would lose much of their income, says the faddist, if people were allowed to know that processed foods cause disease and that natural foods rather than drugs are the only effective cures. "Your health, your very life," utters the quack, "is being sacrificed to preserve the wealth and prestige of the medical-industrial-educational power structure." Against these groups, of course, the faddist presents himself as a martyred savior, morally obligated to fight on despite oppression.

Exploitation of human insecurity

The vague feelings of guilt, inadequacy, and uncertainty common to all people are shrewdly capitalized on by the faddist. The only way to be *sure* that a child is well nourished, a husband is protected against heart disease, an aging parent enjoys a long life span, or an ailing family member recovers is to turn to the product sold by the faddist. This may be a book or other publication filled with useless or even dangerous misinformation; a special blender or a set of pans which mysteriously "improves the nutritional value of foods"; a bottle of pills, capsules, or liquid supplying nutrients of "superior value"; organic foods; or a number of other products.

To the objection that these products may not be worth the money, the invariable response is: "How can a price be set on health, peace of mind, even life itself?".

Invention of new diseases

For people who are satisfied that they are already healthy and therefore have no need for unprescribed treatments, the quack is only too happy to invent a disease or two, which might be known as a "subclinical deficiency." Because "subclinical" refers to the absence of outward signs or symptoms of actual disease, it is difficult for anybody to prove that he or she is, indeed, free of such a condition. Accordingly, some people can be convinced that every vague problem, from stiff muscles following exertion to a reluctance to get out of bed on Monday morning, is caused by an extremely mild degree of nutritional deficiency. And, of course, claims the faddist, only the product "scientifically designed" to treat these mild deficiency states can prevent their progression to a serious and possibly fatal outcome.

Misuse of scientific data

Not bound by the limitations of legitimate scientific research, faddists are therefore free to build up a plausible-sounding interpretation that cannot fail to dazzle many uninformed readers or listeners. Data quoted out of context, interpreted incorrectly and supplemented if necessary by statements that are totally incorrect, allow the faddist to reach any conclusion desired.

An example of the difference between the food faddist's interpretation and that of acceptable scientific sources may be illustrated as follows: It is a fact that severe deficiency of the vitamin, niacin, leads to a form of mental illness which responds to the missing vitamin. The only scientifically valid interpretation of this fact is that niacin is effective in the treatment of those cases of mental illness caused by niacin deficiency—which virtually never occurs in countries such as the United States at present.

Note, however, how the same fact can be handled by the faddist. "Research has shown," he states, "that mental disorders are caused by malnutrition and can be cured by proper diet." First, there are the magic words, "Research has shown"—modern humanity's equivalent of "The Lord sayeth." Second, one specific type of mental illness becomes "mental disorders" in general. Finally, a specific vitamin is illogically replaced with "proper diet," which could imply health foods, any or all nutrient supplements, or even nonnutrients such as *rutin* or *bioflavinoids,* which faddists insist are essentials in human diets.

Results of genuine research do not as a rule make headlines, and are generally not asserted in a manner which leaves no room whatever for doubt. The faddist, unhampered by the need for a cautious interpretation of results, is free to use sensationalism, often reaching extravagant conclusions which many find more interesting than properly handled scientific data.

Use of undocumented case histories

The case histories presented in many faddist publications could almost wring tears from a stone. You may read of a child who died of cancer because the physician refused to use a "miraculous" liver-extract cure; of a woman who gave birth to a retarded infant because she ate refined foods; of a marriage destroyed by the short tempers of a husband and wife suffering from "nervousness" caused by "subclinical deficiencies." However, you will search in vain for these stories in accepted scientific journals, for they are not published there.

Conversely, medical miracles seem to abound for those who accept certain dietary treatments and food fads. The child with encephalitis is cured with vitamin C; the mental patient returns to college after undergoing "megavitamin therapy" based on enormous doses of vitamins and minerals; and one could almost be convinced that the novel, *Love Story,* would have had a happy ending if Oliver and Jennifer had only patronized their friendly neighborhood health food store.

Impressive titles

No legal restraints are imposed upon nonspecialists who choose to call themselves "nutritionists," "health advisors," "diet specialists," or "world-renowned nutrition experts," and certainly the title "Vice President of Research of the New York Nutrition Society" is much more impressive than the accurate description of the same person as "co-owner of a health food store in New York." Many "experts," unacceptable as members of the professional organization of nutritionists, the American Institute of Nutrition, nevertheless manage to impress their followers by joining the "American Academy of Applied Nutrition."

This is a group of persons who are not nutritionists, and have no scientific standing whatever. The average person, however, has no way of knowing the difference between a reputable organization and a disreputable one.

THE CONSEQUENCES OF FOOD FADS AND NUTRITION QUACKERY

Faddism and quackery are intellectually offensive, depending as they do upon statements, interpretations, and practices more akin to medieval alchemy than to established knowledge. On this basis alone, they are objectionable. In addition, however, they can be criticized for two other important reasons: economic and medical.

Economic aspects

Ordinary foods can supply all the nutrients needed except in unusual cases, such as that of a person unable to digest or utilize food normally. In this event, medical treatment, rather than special health foods or supplements, is needed.

The prices of health foods, organic foods, unnecessary and unprescribed nutrient supplements, and similar items are so high that real economic losses accrue to those who buy them, with no actual health benefits in return. "Fertile eggs," for example, may cost twice as much as eggs from the supermarket, although they are of identical nutritional value. "Organic apples" (each of which may contain at least one worm) are priced far higher than apples of better quality available in ordinary markets. Some families give their children a daily vitamin pill in addition to a good diet, yet feel that an annual examination by a pediatrician would be a financial burden. The cost of the vitamin supplement over a year's time, applied to the cost of an examination, could be far more valuable.

Medical aspects

Three distinct medical aspects of food fads can be identified.

First, food fads that recommend enormous doses of nutrient supplements can result in actual toxicity. Many documented cases of poisoning by excess vitamins A and D have been reported, especially in children. As massive doses of other nutrients become popular fads, toxic effects of these may also become apparent, because all substances, including nutrients, are toxic if taken in large enough amounts.

Second, many fads actually cause or encourage nutritional deficiencies. A daily dose of anything, be it honey, wheat germ, or a multivitamin preparation, is no substitute for an ordinary diet which supplies all of the nutrients actually needed. An extreme example of a dangerously deficient fad is the so-called "macrobiotic diet," consisting of virtually nothing but brown rice. Extreme deficiencies and even several deaths have resulted from this diet.

Third, faddists very commonly encourage their followers to diagnose and treat their own illnesses with food, thereby delaying the conventional medical treatment which may benefit the patient. This delay can result in unnecessary suffering or permanent disability in many cases. In diseases such as cancer, often treatable in the early stages but not in later stages, attempts to effect cures with health foods and nutrient supplements can have even more serious consequences. They can, in fact, be quite literally deadly.

SUGGESTED READINGS

Bruch, H. "The Allure of Food Cults and Nutrition Quackery." *Journal of the American Dietetic Association* 57 (1970):316.

Christakis, G., and A. Miridjanian. "Diets, Drugs, and Their Interrelationships." *Journal of the American Dietetic Association* 52 (1968):21.

Council on Foods and Nutrition. "Zen Macrobiotic Diets." *Journal of the American Medical Associaton* 218 (1971):397.

Dykes, M. H. M. "Evaluation of Three Anorexiants." *Journal of the American Medical Association* 230 (1974):270.

Horner, M. "Safe Handling of Foods in the Home." FDA Papers, June 1972, p. 18–25.

Latham, M. C. "Nutrition and Infection in National Development." *Science* 188 (1975):561.

Lee, D. H. K. and P. Kotin, eds. *Multiple Factors in the Causation of Environmentally Induced Disease.* New York: Academic, 1972.

Liener, I. E., ed. *Toxic Constituents of Plant Foodstuffs.* New York: Academic, 1969.

Margolius, S. *Health Foods: Facts and Fakes.* New York: Walker and Company, 1973.

"Food, Science, and Society." New York: The Nutrition Foundation, Inc., 1969.

Pederson, C. S. *Microbiology of Food Fermentation.* Westport, Conn.: Avi Publishing Co., 1971.

Roe, D. A. "Nutritional Side Effects of Drugs." *Food & Nutrition News* 45 (October–November, 1973).

Scrimshaw, N. S., C. E. Taylor, and J. E. Gordon. *Interactions of Nutrition and Infection.* Geneva: World Health Organization, 1968.

Spratt, N. T. Jr. *Developmental Biology.* Belmont, Calif.: Wadsworth Publishing Co., Inc., 1971.

Taussig, H. B. "The Thalidomide Syndrome." *Scientific American* 207 (1962): 29.

Whitten, C. F., M. G. Pettit, and J. Fischhoff. "Evidence that Growth Retardation from Maternal Deprivation Is Secondary to Undereating." *Journal of the American Medical Association* 209 (1969):1675.

8

meeting dietary recommendations

Do the genuine nutrition experts have all the answers? No, admittedly, they do not. However, unlike the self-styled experts, the real ones are *aware* of the limitations of their knowledge, and can therefore base their judgments on what is known rather than on mere dogmatic opinion.

For over a hundred years, nutritionists have made various recommendations for the purpose of attaining certain standards against which human diets could be measured. The dietary standards used today differ from those of the past, as well as differing from place to place throughout the world. A major reason for these variations is that nutrition has been, and still is, a complex and growing science; for example, until well into the twentieth century there could be no recommendations for vitamins because these nutrients were virtually unknown. Even today, with much more known about nutrition than was known even ten years ago, there is still not complete agreement on the calorie and nutrient intakes which should be considered ideal.

One problem is that, even if the ideal intake could be precisely determined at any given time, it might be unsuitable for other times. For example, when hard physical work was common the calorie requirement was necessarily very high. Modern students, office workers, or homemakers would become overweight on the energy intake that was suitable for their less sedentary grandparents.

Also, although recommendations represent admirable goals, allowances must be made for practical matters of fact. For example, nations with relatively little protein available, or with populations which reject many high-protein foods, would probably find it pointless to recommend a protein intake as high as that advocated in the United States.

Six different types of standards related to nutrition are or have been important in this country or in other parts of the world:

The Recommended Daily Dietary Allowances, or RDA. These are recommendations for calories, protein, and certain vitamins and minerals (Table 8–1). They are set by the Food and Nutrition Board of the National Academy of Sciences—National Research Council of the United States, and make recommendations for a number of age categories of people of both sexes.

The Minimum Daily Requirements, or MDR. These were legal nutrient standards set by the United States Food and Drug Administration (FDA) and used until recently by food and drug industries for purposes of labeling products. However, the name was confusing; in many cases the MDR for a nutrient was above the true minimum below which deficiency disease would be probable. Also, they were not revised during the many years after they were set, despite considerable evidence that there was little scientific evidence to support some of them. For these reasons, federal legislation passed in 1973 provided for new nutrient labeling standards by 1975.

The U.S. Recommended Daily Allowances, or U.S. RDA. These are the legal standards which replaced the MDR. Although related to the RDA, they are not identical to them. For most nutrients, the U.S. RDA is equal to or higher than the RDA for adolescent males. As anybody who has ever observed the eating habits of a well-fed teen-aged boy would suspect, the largest amount of almost anything that is needed or consumed will be that needed or consumed by this voracious young male rather than by a person in any other sex-age category. Consequently, the U.S. RDA is greater than the RDA for most people in a family or a population

The Basic Four food group plan. Sometimes referred to as the daily food guide, this is similar to the RDA in that it is a set of *recommendations* rather than legal standards imposed upon industries. In contrast to the RDA, however, the Basic Four plan was set up by the United States Department of Agriculture (USDA) and recommends *foods* rather than energy and nutrients.

In addition to the above four sets of standards, which were developed for use in the United States, two other general types of dietary standards exist:

National standards. These are variously called "standards," "requirements," and "allowances," and have been established by a number of countries for their own populations. In some cases the levels decided upon are those believed adequate for the average person, whereas in other cases the standards include a generous safety factor in addition. The RDA can be compared to the standards of other countries only if it is recognized that levels recommended in different countries may not be intended to accomplish the same goal.

The FAO-WHO dietary requirements. These are recommended intakes of calories, protein, and selected minerals and vitamins. They were developed by the Food and Agriculture Organization and the World Health Organization, both of which are agencies within the United Nations, and were designed for use by nations which have not yet developed their own standards. In practice, they are used mostly by developing countries in which the food supply is much less abundant than in countries such as the United States. They therefore represent estimated average requirements rather than the generous allowances which more affluent nations can afford to recommend.

Some of the differences in dietary standards are shown in Table 8–2. Because the RDA, U.S. RDA, and Basic Four Food Group Plan are the three sets of standards used in the United States at present, each of these will be discussed in greater detail.

THE RECOMMENDED DIETARY ALLOWANCES

Even before the beginning of the twentieth century, it was recognized that certain substances other than water and energy nutrients were necessary in human diets. However, little was known about the amounts needed, and recommendations of intakes of vitamins and minerals obviously could not be made at that stage of knowledge.

Shortly before World War II, the high rate of impaired health among men examined for military service suggested that perhaps some of the diseases in the United States could be the result of nutritional deficiencies. Consequently, the first Food and Nutrition Board of the National Research Council was organized in 1940. This board, consisting of 25 recognized authorities in nutrition, published the first RDA in 1943. Allowances for many nutrients were based on admittedly very incomplete information. Nevertheless, it was believed that the need for

TABLE 8–1
The recommended dietary allowances

Age (years)	Weight (kg)	Weight (lbs)	Height (cm)	Height (in)	Energy (kcal)	Protein (g)	Fat-soluble vitamins: Vitamin A activity (IU)	Fat-soluble vitamins: Vitamin D (IU)	Fat-soluble vitamins: Vitamin E activity (IU)
Infants									
0.0–0.5	6	14	60	24	kg x 117	kg x 2.2	1400	400	4
0.5–1.0	9	20	71	28	kg x 108	kg x 2.0	2000	400	5
Children									
1–3	13	28	86	34	1300	23	2000	400	7
4–6	20	44	110	44	1800	30	2500	400	9
7–10	30	66	135	54	2400	36	3300	400	10
Males									
11–14	44	97	158	63	2800	44	5000	400	12
15–18	61	134	172	69	3000	54	5000	400	15
19–22	67	147	172	69	3000	54	5000	400	15
23–50	70	154	172	69	2700	56	5000		15
51 +	70	154	172	69	2400	56	5000		15
Females									
11–14	44	97	155	62	2400	44	4000	400	12
15–18	54	119	162	65	2100	48	4000	400	12
19–22	58	128	162	65	2100	46	4000	400	12
23–50	58	128	162	65	2000	46	4000		12
51 +	58	128	162	65	1800	46	4000		12
Pregnant					+300	+30	5000	400	15
Lactating					+500	+20	6000	400	15

"Food and Nutrition Board: Recommended Dietary Allowances," 8th ed., Pub. No. 1694, Washington, D.C.: National Academy of Sciences-National Research Council, 1974.

some sort of standard was great enough to justify setting one, even though it would probably need to be revised later. In fact, the eighth edition of the RDA, published in 1974, is the seventh revision of the original RDA.

There were and still are several problems in setting the RDA. First, information is still lacking for some nutrients because requirements in humans are difficult to determine. Minimal requirements are ordinarily determined by finding the smallest amount needed to keep people in good nutritional status, or to prevent or cure deficiency. However, some nutrients are obtained so easily from ordinary diets that it is actually difficult to find humans who do not obtain far more than the actual amount needed. Therefore, very unusual diets must be fed to experimental subjects for long periods of time before any signs of deficiency appear. This type of research is too tedious and time-consuming to

Water-soluble vitamins							**Minerals**					
Ascorbic acid (mg)	**Folacin (μg)**	**Niacin (mg)**	**Riboflavin (mg)**	**Thiamin (mg)**	**Vitamin B_6 (mg)**	**Vitamin B_{12} (μg)**	**Calcium (mg)**	**Phosphorus (mg)**	**Iodine (μg)**	**Iron (mg)**	**Magnesium (mg)**	**Zinc (mg)**
35	50	5	0.4	0.3	0.3	0.3	360	240	35	10	60	3
35	50	8	0.6	0.5	0.4	0.3	540	400	45	15	70	5
40	100	9	0.8	0.7	0.6	1.0	800	800	60	15	150	10
40	200	12	1.1	0.9	0.9	1.5	800	800	80	10	200	10
40	300	16	1.2	1.2	1.2	2.0	800	800	110	10	250	10
45	400	18	1.5	1.4	1.6	3.0	1200	1200	130	18	350	15
45	400	20	1.8	1.5	2.0	3.0	1200	1200	150	18	400	15
45	400	20	1.8	1.5	2.0	3.0	800	800	140	10	350	15
45	400	18	1.6	1.4	2.0	3.0	800	800	130	10	350	15
45	400	16	1.5	1.2	2.0	3.0	800	800	110	10	350	15
45	400	16	1.3	1.2	1.6	3.0	1200	1200	115	18	300	15
45	400	14	1.4	1.1	2.0	3.0	1200	1200	115	18	300	15
45	400	14	1.4	1.1	2.0	3.0	800	800	100	18	300	15
45	400	13	1.2	1.0	2.0	3.0	800	800	100	18	300	15
45	400	12	1.1	1.0	2.0	3.0	800	800	80	10	300	15
60	800	+2	+0.3	+0.3	2.5	4.0	1200	1200	125	18+	450	20
80	600	+4	+0.5	+0.3	2.5	4.0	1200	1200	150	18	450	25

TABLE 8–2
Comparison of dietary standards for energy and selected nutrients

	United States		Canada		FAO	
	Male	Female	Male	Female	Male	Female
Kilocalories	2700.0	2000.0	2850.0	2400.0	3200.0	2300.0
Protein (grams)	56.0	46.0	50.0	39.0	46.0	39.0
Calcium (grams)	0.8	0.8	0.5	0.5	0.4–0.5	0.4–0.5
Iron (milligrams)	10.0	18.0	6.0	10.0	10.0	18.0
Vitamin C	45.0	45.0	30.0	30.0		
Thiamin	1.4	1.0	0.9	0.7	1.3	0.9

Note: The FAO standard designed for use in many developing countries includes a high recommendation for energy. This reflects the greater physical activity of people in developing countries compared to the average American. The FAO standards for essential nutrients are in general lower than the U.S. standards.

attract many investigators, and the diets too unpalatable to attract many volunteers as subjects.

Second, although a great deal of research has been done on some nutrients, different nutritionists disagree on how the data should be interpreted. A tremendous range of requirements may be found among apparently normal people (Figure 8–1). One scientist may believe that the RDA should equal or exceed the needs of 90 percent of the subjects studied, and another may insist that it should be set at a higher level in order to cover the needs of 95 percent or more.

Third, some nutrients have been studied almost entirely in laboratory animals rather than in humans, and whether data from animal experiments can legitimately be used to set nutrient allowances for humans is a matter of controversy. Some nutritionists advocate using animal experiment data simply because it is the only information yet available for some nutrients; others believe that species differences are too great to allow for valid comparison between human and rat requirements.

The following points should be noted regarding the current RDA:

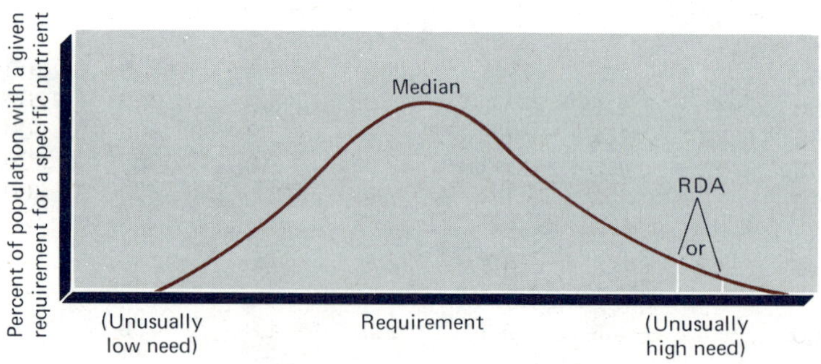

FIGURE 8–1. The range of requirements of normal people.

Recommendations are made for energy and for 17 nutrients: protein, 10 vitamins, and 6 minerals. Although many nutrients other than these 17 are known to be essential in human nutrition, too little information is available even today to set recommendations for all of them.

The RDA for energy does *not* include a safety factor above estimated average need. Calories in excess of need lead to excess weight, which could certainly not be recommended by nutritionists. For this reason, the allowance for calories for each age-sex group is set *at*, rather than above, the estimated energy need.

The allowances for nutrients, however, include a margin of safety above average requirements, and in some cases this margin is generous indeed. The RDA for ascorbic acid, for example, is more than five times the amount necessary to prevent deficiency disease. Safety margins for other nutrients, although less generous than this, are adequate to permit full realization of the potential for growth and productivity in practically all healthy people in the American population.

How should the RDA be interpreted?

In the words of the Food and Nutrition Board, the RDA are intended "to serve as goals for planning food supplies and as guides for the interpretation of food consumption records of groups of people." The allowances should therefore *not* be used as rigid criteria against which the diets of individuals are measured and below which malnutrition is assumed. It is certainly desirable for each person to attempt to achieve the RDA for his or her age-sex group, because whether each individual has higher than average requirements is impossible to determine. However, to judge a person "malnourished" or a diet "poor" solely because the diet does not provide the intakes recommended in the RDA is unjustified.

An example of *misuse* of the RDA is commonly seen in the advertising of certain iron-containing supplements. Diet surveys often show that many women do not obtain the recommended allowance for iron. However, by no means are all of these women suffering from iron deficiency; some of them need far less than the generous recommended allowance because they absorb iron more efficiently than others do, or because they lose significantly less iron in their menstrual periods than other women do. It is therefore obviously incorrect to assume that women who do not obtain the RDA for iron have "iron-deficient diets." This fact, however, is generally ignored by advertisers of iron-containing supplements, so as to imply that their products are needed by practically all women.

The allowance for calories should be used in a particularly flexible manner, for people with below average energy needs *must* restrict their energy intake to a level below the RDA in order to control body weight. The correct standard of energy intake for a given individual is that which results in normal body weight, and people of normal weight are obviously obtaining their own individual calorie need whether or not it agrees with the RDA.

If you meet the RDA in all respects are you *certain* to be well nourished? No, because an occasional person may have unusually high individual requirements which exceed those of "practically all healthy people in the American population." People like these are so rare, however, that there is no justification for the practice of swallowing handfuls of vitamin and mineral supplements on the slight chance that a given person's particular requirements are too high to be supplied by ordinary foods as most people's need are.

Recommendations versus requirements

The word "recommended" in RDA should *never* be replaced by the word "required." If a young adult's daily calcium intake is 600 milligrams, it is valid to state that this is only three-fourths of the RDA, but it is *not* correct to state that it is only three-fourths of the individual's actual calcium requirement.

People who consistently fail to meet their actual nutrient requirements eventually become malnourished. Much has been written, particularly in the popular press, about the extent, location, and causes of malnutrition and poor diets in the United States; many of the conclusions, however, have been based on nothing more than food-consumption data. This is not a correct way to determine the nutritional status of people. Physical examination for signs of deficiencies, biochemical tests of body fluids such as blood and urine, and other methods are necessary in order to determine whether a given individual is well nourished or not. It must always be remembered that the ultimate consumers of the nutrients provided in human diets are the individual body cells, and if the cells receive the kinds and amounts of nutrients needed for optimal functioning, the person is well nourished whether or not the intakes agree with any arbitrary standard.

THE UNITED STATES RDA, NUTRITION LABELING, AND THE CONSUMER

People can use nutrition information on labels in three ways:

1 They can compare the nutritive values of different foods by reading the label statements about the kinds and amounts of nutrients present.
2 They can increase their knowledge of nutrition in general by becoming familiar with many of the nutrients required in human diets.
3 Most important, from a practical point of view, they can plan diets that will provide recommended amounts of nutrients. Those who need special diets, such as low calorie or low cholesterol, can select foods meeting specifications of their diets.

Federal regulations on nutrition labeling, published by the Food and Drug Administration (FDA) in 1973, set rules on what information shall be put on labels and how it shall be presented. Nutrition labeling is *voluntary* in the case of most foods, although competitive pressures may force many processors to use it even if the law does not. However, nutrition labeling is *required* by law if any nutrient has been added to the food or if any nutritional claim is made either on the label or in advertising.

Information is provided in a standard format on a printed *panel,* such as those shown in Figure 8–2. *Required* information includes:

The serving size
The number of servings in the package
Calories per serving
Protein, carbohydrate, and fat per serving, expressed in grams
Amounts of protein, 2 minerals, and 5 vitamins in a serving, expressed as a percentage of the U.S. Recommended Daily Allowance (U.S. RDA)

Optional information includes:

Amounts per serving of 7 vitamins and 5 minerals in addition to those for which information is required, expressed as a percentage of the U.S. RDA
Amounts of saturated and polyunsaturated fats per serving
Cholesterol content per serving
Sodium content per serving

If information on fat and cholesterol is given, it must be accompanied by a statement that this is provided for those who, on a physician's advice, are modifying their intake of these. Otherwise, people might incorrectly assume that the FDA has made a definite decision on the controversy over the role of these nutrients in heart disease.

The U.S. RDA (Table 8–3) were derived from the 1968 RDA which, it will be recalled, are considerably above the actual nutrient requirements of average people. In turn, the U.S. RDA for most nutrients is higher than the RDA for most age-sex categories. In short, the U.S. RDA is in most cases above the RDA for most persons, and even farther above their actual requirements.

Proteins: all are not created equal

Of the nutrients listed on a nutrition information panel, protein is unique in that *both* the amount in grams and the percent of the U.S. RDA are listed. This is because there are two U.S. RDA values for proteins: one for higher quality proteins and the other for those of lower quality. Of the 20 or so amino acids that occur as parts of protein molecules, 8 are essential for adult humans. If all 8 of these are present in adequate amounts, the protein is of high quality and is said to be "complete," or of high biological value. If one or more essential amino acids are lacking, the protein quality is correspondingly decreased. Protein *quality* partly determines the total *amount* of protein needed, for if a

FIGURE 8–2
"Enriched, nutritious, and low-calorie!" is not enough. Nutrition information on product labels must conform to a standard format and appear in a panel (right).

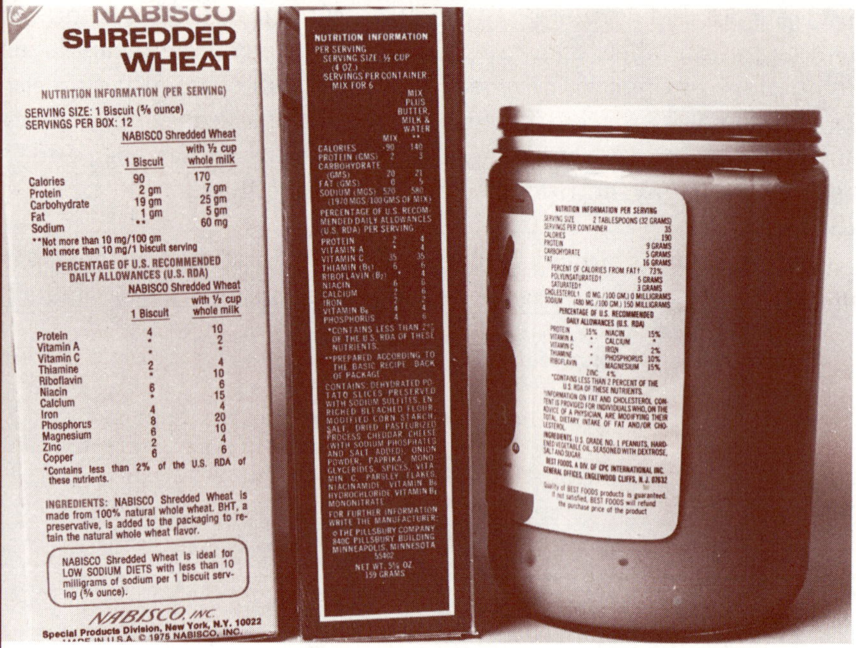

TABLE 8–3
The U.S. RDA used in labeling

Nutrient	U.S. RDA
Protein (grams)	45.0 (or 65.0 depending on quality)
Vitamin A (IU)	5000.0
Vitamin C (milligrams)	60.0
Thiamin (milligrams)	1.5
Riboflavin (milligrams)	1.7
Niacin (milligrams)	20.0
Calcium (grams)	1.0 (1000 milligrams)
Iron (milligrams)	18.0

The above *require* either a listing or a disclaimer on a nutrition label. In addition, the following may be included if the producer wishes:

Vitamin D (IU)	400.0
Vitamin E (IU)	30.0
Vitamin B_6 (milligrams)	2.0
Folacin (milligrams)	0.4
Vitamin B_{12} (micrograms)	6.0 (0.006 milligrams)
Phosphorus (grams)	1.0 (1000 milligrams)
Iodine (micrograms)	150.0 (0.150 milligrams)
Magnesium (milligrams)	400.0
Zinc (milligrams)	15.0
Copper (milligrams)	2.0
Biotin (milligrams)	0.3
Pantothenic acid (milligrams)	10.0

protein is of high biological value, less is needed than if the protein were of lower quality.

The principal milk protein, called *casein,* is used as a standard of comparison. For proteins with quality equal to or higher than that of casein, the U.S. RDA is 45 grams; for proteins of lower quality, the U.S. RDA is 65 grams. Consumers do not have to calculate the percentage of the U.S. RDA for protein because this is done for them and the result is listed on the label. However, it is simple to do so. For foods containing proteins of high biological value, the number of grams of protein is divided by 45; if the protein quality is less than that of casein, the number of grams of protein is divided by 65. Two foods which each contain 15 grams of protein per serving might therefore provide different percentages of the U.S. RDA for protein. The food with high quality protein would provide 33 percent of the U.S. RDA (15 divided by 45), but the one with lower quality would provide only 23 percent (15 divided by 65).

Advantages of using percentages of U.S. RDA

Quantities of protein, vitamins, and minerals are given as percentages of the U.S. RDA rather than in units of weight such as milligrams or grams. This allows consumers to know whether they meet the U.S. RDA without having to refer to a table of standards; they can simply add the percentages for all foods eaten in a day. For example, if 5 servings of food contain, respectively, 10, 25, 4, 8, and 35 percent of the U.S. RDA for a given nutrient, the total intake was the sum of these, or 82 percent of the U.S. RDA. Because most people do not need the full 100 percent for each nutrient, an intake of 82 percent is almost certainly satisfactory.

Percentages of U.S. RDA are expressed as follows on labels:

2 percent increments up to 10 percent
5 percent increments from 10 to 50 percent
10 percent increments above 50 percent

To express them in smaller increments would imply a greater degree of accuracy than can be achieved, because foods, like people, vary in their composition.

Restrictions under FDA labeling regulations

When food industries add enormous amounts of nutrients to their products solely for the purpose of advertising advantages, nutrient "horsepower races" occur. In order to discourage this practice, foods that are fortified to contain 50 percent to 150 percent of the U.S. RDA per serving may be declared to be *vitamin-mineral supplements,* and products containing *more* than 150 percent of the U.S. RDA may be classed as *drugs.* Supplements and drugs are, of course, subject to more rigid legal regulation than are foods.

FDA regulations also restrict health and medical claims on labels and in advertising by *prohibiting* any of the following false statements or implications:

A food can cure or prevent disease.
Adequate nutrition cannot be provided by balanced diets of ordinary foods.
Dietary inadequacies are caused by soil and plant growth conditions such as the use of chemical fertilizers.
Processing of foods causes dietary inadequacies.
Substances such as *inositol, para-amino benzoic acid,* and *bioflavinoids* are of nutritional value to humans.
Synthetic vitamins are inferior to naturally occurring ones.

Because all of the above are false, foods labeled or advertised with such statements can legally be declared to be misbranded, seized, and destroyed.

Exceptions to the nutrition labeling regulations

Some foods are subject to special labeling laws and others are exempt from *all* nutrition labeling requirements, even though nutrients have been added.

Foods for babies and young children. The serving size is naturally smaller than that used for adults, and a special set of U.S. RDA's, lower than the set used for others, is used up to the age of four years.

Foods used for special dietary use. These are used in the dietary management of specific diseases and may be the sole item of the diet for some individuals. They are labeled according to a specific law, which differs from that regulating ordinary foods.

Foods exempted from nutrition labeling laws although nutrients have been added. This category consists of the following:

1 Iodized salt
2 Foods containing nutrients added solely for technological reasons, such as vitamin C added to prevent discoloration of fruits
3 Foods shipped in bulk and used solely in the production of other foods
4 Foods supplied for institutional food service only
5 Standardized foods, either in themselves or as ingredients in other foods, such as enriched white flour, either alone or as an ingredient in a mix

Standardized foods, examples of which are shown in Figure 8–3, have long been exempt from labeling laws which apply to other foods. These are foods for which FDA has established an ingredient list or recipe which must be followed by any producer who labels the product by that name. The original purpose was to prevent cheating in the marketplace, as can easily happen when much of the baking, canning, and preserving is done by industry instead of in the home. Laws that specify the kinds and amounts of ingredients in a food are therefore designed to prevent manufacturers from making an unfair profit by using cheap, inferior ingredients. Legal definitions, called "standards of identity," have been set for approximately 365 food items. Although these foods

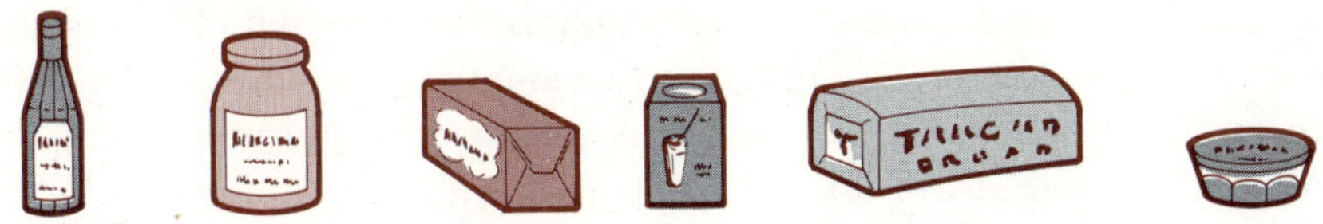

FIGURE 8–3. Examples of "standardized foods," for which standards of identity have been set.

can be labeled as to ingredients and added nutrients, no law *requires* such labeling because the name itself determines the ingredients in the product. However, people can get this information by writing to the company that makes the product.

Misuse of the U.S. RDA

Like any other standard, the U.S. RDA can be used incorrectly. First, a consumer may assume that malnutrition is inevitable if 100 percent of the U.S. RDA is not consumed every day; this assumption can arouse an unwarranted degree of concern. Second, the knowledge gained from reading labels may lead some consumers to consider themselves "instant nutritionists," paradoxically making themselves more rather than less susceptible to nutrition misinformation. Third, people may judge foods *solely* by nutrient content, and believe that the only foods worth eating in each category are those with the highest percent of the U.S. RDA. For example, a woman may customarily serve canned pineapple rings with baked ham. However, upon comparing the labels of various canned fruits and vegetables, she may note that canned tomatoes are a much richer source of vitamin A and ascorbic acid, and may therefore choose tomatoes rather than pineapple, even though the family is less happy about the choice. Her decision may not even serve any real nutritional purpose, for if the family has enough other sources of these vitamins, the higher levels in tomatoes compared to pineapple offer no further advantage. They would not, therefore, be the better choice overall; the buyer should have considered the *total* diet, and not just the apparent superiority of one food compared to a food which is better liked.

THE BASIC FOUR FOOD GROUP PLAN

Although the RDA and the U.S. RDA serve as valuable guides in planning nutritionally adequate diets, few people have the time and interest to use them exclusively. In theory, everyone could read the labels on food packages, look up nutrient and calorie values for unlabeled foods, add up all the values, and finally compare the totals to a standard. In practice, hardly anybody would.

In order to facilitate the planning of an adequate diet, it is therefore necessary to have a simple, easily remembered plan which, if followed, insures that the diet will come close to meeting the allowances. Such a plan is based on classifying foods in certain basic groups; each group contains foods that are similar enough in nutrient content to be more or less interchangeable.

The earliest known attempts to set up a food grouping system in the United States were made during World War I. Several years later, the U.S. Department of Agriculture published a plan built around the following five groups:

1 Vegetables and fruits
2 Meat, fish, and milk
3 Cereals
4 Sugar
5 Fat

This publication, entitled *Good Proportions in the Diet,* was widely accepted for years, despite its numerous shortcomings. However, during World War II, when food rationing began and examination of men for military service detected considerable malnutrition, the USDA published the *National Wartime Nutrition Guide* to replace the former system. This time *seven* food groups were specified, and emphasis was placed on selection of alternate foods for those limited by wartime rationing; for example, fat was retained as a separate group, but sugar was not. No definite portion sizes were recommended, and the number of servings daily were left to the individual's discretion. Eating properly had become a patriotic duty, with a true patriot defined as one who ate well enough to remain a healthy citizen, though eating frugally enough to avoid wasting materials needed to support the war effort. The plan was revised in 1946, recommending a given number of servings daily from each food group. For the next decade, this *Basic Seven* food group plan was used in educational programs for the general public, as well as in high schools and colleges.

It was eventually decided, however, that seven groups made for a plan that was too complicated to appeal to many people, and a number of nutritionists suggested that the plan be streamlined. A system similar to that of today, called the *Basic Four Daily Food Guide,* was published in the 1950s and, with slight modifications, has become the guide used today in the United States (Table 8–4).

Advantages of the basic four plan

One important advantage of the Basic Four Plan is that it is simple and fairly easy for people to learn; the names of the four groups can easily be taught to children in kindergarten. Second, it is practical in terms of availability of foods and the eating habits of the majority of Americans. Third, it is flexible, allowing for choices within each group; for example, a person who cannot afford meat every day, or who does not choose to eat meat, could still follow the plan by eating peanut butter, dried legumes (peas and beans), or other foods that are meat alternates. The principal advantage is that the plan insures that people will meet or come close to meeting the RDA for everything except energy (for both sexes) and iron (for women). It is assumed that people can easily meet their need for energy by eating more of everything, including the "additional foods" not included in any of the four food groups. With respect to iron, however, the RDA is set so high for females of reproductive age that there is no practical and acceptable food grouping system that would insure meeting it. A plan recommending frequent generous servings of high-iron foods such as liver could insure meeting the RDA for iron, but needless to say this would be unacceptable to many.

A *disadvantage* of the Basic Four Plan is that, in order to insure meeting the RDA for ascorbic acid (vitamin C) and vitamin A, the vegetable-fruit group must be divided into subgroups. For example, if you ate the four servings of this group, without any regard to the subgroups, your selections might be similar to those shown in Table 8–5. The totals for ascorbic acid and vitamin A value, although not so low as to make actual deficiency disease inevitable, are far below the RDA for adults. Therefore, to insure that the RDA for ascorbic acid and vitamin A are met, the vegetable-fruit group is further divided into four subgroups.

In effect, then, the more complete form of the Basic Four Plan actually has seven rather than four categories. This is suitable for use with people who are capable of benefitting from it, whereas the less complicated version, consisting only of the four major groups, with no subcategories, is appropriately used as a guide for others.

The main nutritive values of the various food groups

Although all four food groups supply *some* of almost all nutrients, each individual group makes particularly significant contributions in only some respects, and each is significantly lacking in at least one nutrient. Although a discussion of the nutritive value of the food groups will become fully meaningful only after the individual nutrients have been studied in some detail, the study of the nutrients can be more meaningful in light of an early introduction to the nutrient contributions of the various food groups.

THE ENRICHED AND WHOLE GRAIN BREAD AND CEREAL GROUP

Bread is easily identified; it is "the staff of life," the filler to be used to appease hunger when everything else on the table is in short supply, the supporting structure and superstructure of the ubiquitous sandwich. But other words, *cereal, enriched,* and *whole grain,* may all be occasionally misunderstood.

TABLE 8–4
Outline of the Basic Four Food Group Plan

Food group	Minimum amount recommended daily: Number of servings	Minimum amount recommended daily: Approximate size of serving for people age 7 and older
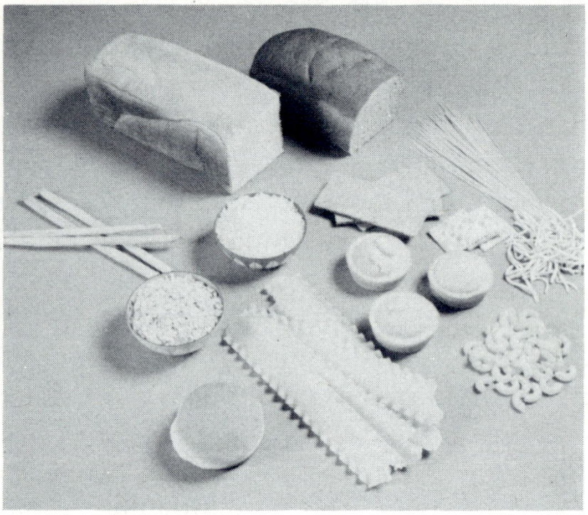		
Breads and cereal products, enriched or whole grain	4	1 slice bread 1 cup flaked cereal ½–⅔ cup cooked cereal 1 muffin or roll 1 pancake ½ hamburger bun
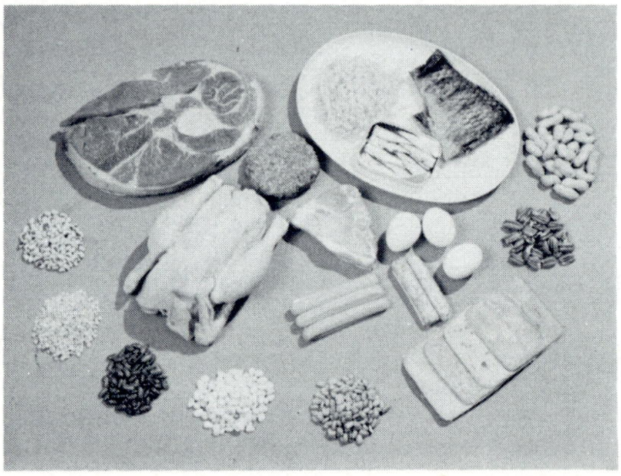		
Meat and meat alternates	The equivalent of 4 ounces cooked meat* (not counting fat or bone)	

* The equivalent of 4 ounces of cooked meat can be obtained from meat or from various combinations of the following, *each* of which is equivalent to 1 ounce of meat:
 1 egg
 1 ounce of nuts
 2 tablespoons peanut butter
 ½ cup cooked dried legumes (such as baked beans)
 1 ounce of cheese (if not counted in milk group)
 ¼ cup of cottage cheese (if not counted in milk group)

	Minimum amount recommended daily	
Food group	Number of servings	Approximate size of serving for people age 7 and older

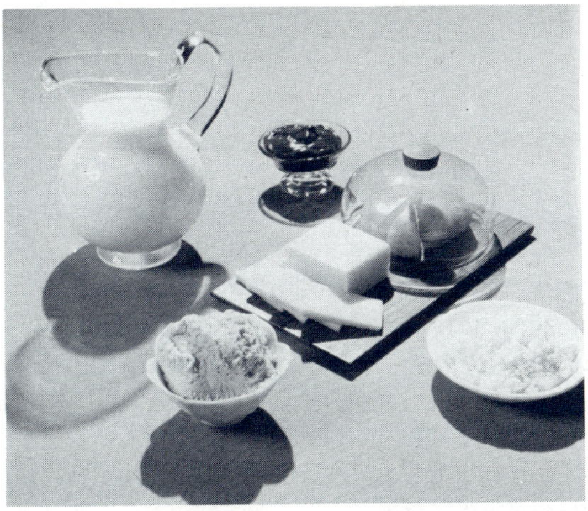

Milk and milk products	2 (age 18 and up) 4 (age 11 to 18) 2 (age 7 to 10)	1 cup milk or light cream 1½ ounce hard cheese 2 cups ice cream 1⅓ cup cottage cheese

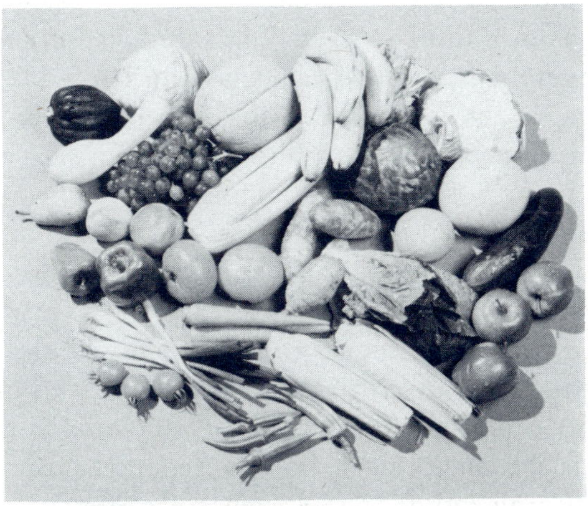

Vegetable—fruit group:		If whole, 1 medium If raw, ⅔ to 1 cup If cooked, or juice, ½ cup
a. Dark green and deep yellow vegetables and fruits	a. 1 every other day	
b. Good vitamin C sources	b. 1 good or	
c. Fair vitamin C sources	c. 2 fair	
d. Other fruits and vegetables	d. Variable; to total of 4	

TABLE 8–5

Low vitamin C and A intakes possible with four servings of vegetables and fruits

	Vitamin C milligrams	Vitamin A value, IU
Yellow corn, canned, ½ cup	7	345
Apple, raw, 1 medium	3	50
Lettuce, chopped, 1 cup	9	950
Fruit cocktail, canned, ½ cup	3	180
	22	1525

To Americans, cereal may mean no more than flaked or puffed breakfast foods. To the majority of the world's people, however, cereals (or grains) are of enormous importance. In fact, the origin of the word *cereal* itself suggests how basic these foods have been to human life. Ceres, the Roman goddess of agriculture, was so distraught when her daughter was carried off to the Lower World that the plants under her care died. At last the god Jupiter decreed that the daughter could spend six months of each year on earth with Ceres, returning to the Lower World for the other six. Thus the ancients explained the seasons, with grains growing high during part of the year and lying dormant in the soil during the other half.

Even today, in some parts of the world cereals may supply 80 percent or more of the total calorie intake, as well as valuable amounts of essential nutrients. In developed countries such as the United States, grains are often used less directly, being fed to animals; the animals and their milk or eggs are then consumed by humans. Even so, cereals consumed directly constitute at least a part of almost everybody's daily diet. For this reason, real nutritional differences result depending upon whether you use enriched and whole grain products or products made from unenriched refined grains.

The bread and cereal group includes enriched and whole grain flour, bread, cornmeal, grits, rice, and products such as macaroni and spaghetti. It does *not,* to many people's surprise, include enriched breakfast cereals. This is because there are no federal enrichment standards for breakfast cereals other than farina and grits. Although manufacturers are required to list the amounts of all added nutrients on the cereal box, they are not required to use, or to list, the same kinds or amounts of nutrients required for products such as enriched bread. Producers may therefore choose to add large amounts of many nutrients, or to add none at all. *Enriched* breads and cereals are those to which have been added *certain nutrients in amounts specified by U.S. federal government standards.* It is not enough that food processors add the nutrients they choose in any amounts they desire. If they do this, they are free to sell the resulting product, but they cannot label it "enriched," for it does not meet specifically defined standards.

Enrichment standards *require* that three B vitamins—thiamin, riboflavin, and niacin—and the mineral, iron, be added to all grain products labeled "enriched." In addition, they *permit* as options the addition of calcium, vitamin D, wheat germ, and dried yeast.

During World War II, nationwide enrichment of white bread and rolls was required. However, after the war, this requirement was dropped and states were allowed to return to the prewar practice of making enrichment compulsory only if they chose. At present about thirty states have passed legislation making enrichment of bread compulsory, but even in some states with no such laws processors voluntarily enrich much of their flour and bread.

Grains are the seeds of grasses such as wheat, rice, barley, and oats; corn is considered a grain when it is dried and used in making bread and similar products, but is considered a vegetable when it is prepared in other ways. Botanically, of course, such a classification is meaningless. Whole grain products are those made from grains which have not had the germ (embryo) and outer coats (bran) removed. Because a high proportion of the essential nutrients of grains are removed when these parts are removed by milling, products made from lightly milled grains are *restored* to natural levels or higher, and products made from highly milled grains are *enriched* according to the standards discussed previously.

Enriched white bread seems to be one of the special hates of certain people, who insist that every food must be eaten in its unsullied natural state. These people reject enrichment as an attempt to perpetuate a great hoax on the American public. After all, they point out, many nutrients are removed by milling, but only a few are returned by enrichment. The fact that the majority of the ones removed are of absosolutely no practical nutritional concern in American diets seems to escape their attention.

The proclivity of certain nonnutritionists to confuse important with insignificant differences in nutrient content was demonstrated by the rating of various breakfast cereals several years ago. The rater, a civil engineer, evaluated these products solely on their ability to supply, in one serving, given amounts of a number of nutrients. Among these were vitamin A, vitamin C, calcium, and other nutrients which are not normally present in significant amounts in cereals. Therefore, and not surprisingly, whole grain cereals such as shredded wheat came out far behind many of the highly fortified cereals which are advertised as supplying "all your vitamin needs for the day." This is an example of an absurd method of evaluating foods. Few people expect to eat nothing but a bowl of cereal each day, yet they may be very impressed by the breakfast cereal box label that implies that the product inside is a meal in itself, or even a day's meals in itself. The nutrient content of the *total* intake, not of one single food, is the point which deserves attention.

THE MEAT AND MEAT ALTERNATE GROUP

The meat group includes all forms of flesh: beef, veal, pork (including sausage), chicken, duck, goose, lamb, mutton, fish, shellfish, organs such as liver, kidney, and heart, and so on. As alternates to these, eggs, nuts, peanut butter, dried mature peas and beans (collectively called legumes), plus extra servings of milk and milk products can be used.

The principal nutritive values are in supplying proteins of high biological value; the minerals, iron and phosphorous; and the group of vitamins known as the B vitamins; organ meats are particularly rich in iron and B vitamins. Most meats, even lean ones, contain considerable fat, and legumes are high in carbohydrate. The most significantly lacking nutrients in this food group are calcium, vitamin C, and vitamin A. Liver is the only meat group item that contains significant amounts of ascorbic acid, and vitamin A in this group is confined to liver, kidney, eggs, and extra milk servings that may have been counted here.

If extra servings of milk can be counted in the meat group, can extra meat servings be placed in the milk group? The answer is that they cannot, because the milk group is the *only* one rich in calcium. Therefore, although all of the nutritive values of the meat group can, with careful planning, be provided by other foods, the calcium provided by milk is not likely to be supplied even by judicious choices from meat or other groups. The one situation that is the exception is that in which bones are eaten, as are the bones of small fish such as sardines and the pieces of bone found in canned salmon. However, although fish bones are a significant calcium source in some cultures, they are not in the United States. Therefore, foods in the meat group are in general far too low in calcium to be considered equivalent to milk.

Certain foods sometimes considered equivalent to meat are actually *not* included in this group. Bacon and salt pork (fatback) are much too high in fat to be considered the nutritional equivalent of meat. Gelatin, although it is 100 percent protein and is derived from the connective tissues of animals, is an incomplete protein of little nutritional value, and is therefore excluded from the meat group.

THE MILK GROUP

Milk is a complex fluid produced by the mammary glands of mature female mammals and used to feed their young. Although cow's milk is by far the most commonly used type in the United States, the milks of various other mammals, including sheep, goats, horses, and camels, are used in other cultures. Whole milk, low-fat milk, skim milk, buttermilk, canned milk, dried milk, yoghurt, cottage cheese, ice cream, ice milk, light or "thin" cream, and hard cheeses such as cheddar, Swiss, and American are all included in the milk group, as are any of these products used in cooking, such as milk or cream used in puddings, sauces, and cream soups.

Many people think of milk as being synonymous with calcium, and it is true that this group is the only one extremely rich in this mineral. However, milk and milk products make other important nutrient contributions (Figure 8–4). Like the foods of the meat group, they supply

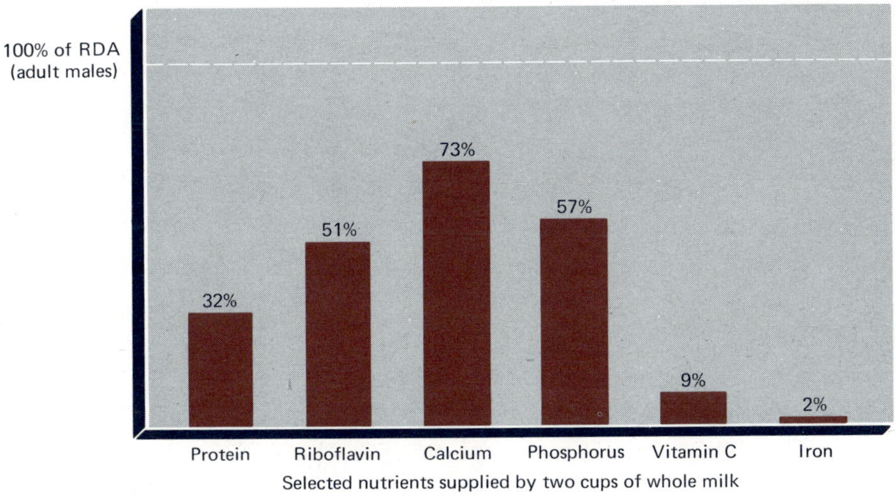

FIGURE 8–4. The nutritional value of milk. Note significant amounts of several nutrients, not just calcium; also note the very low content of iron and vitamin C.

nutritionally valuable (complete) proteins and the mineral, phosphorous. B vitamins are also present in very useful amounts, and in fact milk is the principal source of the B vitamin, riboflavin, in the usual American diet. Another similarity to the meat group is the low ascorbic acid content.

In contrast to the meat group, the milk group is a good source of vitamin D and a fairly valuable vitamin A source. However, this depends upon the type of fortification. All types of milk are naturally low in vitamin D, so if this is present it is because it has been added in order to improve nutrient value. Vitamin A is naturally present in whole milk, but because it is fat-soluble it is removed with the fat when skim milk is produced. For this reason, vitamin A is commonly added to skim milk to replace that which was removed. The label will state whether vitamin A or D, or both, have been added.

Also in contrast to the meat group, milk and milk products are very poor iron sources. Because of this, most nutritionists recommend that extra milk be counted in the meat group only occasionally rather than routinely. However, foods in all of the groups except the milk group can supply useful amounts of iron, so substituting milk for meat will not necessarily lead to a serious iron shortage.

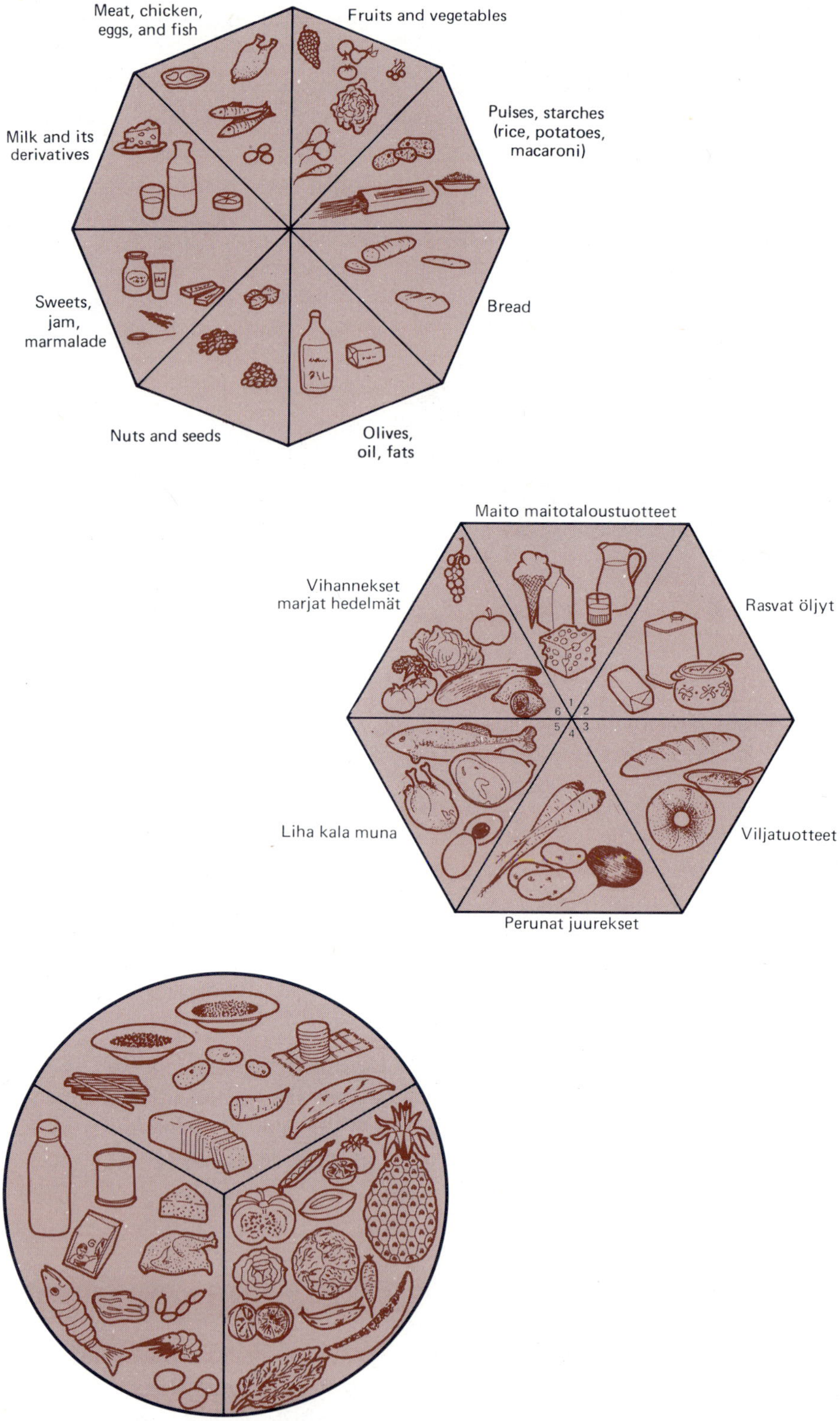

FIGURE 8–5. Food group plans used in other areas of the world: Lebanon (8 groups), Finland (6 groups), and Central America (3 groups).

In some societies, so little milk is consumed that it is impractical to recommend it as a separate group, and milk products may therefore be placed with meats in a general "animal products" group as the only feasible solution. An example is a food group plan used in Central America (Figure 8–5). Even though very little milk may be consumed in such cultures, calcium deficiency may nevertheless be rare. One reason, already mentioned, is the use of small fish containing bones. A second reason is that in some areas lime, a calcium-containing compound, is used in grinding corn into meal. It is possible that calcium intake is increased among some populations by other unfamiliar foods which, although we have not yet recognized them as such, may turn out to be good calcium sources.

The milk group is sometimes called the "dairy product group," and this is acceptable provided that the *absence* of some dairy products is noted. Butter, cream cheese, and heavy cream are much too high in fat to provide the significant amounts of essential nutrients provided by other dairy products relative to the number of calories. For this reason they are all placed in the "additional foods" category rather than in the milk group.

THE VEGETABLE AND FRUIT GROUP

Vegetables and fruits are not the same to the plant specialist as to the rest of us. From the botanist's point of view, fruits are the ripened ovaries of seed-bearing plants. Therefore, many foods which we may consider vegetables, such as the squash, cucumber, and tomato, are actually fruits. In common usage, however, plant parts with a decidedly sweet taste are considered fruits, but those with no pronounced sweetness are generally regarded as vegetables. Foods derived from the ovaries of some plants, as well as from the leaves, stems, roots, tubers, and flowers of all edible plants, are therefore classed as vegetables. And no less an authority than the United States Supreme Court has declared the tomato a vegetable.

Because individual fruits and vegetables vary greatly as sources of ascorbic acid and vitamin A value, this group is divided into four subgroups:

1. *Dark green and deep yellow vegetables and fruits* are important primarily for vitamin A value. The foods in this subgroup are:

Apricots
Broccoli
Cantaloupe
Carrots
Dark green leaves: spinach, beet leaves, chard, collards, cress, dandelion leaves, endive, kale, mustard greens, turnip leaves
Persimmon
Winter squash: hubbard, butternut, acorn; also pumpkin

Two points should be noted. First, the foregoing list does not consist simply of a few examples; it includes virtually all of the items usually available in American markets that could be placed in this category. Second, the recommendation for this subgroup, unlike any other recommendation in the Basic Four Plan, is for one serving *every other day*, or an average of three to four servings per week.

2. *Good vitamin C sources* are those so rich in the vitamin that one serving daily insures meeting the RDA. The foods in this subgroup are:

Broccoli
Brussels sprouts
Cantaloupe
Grapefruit (or juice)
Orange (or juice)
Pepper (green or sweet red)
Strawberries, fresh or frozen

3. *Fair vitamin C sources* are those which, in one serving, contain at least one half of the RDA for ascorbic acid for adults. For this reason, *two* fair vitamin C sources can replace one good source. Fair sources are:

Asparagus tips
Cabbage, *if raw*
Cauliflower
Dark green leaves: see dark green-deep yellow subgroup
Melons other than cantaloupe
Potato *if cooked in skin*
Sweet potato *if cooked in skin*
Tangerine
Tomato

4. *"Other vegetables and fruits"* include all that are not listed in the first three subgroups. Almost all of the common vegetables and fruits we eat most often are in this category: apples, bananas, beets, celery, corn, green peas, green beans, lettuce, peaches, pears, potatoes (unless cooked in their skins), and many others.

Note that two foods, broccoli and cantaloupe, are in both the "dark green and deep yellow" and "good vitamin C sources" subgroups. Also, several foods, such as dark green leaves, are in both the "dark green and deep yellow" and "fair vitamin C sources" subgroups. A serving of these foods can be counted in both subgroups for purposes of evaluating a diet, but of course will be counted only once toward the total number of four servings of fruits and vegetables recommended daily.

In addition to vitamins A and C, the major nutrient contributions of this food group are other vitamins, minerals, cellulose, and variable amounts of starch and sugars. In general, vegetables and fruits contain small amounts of protein, which is not at any rate of high nutritional quality. Except for olives and avocados, the fat content of this group is low.

FOUNDATION FOODS AND ADDITIONAL FOODS

Foods that are included in any of the four groups are called *foundation foods,* because when eaten in specified amounts they form the foundation of an adequate diet. In general, they offer valuable amounts of essential nutrients relative to their calories. Of course, not all of the foundation foods within a group are exactly the same in nutritional value. Ice cream, for example, is a less concentrated source of essential nutrients than milk is; pork is a richer source of thiamin than other meats are; and bananas are very rich in Vitamin B_6 compared to other fruits or vegetables. It is the same as the situation in which grades are assigned; a student with an average of 91 has not performed in exactly the same manner as one with an average of 100, but both may be put in the same category, namely "A students." Also, two students may each earn a score of 91 (or any other number) for different reasons, and not for having performed identically.

Additional foods, sometimes called *not listed* foods, are those which are not in any of the four food groups. Because of this, some people incorrectly assume that nutritionists consider them totally devoid of value and would prefer that people avoid them entirely. This is incorrect for the following reasons:

1. They provide calories. Many people who seem to struggle almost continually to control their weight might find it hard to believe that this is a value. However, the amount of energy provided by the recommended minimum number of servings from the four food groups is ordinarily only about 1200 calories. This can vary somewhat depending upon the individual choices made within each group, but most people need more energy than is provided by the minimum recommended servings of foundation foods. One can, of course, obtain extra calories by eating more or larger servings of foundation foods, but most people will choose to eat at least some of the foods not listed in the Basic Four.

2. Some of the additional foods provide valuable amounts of essential nutrients. Iodized salt provides the mineral, iodine; butter and margarine add significantly to the vitamin A intake; bacon supplies fairly useful amounts of several nutrients including the vitamin, thiamin; and many vegetable oils are very good vitamin E sources. Even foods such as potato chips, which are so often used as a prime example of a high-calorie, low-nutrient food, supply at least small amounts of essential nutrients which can help to meet total needs.

3. Finally, the additional foods are enjoyable. Nutritionists are not self-righteous moralists who equate good nutrition with avoidance of anything that tastes good. On the contrary, some of the most unpalatable items imaginable are bought by "health food" believers from their "special" stores. Reputable nutritionists recognize the social and psychological value of many items, not all of which are in the four food groups. It is exactly because these foods are enjoyable that some people use them *in place* of foundation foods. Nutritionists simply recommend that they be used in *addition to* the recommended amounts of foods which are more concentrated sources of essential nutrients.

NONUSE AND MISUSE OF THE FOOD GROUP PLAN

If the Basic Four Plan provides a simple, practical way to meet the RDA, why do some people use it incorrectly and some not use it at all? Reasons include the following:

Physical inability to eat certain foods. Lactose intolerance, for example, or allergy to the proteins in all available types of milk, will necessarily limit consumption of this group. However, inability to tolerate all of the foods in an entire group is very unusual.

Multiple food dislikes. People with a very narrow range of food likes, such as the "beef, potatoes, and pie" man, may reject entire groups or most of the foods within groups. Because different foods in each group vary in nutrient value, variety is more likely to provide maximum nutritional value than is a choice restricted to very few foods.

Lack of interest or knowledge in nutrition. Althouh many people have the interest and opportunity to learn about nutrition and to apply it, it would be naïve to think that this is true of everybody. Particularly in low-income groups, there may have been little opportunity to learn, or the plan may have been presented in an uninteresting or incomprehensible way.

Individuality and desire for novelty. Conventional patterns do not appeal to all, and some people prefer to devise their own. However, almost any plan which provides recommended nutrient intakes will end up being similar or identical to the Basic Four. Vegetarians, if they accept milk, can substitute legumes and nuts for meat and may accept eggs as well. Vegans, strict vegetarians who reject *all* foods of animal origin, will not accept any foods in the milk group, and it is very unlikely that their diets can provide recommended nutrient intakes.

Errors in classifying foods. Dried legumes are properly classed as meat alternates, not as vegetables. Lemons and lemon juice are not classed as either good or fair vitamin C sources because the usual serving size is too small. Bacon is not a meat; corn, lettuce, green peas, and green beans are not dark green or deep yellow vegetables; and fruit-flavored artificial drinks, beverage powders, and diluted sweetened juice drinks are not nutritionally equivalent to fruit juices, even if the astronauts did take them on space flights. As larger numbers of simulated foods such as nondairy milk and soybean meats are fabricated, classifying will become even more complicated than it is at present.

Mistakes in serving sizes. One cup of ordinary fluid milk is one serving; one cup of *evaporated* milk is two servings; and one cup of dried milk *powder* is three to four. The number of servings is determined by the total volume after water is added to the evaporated or dried milk to dilute it to the equivalent of fluid milk.

A light sprinkling of grated cheese, a scrap of lettuce on a sandwich, the lone radish or carrot stick used as a garnish, a splash of milk in coffee, and other small amounts of food constitute fractions of a serving, and they should not be counted as full servings.

Consideration of calories. "If I ate all of that, I'd gain weight" is a common and incorrect objection to the kinds and amounts of foundation foods recommended. Ordinary choices result in a total of approximately

1200 Calories daily: careful choosing can bring this figure down to 1000 or even less.

Prices. Objection to the cost of the Basic Four Plan is valid only for those who cannot afford enough food of any kind. Fresh fruits out of season, expensive cuts of meat, and other high-priced foods can indeed make the cost of eating uncomfortably high. However, neither meat nor fresh fruit is specifically recommended. Within each group are numerous low-cost foods, some actually more nutritious than higher cost choices in the same group. In general, the most expensive foods relative to nutrient value are the additional foods, such as soft drinks, chips, and many desserts, rather than the foundation foods.

Objections based on erroneous ideas about health. Among objections by health food enthusiasts are the following: The plan does not specify certain "miracle foods" such as wheat germ and brewer's yeast. Sweeteners such as honey and molasses are placed in the same category (additional foods) as refined sugar. Whole wheat bread is considered equivalent to enriched white bread. The entire plan, in fact, is based on what faddists refer to as the "pathetically low" RDA rather than the much higher levels which health food enthusiasts insist are needed for "real" health.

These objections are based on emotions rather than facts. For example, milk and honey are often imbued with mystical significance because these are the only two foods specifically "designed by Nature" to be consumed by living things, young mammals in one case and the larvae of bees in the other. However, the Basic Four Plan is intended to meet the nutrient needs of people, and must therefore be based on the facts regarding the nutritional values of foods, not on emotional values which people may attach to certain foods. The fact is that milk is highly nutritious for humans and honey is not, despite whatever design Nature may have had in mind.

SUGGESTED READINGS

Feeney, M. C. "Nutritional and Dietary Management of Food Allergy in Children." *American Journal of Clinical Nutrition* 22 (1969):103.

Food and Nutrition Board, National Research Council–National Academy of Sciences. *Recommended Dietary Allowances,* eighth edition. Washington, D.C., 1974.

Hegsted, D. M. "Problems in the Use and Interpretation of the Recommended Dietary Allowances." Ecology of Food and Nutrition 1 (1972):255.

Leverton, R. M. The Paradox of Teen-Age Nutrition. *Journal of the American Dietetic Association* 53 (1968):13.

Peterkin, B., J. Nichols, and C. Cromwell. "Nutrition Labeling—Tools For Its Use." USDA: Agricultural Information Bull. No. 382, Washington, D.C., 1975.

Stewart, M. R. "Nutrition Labeling." USDA: *Nutrition Program News,* Washington, D.C., July–August 1972.

Wolff, R. J. "Who Eats for Health?" *American Journal of Clinical Nutrition* 26 (1973):438.

9

hunger and malnutrition: causes and consequences

We do not need to demonstrate intellectual impairment or any of the other possible negative consequences of hunger or malnutrition to know that permitting children to be hungry in the midst of affluence violates crucial moral norms (those norms which are necessary for the preservation of the essential forms of our society). A violation of these moral norms reduces the probability of the society surviving in its present form. The persistence of hunger in the midst of affluence may well create as well as reflect attitudes and values among the affluent which are at serious variance with the values of democracy and equality. The final question then is not the impact of hunger on the hungry but on the nonhungry—the affluent. What are the consequences for an affluent society of permitting children to go hungry? The answer is unknown, but critical.

–David J. Kallen, "Nutrition and Society," *Journal of the American Medical Association,* **215**:94, 1971.

A great deal of attention has been focused in recent years on the problems of hunger and malnutrition, in developed countries such as the United States as well as in the less developed areas of the world. Nevertheless, as the quotation above states, our knowledge of the entire subject is far from complete at present. Although we can state with confidence that hunger and malnutrition are realities in numerous parts of the world, questions that have not yet been resolved include the following:

Causes. Unlike those diseases which can be attributed to a single factor, the complex of diseases known as *malnutrition* are multifactorial

FIGURE 9–1. The multifactorial causes of malnutrition.

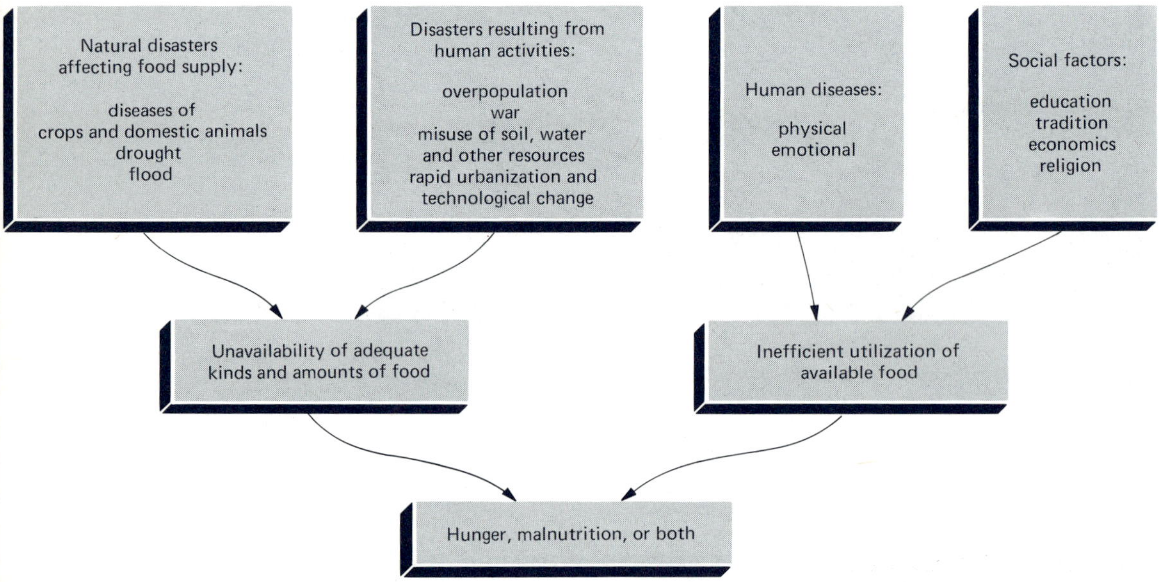

(Figure 9–1). The roots may lie in unavailability of food in some cases; in other cases, failure or inability to use available food to best advantage is responsible. In turn, multiple explanations can be offered for each of these.

Incidence and severity. How commonly hunger and malnutrition occur, and the degree to which they are manifest, are unknown; conclusions regarding hunger and malnutrition are often based entirely on hypotheses and assumptions rather than on experiments and observations. The problem has been overdramatized and exaggerated in some instances, and minimized in others. Although we can safely discount extreme statements that say, in effect, that most Americans are malnourished or that severe hunger and malnutrition are common in the United States, we can equally discount statements that these problems do not exist at all except in certain developing countries. Many more studies on nutritional status are needed in order to make more definite estimates.

Distribution. A priori assumptions are commonly made that certain groups are more vulnerable to hunger and malnutrition than others. The very young and the elderly, for example, are assumed to have special nutritional needs which often may not be met. It is sometimes taken for granted that low-income groups are significantly less well fed than are those in more favorable economic circumstances, and that adequate income generally insures adequate nutrition. Although these are reasonable-sounding assumptions, the extent to which particular segments of different populations actually experience hunger or malnutrition has not been established with certainty.

Consequences. It is in this area that the most extreme views are expressed. In the opinion of some, hunger and malnutrition are major contributing factors in a number of diseases and constitute medical and social problems of great urgency. Others believe that, except for the extreme degrees—such as those found in certain areas of the developing countries—hunger and malnutrition are relatively mild impediments to reaching maximum potential. Obesity, or excess accumulation of body fat, is an outstanding example of a form of malnutrition that is not taken seriously by large numbers of people; it is, in fact, literally a joke in the minds of many.

What are the reasons for the confusion surrounding this subject? They can be found in two general areas. One is the extremely common practice of using the terms *hunger* and *malnutrition* imprecisely or obscurely. This may be done deliberately in order to sell a product or to gain publicity, or it may be done innocently by well-meaning but uninformed people who sincerely wish to improve the lot of those who are hungry and malnourished. An understanding of these and related terms is therefore a prerequisite to an understanding and solution of the problems.

The second reason is the paucity of agreed-upon factual knowledge upon which more reliable conclusions could be based. Of the billions of people living in the world today, the nutritional status of only a very minute proportion has actually been studied. Some studies have yielded equivocal results, or results which conflict with those of other investigators. Even a single given study may be interpreted in various ways by different people, because of differences in personal bias or in degree of understanding of the study. The purpose of the following discussion is to examine certain aspects of what is currently known regarding hunger and malnutrition. When controversy and uncertainty exist, they will be so identified. Statements such as those commonly presented in the popular press, which have often been based largely on emotion rather than on evidence, will be included as tentatively acceptable hypotheses rather than as firm conclusions. Finally, present attempts to alleviate the hunger and malnutrition which are actually known to exist will be summarized.

HUNGER AND MALNUTRITION

Hunger is a subjective feeling of desire for food. It may range from a mildly uncomfortable sense of unease to a sensation of actual pain. Although it is common to assume that those who are hungry are also malnourished, this is not necessarily the case. Only when hunger is caused by a more or less prolonged lack of food actually needed will malnutrition be inevitable. For example, the person who eats less than desired in order to control weight may often be hungry, but will not necessarily be malnourished; in fact, such a person would become malnourished (obese) if the sense of hunger were to be satisfied each time it was felt.

Conversely, lack of hunger does not necessarily insure adequate nutrition. More than the feeling of a full stomach is necessary, because the kinds of food, as well as the amount, contribute to nutritional status. In fact, certain forms of malnutrition, such as some vitamin deficiencies, are characterized by a spontaneous *loss* of the sense of hunger. People with diseases such as these may feel completely free of hunger precisely because they are suffering from a form of malnutrition.

MALNUTRITION, PRIMARY AND SECONDARY

Malnutrition simply means *poor nutrition.* It is often considered to be identical to nutritional deficiency, or *undernutrition,* and certainly on a worldwide basis lack of nutrients or of total food is more widespread than excesses are. However, extremes above normal nutrition also constitute malnutrition. The term *overnutrition,* used to describe the condition resulting from excess calories or nutrients, is sometimes misinterpreted by those who assume that more than adequate nutrition must be even better than that which is merely adequate. On the contrary, in developed countries such as the United States, nutritional diseases caused by excesses are more common than are diseases of undernutrition.

Primary malnutrition results when average people eat diets that are inherently too low or too high in energy or in one or more nutrients. An example of a primary *deficiency* is the iron-deficiency anemia commonly seen in infants or children who drink milk to the exclusion of foods needed as iron sources. An example of a primary form of *overnutrition* is vitamin toxicity, generally resulting from overuse of vitamin supplements.

Secondary malnutrition results when an ordinarily adequate food intake is ingested by a person whose individual characteristics make the usual intake unsuitable. Those who produce abnormally large amounts of the hormone *aldosterone* retain abnormal, perhaps toxic, amounts of sodium, even though their sodium intakes may be no greater than those easily tolerated by others; conversely, one who secretes an abnormally small amount of the hormone suffers from sodium deficiency on ordinary diets. Secondary deficiencies of fat-soluble vitamins can occur in people who are unable to secrete normal amounts of bile, a digestive fluid necessary for absorption of fat-soluble vitamins; diets containing normally adequate amounts of vitamins are therefore deficient for these individuals. People who lose excessive amounts of blood, through internal hemorrhage or abnormally large menstrual losses, can suffer from iron-deficiency anemia even though their diets supply enough iron to meet the needs of average people.

Severe, prolonged *emotional* stress, as well as *physical* abnormalities, may precipitate malnutrition in people who would otherwise be well nourished. For example, stress can result in endocrine changes which in turn lead to an increased breakdown of amino acids by the cells; some individuals react to stressful situations by excreting larger amounts of calcium in the urine. The diet previously adequate may then become deficient if additional nutrients are not supplied to replace these extra losses.

The Recommended Dietary Allowances include safety factors to cover the increased needs during common stresses, so that the intakes ordinarily recommended will not suddenly become inadequate as the result of short term or mild stresses and anxieties. Therefore, increased nutrient intakes are not demanded each time final examination week looms on the horizon or because of a disappointment in love. However, the RDA are *not* set high enough to cover the needs of the small minority whose special physical or emotional problems interfere with normal nutrient utilization. Medical treatment of the underlying causes of the secondary malnutrition is necessary for good nutrition in these people.

The development of primary and secondary malnutrition is shown in Figure 9–2. Admittedly, not all forms of malnutrition are known to

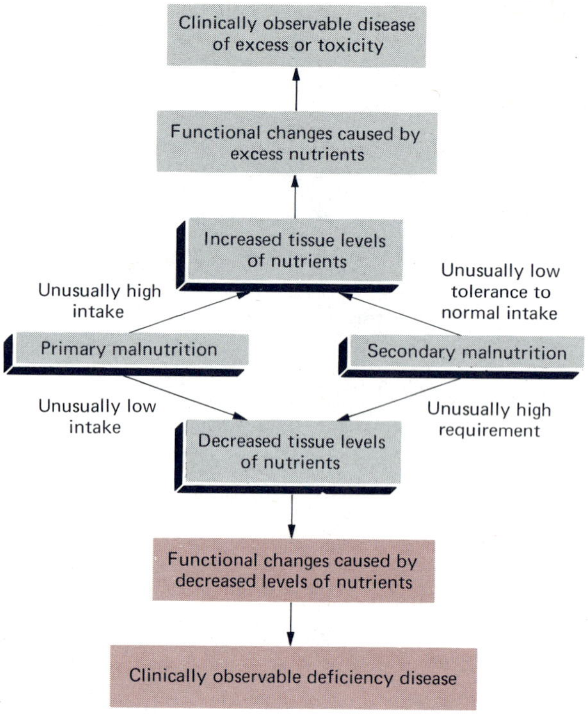

FIGURE 9–2. Development of primary and secondary malnutrition.

proceed through all the steps exactly as outlined. For example, in the development of obesity, tissue levels of energy nutrients increase and excess body fat accumulates, but there is little evidence that functional changes occur prior to obvious and clinically observable obesity. In general, however, a nutritional disease occurs as shown in the diagram. First, tissue levels of the nutrient itself become abnormally low or high. Next, functional changes occur because of changes in enzymes or other cell constituents, normal amounts of which depend upon normal levels of the nutrient. Finally, outwardly visible disease, called *clinical disease,* occurs if malnutrition is extreme enough and prolonged enough.

How much time is required for the appearance of obvious disease? No definite answer can be given, for the time varies greatly from one form of malnutrition to another as well as from one person to another. Clinical scurvy may occur within a few months on a diet devoid of vitamin C, whereas a year or more on a diet free of vitamin B_{12} may be too short a time for the signs of deficiency disease to develop.

In the case of some nutrients, clinically detectable disease is rare or nonexistent in humans. Copper toxicity, for example, is almost exclusively a secondary form of malnutrition seen in individuals with a genetic disease which causes the mineral to accumulate in abnormally large amounts in their tissues. Unless taking large amounts of copper in the form of supplements becomes fashionable, primary copper toxicity will probably continue to be a rare problem. Also, some nutrients can be taken in amounts far exceeding recommended amounts without toxicity occurring, because the body rejects excesses of many nutrients by excreting them in the urine. However, even this protective device may fail if the overabundance is extreme enough, because above some level, any nutrient can be toxic. Fortunately this level is so high for some nutrients that only the most enthusiastic supplement takers are likely ever to exceed it.

The final results of malnutrition are the same regardless of whether it is of a primary or secondary type. However, the differences in causes will of course determine the treatment. Some examples may help to clarify this point:

People can become obese only as a result of energy intake in excess of needs. For this reason, treatment is *always* directed toward an intake below actual needs so that body fat must be consumed. However, this does not necessarily mean that decreased calorie intake alone is invariably the preferred solution. A person's calorie intake may be no greater than that of the average person, yet the individual may still become overweight because of a lack of exercise. Two possibilities are then apparent. The individual can *decrease calorie intake* to below that of the average person, or can *increase physical activity* to average or above average levels.

Similarly, anemia caused by a low-iron diet is medically indistinguishable from iron-deficiency anemia caused by excess blood loss. However, the treatment would be very different in the two situations. Increasing the dietary iron intake would be the solution in the first case. Treatment of the underlying causes of blood loss, or replacement of lost blood, would be necessary in the second.

STUDYING THE CONSEQUENCES OF HUNGER AND MALNUTRITION

One of the most important questions regarding hunger and malnutrition is "What are their effects or consequences?" We assume that hunger is undesirable, that adequate nutrition is one factor in health, and that both deficiences and excesses are detrimental. To justify these assumptions, however, it is necessary to demonstrate that there are significant differences between those who are, and those who are not, hungry or malnourished. Any differences identified must be described and, if possible, explained. Finally, it should be demonstrated that certain characteristics of hungry or malnourished people are the direct result of the hunger and malnutrition rather than of other unfavorable conditions which often occur concomitantly. Differences in nutrition are often associated with great differences in other factors such as medical care, educational and recreational opportunities, and social stimulation, and attempts at prevention of consequences are certain to fail if the causes of observed end effects are not clearly defined.

Basically, four different methods or types of studies have been used to determine the effects of hunger and malnutrition. These are:

1 Controlled experiments using nonhuman species
2 Deliberate alterations of human diets
3 Studies of populations under normal living conditions
4 Studies of populations under unusual nutritional stresses

It must be recognized that each of these methods has certain limitations as well as certain values. However, emphasizing their limitations does not obviate their usefulness. Rather, it sounds a precautionary note in pointing out the ease with which studies can be misinterpreted, or interpreted far beyond the legitimate limits of the results.

ANIMAL STUDIES

The importance of animal experiments in nutrition can hardly be overemphasized. Animals have been used to elucidate the biochemical roles of nutrients by showing what particular enzymes, cells, and biological functions are most likely to be affected by excesses or deficiencies. To obtain estimates of the amounts of nutrients necessary to prevent or cure deficiency diseases in humans, animals are often used in preliminary studies. A major advantage of using subhuman species as experimental subjects is that their environment can be rigidly controlled so that only the diet is altered. Such a degree of control over human subjects would be extremely difficult to achieve.

Of the animals which have been used in experimental work, the rat is overwhelmingly the animal of choice. It is inexpensive and small enough to be fed, caged, and handled easily. Because they are omnivorous, as humans are, rats readily accept diets resembling those of humans, an obvious advantage considering the difficulty of getting cats or cattle, for example, to accept diets similar to those ordinarily eaten by humans. In addition, rats produce large litters, thus allowing the experimenter to use littermates, which are genetically very similar, in the various experimental groups. This eliminates differences which could occur as the result of greater genetic variability. Some of these points are illustrated in Figure 9–3.

A major *disadvantage* of using nonhuman species in nutrition experiments is that it is rarely possible to extrapolate the results directly from these animals to humans. For example, the effects of a given kind and degree of malnutrition on newborn rats may be very different from the effects on newborn humans. Rats are considerably less mature at birth than human babies are, and malnutrition affects less mature organisms far more severely than it affects more mature ones. Thus newborn rats can be subjected to extreme malnutrition when their stage of development is comparable to that of a human

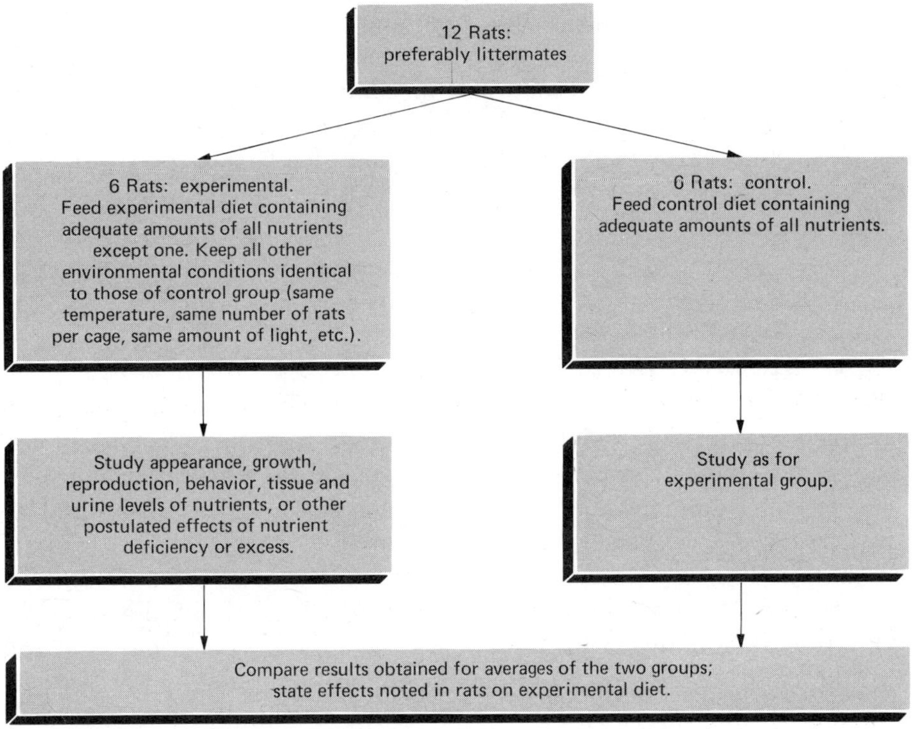

FIGURE 9–3. How a properly controlled animal experiment is done.

some time before birth, at which stage the fetus is largely (although not entirely) protected by the maternal organism. Complete withholding of nutrients, possible with the newborn rat, is not possible with the human fetus, for even if the pregnant woman is completely starved the fetus will derive at least part of its nutrient needs from her.

When it comes to studying the effects of hunger or malnutrition on behavior, extrapolation from animals to humans is on even shakier grounds, for humans are even less similar to other animals in their social and psychological traits than in their physiological characteristics. For example, severe early malnutrition in young rats and pigs has been shown to result in later slowness in learning, as in running mazes or avoiding an electric shock. Superficially, this appears to be similar to human mental retardation, in which intellectual potential is restricted. However, this assumption presents several difficulties. First, humans attain a much higher level of mental development, particularly with respect to the ability for abstract thinking, than do other species; socially and emotionally, also, people are more complex than are rats or other experimental animals. Second, the maximal growth rate of the brain occurs shortly *before* birth in humans, while there is still protection by the maternal orgainsm, but occurs *after* birth in rats. Finally, learning ability is not rigidly fixed and innate, but is determined by a variety of environmental agents as well as by the inherent intellectual ability (Figure 9–4). Considering these multiple factors in human learning, it is obvious that animal experiments in themselves cannot provide proof of cause-and-effect relationships between malnutrition and impaired learning in humans. Social scientists as well as nutritionists have much to contribute to the solution of this complex problem, and too much remains unknown to justify dogmatic or unambiguous conclusions at present.

EXPERIMENTAL MANIPULATION OF HUMAN DIETS

"Will You Starve That They Be Better Fed?" This question was asked on the cover of a booklet calling for volunteers to take part in the Minnesota study of semistarvation during World War II. The purpose was to determine the effectiveness of various diets in rehabilitating the large numbers of severely undernourished people known to exist as the result of the war.

During the first three months of the year-long study, the subjects, 36 normal men between the ages of 20 and 33, were given physical and mental tests, results of which were to be compared to those later obtained during starvation. In the following six months, the daily food intake was reduced to a level that resulted in an average loss of almost one-fourth of the original body weight. Following this, three months were spent in rehabilitation under controlled conditions of increased food intake.

The Minnesota experiment yielded a great deal of valuable infor-

FIGURE 9–4. The multiple factors that determine learning.

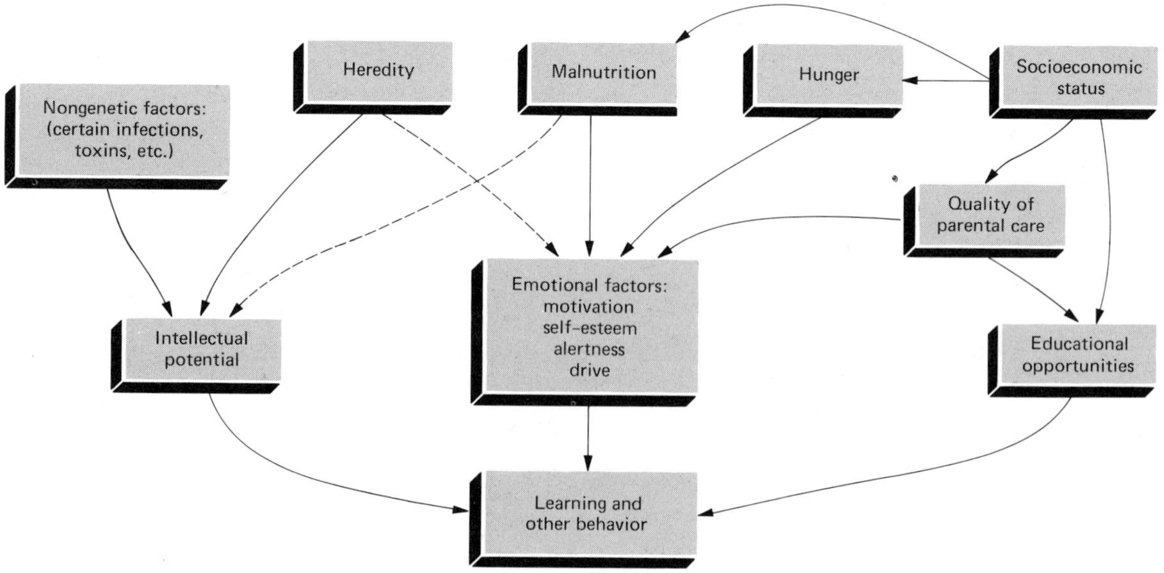

mation which could not have been obtained in any other way. As would be expected, the subjects focused their concern almost entirely on food, which became the main topic of conversation, reading, plans, and daydreams. A few men, however, reacted against this "tyranny of food," one man describing such engrossment as "nutritional masturbation." In activities not related to food, interest deteriorated; many of the men neglected grooming almost completely, became egocentric and irritable, and ceased to participate in group activities. Humor, except for the sarcastic variety, virtually disappeared, and sexual interest and activity declined until they were practically absent. As one man described himself, he had "no more sexual feeling than a sick oyster."

The men complained of intellectual inefficiency, and some concluded that they had actually lost part of their mental ability. However, performance as measured by intelligence tests showed no change as the result of starvation. The subjects' opinions of their own mental changes therefore appear to have been the result of emotional factors and physical weakness, which led to apathy and lack of interest; these in turn gave the *appearance* of an actual intellectual deficit. As one subject stated it: "I can talk intellectually, my mental ability has not decreased, but my will to use the ability has. So my talk is of food and past memories, or future ambitions mostly in the cooking or eating line."

Although controlled studies such as the Minnesota study are of unquestioned value, there are several built-in shortcomings. The serious moral question of performing experiments which may result in permanent impairment of humans tends to discourage investigators from performing studies using human subjects. In addition, the human is a poor experimental animal in many respects, being large, ill-tempered in confinement, and vocally abusive in its complaints. It is even possible that effects seen under controlled laboratory conditions are not really comparable to those occurring as the result of "natural" starvation. As one volunteer vividly expressed it after completion of the Minnesota study:

> **"I look back to those days . . . and recall my feeling of apathy. Yet that was starvation** *only*, **for I had warm clothes and living quarters. I was free from disease and could keep clean; but I think of Europe and Asia and I see bodily discomfort increased multifold with the addition of disease and cold and filth. I see mental torture multiplied because of bitterness and sorrow from war's devastation, and the constant wonder if the day will ever come when food will again be plentiful."**

Because of considerations such as these, studies with human subjects more commonly involve manipulating diets in the direction of *improvement* rather than in the direction of decreased intakes. The results of some of the many studies that have sought to investigate the effects of diet improvement upon growth, reproductive efficiency, resistance to disease, and other aspects of human health will be presented in later sections. For the time being, certain criticisms of these can be made as follows. First, many were quasi-experimental, in that they were not performed in a laboratory setting and were not, therefore, rigidly controlled; in a well-controlled nutrition study, *all* environmental factors are held constant except for the diet. In some of the studies which have claimed to demonstrate some type of improvement as a result of specific improvements in nutrition, factors other than nutrition were altered at the same time. Obviously, any improvement in health which is noted after simultaneous improvements in medical care, housing, environmental sanitation, and emotional climate as well as in nutrition should not be attributed to nutritional improvement alone, as has sometimes been done.

A second problem with studies such as these is that expectations of nutritional improvements may affect the subjects' responses more than the nutrients themselves do. This effect is so well known that all nutrition studies on humans should include a control group which receives a placebo—an inert substance identical in appearance and taste and therefore indistinguishable from the active material. If the control group receiving the placebo responds in the same manner as the experimental group does, the response obviously cannot be explained on the basis of nutritional improvement. Thus one report, that a large group of university students receiving vitamin C supplements had fewer colds than during the previous winter, is less impressive in light of the fact that students taking placebos showed the same reduction in number of colds!

A final problem is that of the expectations of the experimenter. Hypothetically, the spirit of objective scientific inquiry insures that investigators are entirely unbiased. In fact, not all are entirely free of the temptation to emphasize those results that are compatible with the original hypothesis and to ignore or rationalize away those that are not. For this reason, studies designed in a *double-blind* manner, in which neither the investigator *nor* the subjects know who is getting a placebo and who is getting the actual treatment until the study is completed, are particularly valuable.

The tendency to look at many results but to see only the ones desired has unfortunately colored the outcome of numerous studies. Eventually, of course, it becomes obvious that this has happened, because later studies fail to confirm the earlier ones. However, the earlier results may have become so firmly entrenched by then that it is very difficult to correct the former erroneous conclusions. A classic example of this is a series of studies done in the 1940s on the effects of thiamin supplementation on children's physical and mental abilities. From the start, some of the results were greeted with justifiable skepticism. For example, it was claimed that thiamin caused a marked improvement in visual acuity of the right eye but deterioration in visual acuity of the left! However, despite such dubious claims, these studies have been accepted uncritically by many, and even today textbooks of education and psychology occasionally state that thiamin has been demonstrated to improve both the intelligence and the physical abilities of children. Therefore, although the studies have long been discounted because nobody has succeeded in reproducing the spectacular original results, the earlier impressions remain and continue to create false impressions.

CORRELATIONS BETWEEN ORDINARY NUTRITIONAL DIFFERENCES AND POSSIBLE REPERCUSSIONS

Observations are often made on subjects who consume ordinary diets, with no attempt made to manipulate the diets either for better or for worse. Because the investigator can concentrate on obtaining information on the subjects rather than on changing their diets, large numbers of people can be studied. It is the relative ease of this method that accounts for its being used far more commonly than controlled studies are.

Two major areas of the subjects' lives are studied. First, the diet or level of nutrition is investigated in an attempt to estimate the dietary ratings of the various subjects. Second, the investigator looks for the presence of postulated effects of dietary differences. Findings are then expressed as associations or correlations. If the two variables, diet and postulated effects, change in the same direction, they are said to be *positively* correlated; if one variable increases as the other decreases, the correlation is said to be *negative* (Figure 9–5).

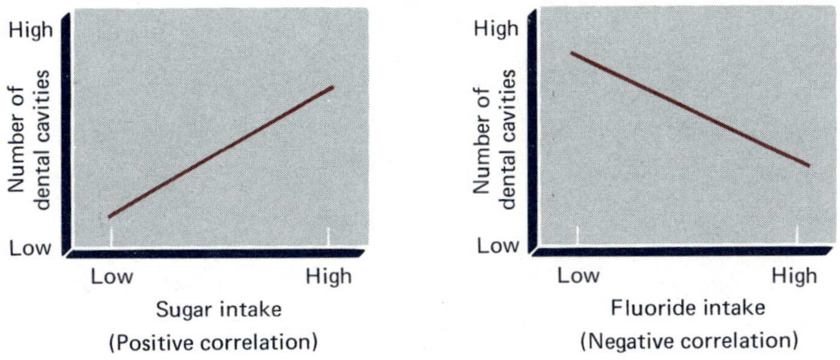

FIGURE 9–5. Correlation of two factors: positive and negative.

Statements such as the following are representative of this type of study.

Small food intakes are associated with small body size and slow growth in children.

High food intakes in pregnant women are correlated with above-

average birth weights in their infants, and low food intakes with below-average birth weights.
Low fluoride intakes are correlated with high rates of dental caries, or cavities.

The main problem inherent in this type of study is that people tend to confuse correlation with cause-and-effect relationships. *The fact that two findings generally occur together does not prove that one causes the other.* In fact, there are four possible explanations or interpretations (Figure 9–6).

1 Two findings may occur together by pure coincidence. This is particularly likely in studies involving small numbers of subjects. If a coin is flipped four times, it might by chance land heads up each time, but it could hardly be concluded from this that flipped coins *always* land heads rather than tails. Obviously, more trials will be needed to answer the question of whether the results were fortuitous.
2 If two findings, A and B, are correlated, it *may* signify that A causes B. In the example of children's food intake and body size, for example, the small food intake (A) might be the cause of slow growth and consequent small size of the children (B).
3 The correlation of A and B might also, however, mean that B is the cause of A. Using the same example of food intake and body size, the small size (B) could be the cause of the small food intake (A); a child genetically destined to become a small adult does not need, and is not likely to eat, the amount of food appropriate for children destined to grow into large adults, any more than a toy poodle puppy is likely to have the appetite of a St. Bernard puppy.
4 The final possibility is that A and B are only indirectly related, in that a third factor is causally related to both. With respect to food intakes of pregnant women and birth weights of infants, for example, a third factor is commonly the underlying cause. This third factor,

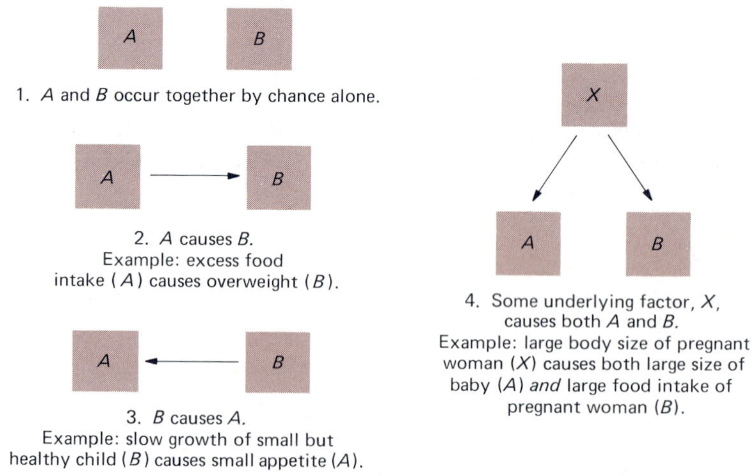

FIGURE 9–6. Various possible explanations for an observed correlation between two factors.

under everyday conditions of nutritional differences, appears to be the body size of the pregnant woman; in general, larger women eat more, and also have larger babies, than smaller women do. Thus large food intakes do not generally cause large babies, any more than the presence of an unusually large fetus stimulates the pregnant woman's appetite. Rather, both food intakes and birth weights of infants commonly vary as the result of differences in the sizes of women.

Is there, then, any value in seeking correlations if these are open to so many different interpretations? The answer is that correlations are of great value in pointing the way to *further* studies, which can determine whether or not a cause-and-effect relationship exists. The relationship between fluoride intake and dental caries is a well-known example. Since the early part of this century, it had been repeatedly observed that a high level of fluoride in the drinking water was associated with a low incidence of caries. Although these observations in themselves did not establish fluoride deficiency as one of the causes of tooth decay, they suggested that this was a reasonable hypothesis and eventually led to controlled studies in which fluoride was added to the water supplies of selected cities. In this way, it was established that optimal levels of fluoride can reduce the incidence of caries in children by approximately 50 percent or more. The conclusion can therefore now be stated in terms of cause-and-effect relationships: Fluoride deficiency is one cause of tooth decay, and optimal fluoride intake causes increased resistance to decay.

Studies which seek correlations between factors are of great value in suggesting future avenues of controlled research; it is therefore unfortunate that people so commonly make the mistake of assuming that the correlations, in themselves, constitute proof of causal relationships.

STUDIES OF POPULATIONS UNDER SEVERE NUTRITIONAL STRESSES

In circumstances such as famine and war, humans are subjected to extremes of hunger and malnutrition seldom seen in normal times. Understandably, people are not primarily concerned with record-keeping during crises, and for this reason detailed data is not always available either on diets or on possible effects. In some cases, however, medical records and statistics on births, deaths, and diseases are available for populations known to have endured severe nutritional privation.

This type of study can be illustrated by a specific example that occurred during World War II in the Netherlands. The cause of the famine was a transport embargo imposed by the Nazis in retaliation against the Dutch cooperation with the British. The degree of undernutrition was severe; many subjects lost as much as one-fourth of total body weight, and many deaths in the famine area were shown to have been caused by starvation. However, complete breakdown of the social system did not occur as it sometimes does under extreme stress, and accurate records were therefore available for study after the war.

Studies of intelligence of adults born between early 1944 and the end of 1945 have sought to establish relationships between the known severity of malnutrition and later effects on mental ability. Adults were divided into various groups, depending upon whether they were conceived or born before, during, or after the famine period. No effects could be found on the frequency of mental retardation or on intelligence as measured by standardized tests. The conclusion therefore appears to be that, even in extreme maternal malnutrition, the human fetus is not damaged with respect to later intellectual performance. However, this conclusion may not necessarily apply to famine conditions in general. Most of the women in the Dutch population were well nourished prior to pregnancy, and most of the babies born during the famine were well nourished after this period; for these reasons the findings of the Dutch famine may not represent the repercussions of chronic famine conditions.

In particular, famine lasting for a sharply circumscribed period of time may be totally unlike the situation in many developing countries, where women may enter pregnancy in poor nutritional status as well as being at risk of periodic times of extreme food shortages during pregnancy. This may at least partly explain the conflict between the findings of the Netherlands study and the findings of studies from many developing countries, in which impaired learning has been reported in previously malnourished children. However, an alternate possibility is that in developing countries severe malnutrition generally occurs disproportionately in the lower social classes, in which people suffer many deprivations other than malnutrition. Later "intellectual impairment" of offspring may then be the result of *social* factors associated with malnutrition rather than of malnutrition itself.

Another point that may be relevant is that genetic inheritance may be an underlying factor in both intelligence and nutritional status. Although this is a sensitive point, which some investigators avoid, the possibility remains that individuals with low intelligence may be less capable than others of coping with stress, including severe nutritional stress. The findings of some studies—that malnourished children appear to be intellectually impaired—may therefore represent the influence of parents with low intelligence on both the nutrition *and* the inherited mental ability of their children.

A final point that deserves emphasis is that the psychological trauma of famine or war may have effects which are as extreme as the physical damage. Although this was not the case in the Holland famine, the loss of social ties, emotional tension, social disintegration, and anxiety regarding homes and families, superimposed upon the fear of starvation, can provoke effects which may be more severe than those of starvation alone. Under these conditions, some of the effects on physical and mental health may be caused only indirectly by food shortages during famine or war, with the direct cause attributable to the human response to these tragic circumstances.

SUGGESTED READINGS

Cattell, R. B. *Abilities: Their Structure, Growth, and Action.* Boston: Houghton-Mifflin, 1971.

Subcommittee on Nutrition, Brain Development, and Behavior. Food and Nutrition Board, National Academy of Sciences–National Research Council. "The Relationship of Nutrition to Brain Development and Behavior." Washington, D.C., 1973.

Frisch, R. E. "Present Status of the Supposition that Malnutrition Causes Permanent Mental Retardation." *American Journal of Clinical Nutrition* 23 (1970):189.

Keys, A., J. Brozek, A. Henschel, O. Mickelson, and H. L. Taylor. *The Biology of Human Starvation,* Vol. 2. Minneapolis: University of Minnesota Press, 1950.

"Guidelines for a National Nutrition Policy." *Nutrition Reviews* 32 (1974):153.

10

nutritional status in the world today

In order to study the relationships of nutritional differences and human well-being, we must have methods of detecting differences in nutritional status. Although severe malnutrition can generally be detected fairly easily, in borderline cases it may be very difficult to answer the seemingly simple question: Is this individual or this group well nourished? For this reason, a combination of various methods, shown in Table 10–1, is commonly used; the information gained from a variety of them is considered in making a final evaluation.

Many of the principles of evaluating nutritional status are similar to those used in medical practice for the diagnosis of disease. Techniques include the study of the individual's dietary intake; physical examination; and the use of appropriate laboratory tests. In the evaluation of large numbers of people, statistics such as data on deaths, births, and the incidence of nutrition-related diseases may also be useful.

The development of malnutrition was discussed previously and illustrated in Figure 9–2. Some of the methods of detecting changes which occur as malnutrition develops will now be discussed.

ASSESSING NUTRITION STATUS

Clinical evaluation

A clinical evaluation (commonly called a physical exam) is the method most generally used when the nutritional status of large groups of people must be assessed with the minimum expenditure of time and money. The routine evaluation may include anthropometric measurements—the determination of the size of the body or parts of the body—as well as inspection of outwardly visible body parts. Parameters such as height, weight, and fat-layer thickness are examples of anthropometric measurements. Information obtained from this type of assessment includes the following:

Eyes. Deficiency of vitamin A causes dryness of the cornea and the formation of visible lesions known as *Bitot's spots.* In extreme deficiency, the cornea becomes opaque and extremely susceptible to infection, with total irreversible blindness as the ultimate result. Riboflavin deficiency also leads to visible changes in the eyes, but instead of dryness and clearly demarcated spots, infiltration of blood vessels into the cornea occurs. An experienced observer can therefore readily distinguish the eye changes characteristic of vitamin A deficiency from those typical of riboflavin deficiency.

Skin. The skin is the covering of the body, subjected to continuous battering, and must therefore continuously renew itself by forming new cells from beneath. Because rapidly dividing cells in general have greater nutrient needs and are more severely affected by malnutrition than slowly growing cells are, it is not surprising that the skin readily reflects the individual's nutrition. *Dermatitis* is the term commonly used to designate various forms of skin lesions or disorders, whether or not they are of nutritional origin.

Vitamin A deficiency can cause a rough, dry skin with characteristic changes at the bases of hair follicles; niacin deficiency causes a completely different type of skin lesion, which occurs mostly on parts of the body exposed to sunlight; tiny hemorrhages under the skin can occur in vitamin C deficiency. Numerous other skin changes caused by other forms of malnutrition can be identified by a skilled observer who is familiar with the various diseases.

Mouth. Changes in the lips and cracks at the corners of the mouth are characteristic of deficiency of the vitamin, riboflavin. The color of the tongue may change, becoming scarlet in niacin deficiency or purplish in riboflavin deficiency. Gums which bleed easily are seen in vitamin C deficiency.

Teeth. The presence of dental caries (decay), or the absence of teeth which should be present, is expressed as a DMF (decayed, missing, filled) index. This index may reflect current dietary factors such as excess sugar as well as previous nutrient deficiencies. Mottling of the teeth can indicate that fluoride intake was excessively high while the teeth were forming.

Mucous membranes. In many of these thin coverings and linings, the blood vessels are so close to the surface that the color of the membranes reflects the color of the blood circulating beneath. Pale membranes are commonly seen in those who are anemic, even though the degree of anemia may be too mild to cause obvious pallor of the skin. Anemia, although very commonly caused by iron deficiency, can also be caused by deficiency of any one of a number of other nutrients, or by loss of blood.

Ankles and feet. Swelling due to accumulation of fluid, called *edema*, is seen in individuals who are severely deficient with respect to protein or thiamin or who are retaining sodium and water for some other reason. In some cases, the edema is not confined to the lower extremities, but is generalized over the entire body or obvious in the area of the abdominal cavity.

Bones. Although bones themselves cannot be observed directly, certain bone changes can be detected by outward inspection. Examples are the bowed legs and the "beading" of ribs seen in the vitamin D-deficiency disease, rickets.

Thyroid gland. Unlike other endocrine glands, the thyroid gland may enlarge until the swelling is outwardly visible. The enlarged gland, known as a goiter, can be caused by lack of the mineral, iodine, as well as by other factors.

Hair. In severe protein deficiency, the hair may be smaller in

TABLE 10–1
Assessment of nutritional status

Sources of information	Nature of information obtained	Nutritional implications
Clinical nutritional surveys	Physical signs	Deviation from health owing to malnutrition
Anthropometric studies	Physical growth and development	Effect of nutrition on physical growth and development
Biochemical studies Tests of function	Levels of nutrients, metabolites and other components of body tissues and fluids	Nutrient supplies in the body Impairment of biochemical function
Dietary surveys	Food consumption	Low, excessive or unbalanced nutrient intake
Agricultural data Food balance sheets	Gross estimates of agricultural production Agricultural methods Soil fertility Predominance of cash crops Overproduction of staples Food imports and exports	Approximate availability of food supplies to a population
Socioeconomic data Information on marketing, distribution and storage	Purchasing power Distribution and storage of foods	Unequal distribution of available foods between the socioeconomic groups in the community and within the family
Food consumption patterns Cultural–anthropological data	Lack of knowledge, erroneous beliefs and prejudices, indifference	
Special studies on foods	Biological value of diets Presence of interfering factors (e.g., toxins) Effects of food processing	Special problems related to nutrient utilization
Vital and health statistics	Morbidity and mortality data	Extent of risk to community Identification of high-risk groups
Additional medical information	Prevalent disease patterns, including infections and infestations	Interrelationships of state of nutrition and disease

Slightly adapted from "World Health Organization Technical Report Series No. 258," Report of Expert Committee on Medical Assessment of Nutritional Status, Geneva, 1963.

diameter than normal, lacking in normal pigmentation, and dull in appearance.

Anthropometric measurements. Body measurements that are used in assessing nutritional adequacy include height and weight, which are almost invariably part of a physical examination. Other measurements, such as head circumference and chest circumference, are less often taken, largely because they are believed by many to be much less related to nutritional status than height and weight are.

Simple above-average or below-average weight in relation to height may not necessarily mean excess body fat or underweight, because the scale does not distinguish between the weight of body fat and the weight of bones, muscles, and other body components. For this reason, the thickness of the subcutaneous fat layer is commonly measured with the use of calipers. The thickness of a skinfold at one or more sites of the body, along with data on height, weight, and arm and thigh circumference, can be useful in the diagnosis of obesity as well as undernutrition.

Growth rate. In the young, who have not yet completed their growth, the *growth rate* may be used as a measure of nutritional adequacy. A rate *always* involves the measurement of time as well as two or more measurements of height or weight. The difference between two measurements is divided by the time which elapsed between the two, and the growth rate is then expressed as the increase in height or weight per unit of time. An infant weighing only 8 pounds at the age of one month could be considered underweight. If, however, the weight at two months is 9¾ pounds, the *rate* of gain (approximately 1 ounce per day) is entirely satisfactory at this age. Growth rate is thus a better indicator of current nutritional adequacy than is a single measurement.

Behavior. Numerous forms of malnutrition are characterized by marked behavioral changes. Severe deficiency of protein results in irritability and apathy, whereas starvation, or lack of total calories, may be characterized by an appearance of abnormal alertness. In many vitamin deficiencies as well as in anemia, the individual may display fatigue out of proportion to activity. The extreme example of behavioral abnormalities resulting from malnutrition is seen in the case of the niacin-deficiency disease, *pellagra*. This deficiency can cause a type of mental illness, *schizophrenia*, which responds dramatically to niacin administration. This does not, of course, mean that niacin or any other nutrient is effective in treating the vast majority of cases of mental illness, which are caused by factors other than malnutrition.

Shortcomings of clinical evaluations

Despite the relative ease with which data are obtained, several general disadvantages are inherent in clinical evaluations.

As was seen in the figure illustrating the development of malnutrition (Figure 9–2), clinically observable diseases are the most extreme manifestations of nutrient deficiencies and excesses; milder degrees of malnutrition, although able to produce functional changes in cells and organs, can exist for long periods of time without becoming outwardly obvious. Therefore, clinical observations are of no value in the diagnosis of the milder forms of malnutrition which, particularly in Western countries, are far more common than frank deficiency diseases.

A second disadvantage is that the observations are made by human beings whose judgments are necessarily subjective. One physician may consider a thyroid gland definitely enlarged, but another considers the same gland within normal limits; one examiner may declare a child to be somewhat pale, and another may not. Because even well-trained observers may differ in their opinions regarding the presence or absence of clinical signs of disease, the untrained person is, of course, completely unqualified to diagnose the majority of nutritional diseases either by self-examination or in others.

The third weakness of this method, and the most serious one, is that clinically detectable signs of malnutrition are nonspecific; that is, they can result from other causes as well as from malnutrition. Rough, dry skin is not necessarily the result of vitamin A deficiency; it can also be caused by exposure to weather, adverse reactions to cosmetics or other chemicals, lack of cleanliness, or many other factors. Behavioral changes can occur as the result of various forms of physical disease as well as emotional stresses; impaired growth may originate in genetic or hormonal factors, infectious diseases, or a host of other agents; pallor of the mucous membranes and skin is seen in many who are not anemic. In short, of all forms of clinically detectable malnutrition, obesity and underweight are the only ones which are always caused by malnutrition alone. In order to interpret the results of clinical examinations, therefore, we must consider possible non-nutritional causes of each sign or symptom, as well as possible nutritional origins.

Laboratory tests

Evaluating nutritional status by laboratory tests involves estimating the amounts of nutrients or related substances in the person's body. Tests are commonly done on blood and urine samples, which are easily obtained and presumably reflect the biochemistry of cells, tissues, and organs; tests can also measure a person's ability to perform certain functions which depend upon an adequate supply of a nutrient. Some tests are so common that they may be performed routinely, as part of the physical examination; others are so rarely used that the average physician may never perform them in a lifetime of practice. In the case of many nutrients, laboratory tests for adequacy have not yet even been developed.

Two tests performed very commonly are the *hemoglobin determination* and the *hematocrit*. An abnormally low concentration of hemoglobin, an iron-containing protein in the red blood cells, indicates anemia, most often caused by a lack of the iron needed for hemoglobin synthesis. The hematocrit, which represents the percent of whole blood consisting of red blood cells, has the advantage of being performed so easily that even an inexperienced assistant can usually do it correctly, and for this reason is very often done as a routine part of a medical examination.

Other tests are generally performed only if there is some indication that the results are necessary for diagnostic purposes. Examples of measurements which can be made are the levels of certain vitamins in blood or urine; the growth and maturation of bones as estimated from x-ray photographs; the ability of the eyes to adapt normally to dim light; and the urinary excretion of an administered dose of certain vitamins. This last method, called a *load test,* is done by administering a standard dose of the vitamin and then measuring the amount of the vitamin which is excreted in the urine. If the person is deficient with respect to the vitamin, the tissues will take it up avidly, and therefore only a small fraction of the dose will be excreted. By contrast, if the person is already well nourished, the dose will represent an excess over his or her needs and a large proportion will therefore be excreted.

Compared to clinical examinations, laboratory tests have two distinct advantages. First, they yield objective results rather than results based on subjective evaluations and human judgment. For example, findings can be expressed as "11 grams of hemoglobin per 100 milliliters of blood," or "0.4 milligrams of ascorbic acid per 100 milliliters of serum." Definite numbers such as these, obtained by the use of laboratory instruments, are uninfluenced by surmise or personal prejudice. The second advantage is that abnormal levels of nutrients or of compounds related to nutrients can generally be found long before overt signs of nutritional disease can be detected. People with *mild* degrees of malnutrition can therefore be identified, and treatment can be initiated in order to prevent more serious malnutrition.

One *disadvantage* of laboratory tests is the difficulty and consequently the expense of performing some of them. They may require the use of equipment that is available only in special research centers, or they may be so difficult to perform that only highly skilled technicians can do them accurately.

A second disadvantage is that, although the results are objective, the interpretations are subject to considerable differences of opinion, because there is not complete agreement on the standards that should be used to define the range of nutritional adequacy. Some physicians consider a woman anemic if her hemoglobin concentration is less than 12; others would set the standard at 11; still others would accept even lower levels as within the normal range. Thus, although the tests themselves are highly objective, the interpretation of them often is not.

Food group	Name of food eaten	Amount eaten: Measure	Amount eaten: Servings (equiv.)	Total servings eaten in group	Servings short of basic four recommendations	
Vegetables and fruits						
Dark green and yellow	cooked carrots	$\frac{1}{2}$ c.	1	1	0	1
Good and fair vitamin C sources	orange juice, canned	$\frac{1}{2}$ c.	1	1	0	
Other	lettuce, chopped	1 c.	1	1	0	
Whole grain and enriched breads and cereals	enriched white bread	3 sl.	3	3	1	
Milk and milk products		Equivalents in cups of milk				
	vanilla ice cream	$\frac{1}{2}$ c.	$\frac{1}{4}$	approx. $1\frac{1}{2}$ c.	approx. $\frac{1}{2}$ c.	
	American cheese	1 oz.	$\frac{2}{3}$			
	skim milk	$\frac{1}{2}$ c.	$\frac{1}{2}$			
Meat and meat alternates		Equivalents in ounces of meat				
	cooked hamburger patty	2 oz.	2			
	boiled egg	1	1	$4\frac{1}{2}$	$\frac{1}{2}$ oz. over	
	baked beans	$\frac{1}{2}$ c.	1			
	peanut butter	1 tbsp.	$\frac{1}{2}$			
Other foods	2 tbsp. 1000-island dressing		Omit	Omit	Omit	
	potato chips, 10					
	cola drink, 12 oz.					
	beer, 12 oz.					
	2 tbsp. margarine					

FIGURE 10–1. Comparison of two methods of diet evaluation.

Diet studies and food intake records

Dietary data, properly obtained and evaluated, are an important part of any study of nutritional status. The purpose is to provide a description of food consumption, including eating habits, methods of food preparation, and nutrient intakes.

Basically, diet studies are done by determining what foods, and in what amounts, are eaten by an individual or a group, and then comparing the data to a standard. The foods themselves may be compared to a food grouping plan such as the Basic Four, or the energy and nutrient content of the foods may be calculated and the totals compared to a standard such as the RDA. These two methods of comparison are shown in Figure 10–1.

Indirect methods: food balance records and vital statistics

Evaluation of the food intake of a very large group, such as a nation, must be done in indirect ways. One method is to estimate the total

Figure 10–1 (continued)

NAME__________ AGE______ SEX______

FOOD AND AMOUNT	APPROXIMATE ENERGY VALUE AND CONTENT OF SELECTED NUTRIENTS								
	Energy, kilocalories	Protein, g.	Vitamin A, I.U.	Vitamin C, mg.	Niacin, mg.	Riboflavin, mg.	Thiamin, mg.	Calcium, mg.	Iron, mg.
½ c. cooked carrots	22	0.5	7600	5	0.4	0.04	0.04	24	0.5
½ c. canned orange juice	60	1	250	50	0.4	0.03	0.08	12	0.5
1 c. chopped lettuce	10	1	950	9	0.2	0.04	0.03	34	0.7
3 sl. enr. wh. bread	210	6	trace	trace	1.8	0.15	0.18	63	1.8
½ c. vanilla ice cream	130	3	300	1	0.1	0.14	0.03	95	0.05
1 oz. American cheese	105	7	350	0	trace	0.12	0.01	198	0.3
½ c. skim milk	45	4.5	5	1	0.1	0.22	0.05	150	0.05
2 oz. cooked hamburger	180	14	20	—	3.1	0.12	0.05	6	1.8
1 boiled egg	80	6	590	0	trace	0.15	0.05	27	1.1
½ c. baked beans	155	8	165	3	0.8	0.04	0.10	70	2.3
1 T. peanut butter	95	4	—	0	2.4	0.02	0.02	9	0.3
10 potato chips	115	1	trace	3	1.0	0.01	0.04	8	0.4
12 oz. cola drink	145	0	0	0	0	0	0	—	—
12 oz. beer	150	1	—	—	2.2	0.11	0.01	18	trace
2 T. 1000-island dressing	160	trace	100	trace	trace	trace	trace	4	0.2
2 T margarine	200	trace	940	0	—	—	—	6	0
TOTALS	1860	57	11,270	72	12.5	1.19	0.69	724	10
RDA for Age-Sex Group	2000	46	4000	45	13	1.2	1.0	800	18
Total compared to RDA	− 140	+ 11	+ 7270	+ 27	− 0.5	− 0.01	− 0.31	−76	− 8

amount of food available to the country by examining records of food production, exports and imports, wastage, and use of food for purposes other than for humans—such as feeding animals. This type of rough estimate is a means of determining changes in nutrient availability over a period of time, but of course does not provide specific information on the nutrient intakes of various individuals within a population.

Another indirect method of assessing the adequacy of diets is to study the vital statistics recorded by governments. Statistics on the causes of morbidity (illness) and mortality (death) may reveal that nutrition-related diseases are present in a population. The value of this method, however, depends upon the accuracy with which vital statistics are recorded, and those countries with the greatest nutritional problems unfortunately also tend to have the least accurate systems of reporting and recording vital statistics.

Direct methods: food inventories and individual food consumption records

Direct methods of food intake are used in studying those in relatively small units, such as a hospital, a college living group, a family, or a single individual.

The *food inventory* involves keeping a record of all food purchased, grown, or otherwise made available to a group for consumption while the study is in progress, and then calculating the nutritional value of the food. The most serious drawback of this method is that it does not determine the distribution of food *within* the group. For example, if a family of four consumes two quarts of milk daily, this *may* indicate that each person drinks approximately one pint of milk daily; on the other hand, it may indicate that one person consumes milk to the virtual exclusion of all other foods, although the other three drink no milk at all. A second problem is that the very fact of recording information on food availability may change the kinds and amounts of foods obtained; the homemaker who customarily buys large amounts of soft drinks, beer, and potato chips may begin to buy fruit juices and other nutritious foods instead, in order to impress the person who records the inventory.

The *diet history* is used to obtain general, rather than specific, information on an individual's food habits over a fairly long period of time. The interviewer asks questions such as those shown in Figure 10–2. Depending upon the skill of the interviewer and the accuracy of the subject's responses, general trends of food consumption can be detected. A major disadvantage is that considerable time is required for the interview. Also, some subjects may be unwilling to give honest answers to certain questions, such as those relating to weight and alcohol consumption.

A cursory diet history, consisting of a few key questions, can be obtained in a few minutes, but the information obtained may be so incomplete as to be useless, as the following actual example shows:

A pale, listless eighteen-month-old boy was examined by a pediatrician and found to be anemic. The physician asked the mother three questions:

How often does he eat meat?
How often does he eat eggs?
Has he been weaned from the bottle?

The mother replied that the child ate meat and eggs daily, and had only an "occasional" bottle of milk. The physician assumed, therefore, that the anemia must be secondary to some physical disease in the child rather than the result of a low iron intake. However, further tests over a period of weeks failed to disclose any possible reason for the anemia.

Eventually, more probing questions revealed that the child's "meat" intake consisted of a single strip of bacon each morning; that the boy ate only the whites of eggs because he disliked the yolk (which contains the iron); and that the "occasional" bottle of milk was given each time the child appeared to be hungry, tired, or upset. As a result, five or six 8-ounce bottles of milk were a common part of a day's diet, leaving very little appetite for other foods which would have supplied the iron he needed. The information originally obtained was of practically no value because the mother had not been asked *specific* questions regarding the *actual kinds and amounts* of foods included in her child's diet.

In the *recall method,* the interviewer asks the subject to recall the specific kinds and amounts of foods eaten during a recent period of time, most commonly the past 24 hours. Standardized props, such as different sizes of glasses, cups, bowls, and spoons, or models of common foods, can help the subject to identify amounts of food accurately. After the food intake is described, the interviewer can ask further questions on items which people commonly overlook or forget: additions such as butter or margarine on bread, vegetables, or other foods; chocolate or other flavorings in milk; methods of preparation, such as fried, baked, broiled; and so on.

How questions are asked can be as important as *which* questions are asked. A subtle suggestion as to the "right" answer, or a show of approval or disapproval by tone of voice or facial expression, can intimidate a subject into giving the answers that seem to be wanted, rather than the accurate responses. With a trained interviewer, however, the recall method has the advantage of drawing forth a more accurate picture of an individual's food intake than the person would be likely to accomplish without the interviewer's questioning.

Written *food intake records,* kept by the subjects themselves, are far less costly than are methods which require the use of an interviewer. Obviously, they can be used only by those who are literate or who can get someone to write down the information for them. The

Name ______________________ Date ____________

____

We would like to have the following information about YOU.

1. What is your occupation? ______________________

2. How tall are you? __________ What is your weight? __________

3. Have you ever been on a diet? ______ If so, for what purpose? __________

4. How many family members do you live with? __________ Who does the cooking? ______________________

5. Please write a sample menu for your first daily meal, indicating how many eggs, type of milk, other beverages, etc. Where do you usually eat this meal? ______________________ What time? __________

6. Please write a sample menu for your next meal, indicating the kinds and amounts of food. Where do you usually eat this meal? __________ ______________________ What time? __________

7. Please write a sample menu for your third daily meal, if eaten. Indicating the kinds and amounts of food. Where do you usually eat this meal? __________ ______________________ What time? __________

8. Describe the type of snacks you are in the habit of eating between meals; indicate approximate amounts.

MORNING AFTERNOON EVENING

FIGURE 10–2. A sample Diet History form.

9. List any common foods which you *never* eat: ______________________

10. How much coffee do you drink in a day? ______________________ What do you put in the coffee? ______________________

11. How much tea do you drink in a day? ______________________ What do you put in the tea? ______________________

12. How much milk do you use in a day (including milk used for cooking, on cereal, in coffee, etc.)? ______________________

13. How often do you eat cheese or cottage cheese? ______________________ In what amounts? ______________________

14. How many eggs do *you* eat in a week? ______________________

15. How often do you eat meat or fish or chicken, etc.? ______________________

16. What size serving of meat do you eat (estimated in ounces)? ______________________

____

17. How often do you eat a raw vegetable salad? ______________________ In what amounts? ______________________

18. How much dressing do you use on a salad, and what kind? ______________________

19. How often do you eat a cooked vegetable? ______________________ In what amounts? ______________________

20. How often do you eat fruit or juice? ______________________

21. How much bread do you eat a day? ______________________ How much cereal? ______________________ What kind? ______________________

22. How often do you eat rice, spaghetti, or macaroni, etc.? ______________________

23. Are your vegetables seasoned with butter, margarine, or other fat seasonings?

____

24. Do you drink alcoholic beverages? ______________________ How often? ______________________

25. Do you drink soda pop? ______________________ How often? ______________________

Do you drink other soft drinks (lemonade, Kool-Aid, etc.)? ______________________

Is there anything else you believe we should know about your eating habits?

record includes both the kinds and amounts of foods eaten during a specified period of time. Ideally, the subjects would be so highly motivated and eager to cooperate that they would carry the record with them at all times and write down an accurate description of all foods eaten day after day. In practice, most people lose interest in the project after one or two days, forget to record some items, or actually modify their intake in order to impress the person who will later read the record. For these reasons, records kept by the subjects themselves may be questioned as reliable sources of information.

Evaluation of intake records

It is in the evaluation of food intake records that the most glaring errors in diet studies are made. Information obtained on the foods consumed by an individual or by a group is compared to some standard, and a conclusion may be made that the intake does or does not meet the criteria of the standard (Figure 10–1). On the basis of food consumption data alone, diets are sometimes classed as "poor" and people described as "malnourished." This is completely unjustified. It must always be remembered that the Basic Four Food Group Plan insures that all the RDA, except those for calories and iron, will be met, and that the RDA for each nutrient is set far higher than the average person's actual requirement. Therefore, dietary intakes which are lower than those recommended in these high standards should never be considered equivalent to malnutrition.

A second mistake in interpreting food intake records is the tendency to concentrate entirely on apparent shortages and to overlook the fact that excesses, too, can lead to malnutrition. Thus the diet of a grossly overweight individual may be judged "good" because there are no shortages compared to the Basic Four or the RDA—an obviously absurd evaluation.

Properly interpreted, food intake data can *suggest* that the nutritional status of an individual or group should be evaluated further by a combination of other methods. In themselves, without supporting evidence of nutritional disease detectable by clinical examinations or laboratory tests, intake data should never be assumed to indicate that nutritional needs are not being met.

Evaluation by a combination of methods: some examples

Although severe vitamin C deficiency has long been eradicated as an epidemic disease, it may still occur sporadically and may baffle the physician who is unaccustomed to considering it as a possibility. An example was seen in a recent case of a four-year-old boy admitted to a hospital in Athens, Greece. The child was pale and irritable, and suffered from painful swellings at the ends of the long bones. Treatment with a drug commonly used to relieve rheumatic symptoms proved useless.

Eventually, biochemical tests and x-ray examination of the bones revealed changes typical of the ascorbic acid-deficiency disease, scurvy. A diet history showed that, because of behavioral problems, the child for months had refused almost all foods except for milk and bread coated with olive oil and sugar. On the basis of these findings, nutritional treatment was begun in the form of a normal diet supplemented with additional vitamin C. The response was dramatic; the pain regressed within one week, the child began to gain weight, the level of vitamin C in the blood rose to normal, and bone lesions improved, as demonstrated by later x-rays. Thus, although nutritional diseases such as scurvy are now rare, the possibility of their occurrence should be kept in mind, and the tests available for their diagnosis should be used in combination for greatest effectiveness.

A second example, seen very commonly in the developing countries, is the child who is of very small stature for age, who has repeated infectious diseases, and who appears listless and apathetic. If he or she is of normal weight for height, this may be because of edema, or accumulated fluid, rather than because of normal amounts of lean tissue and fat. The skin and hair may show varying degrees of the changes resulting from severe protein deficiency. In such cases, laboratory tests may not even be necessary to confirm the clinical data, and a very cursory diet history may be sufficient to elicit the fact that the child's diet has consisted largely of starchy staples, with few sources of high-quality protein. A feeding trial, using a high protein diet, commonly results in spectacular gains in health and growth, and can attest vividly to the fact that the child was previously suffering from disease caused by protein deficiency.

HUNGER AND MALNUTRITION IN THE UNITED STATES TODAY

Until a few years ago, nutritionists and government officials generally believed that hunger and primary malnutrition had been virtually eradicated in developed countries such as the United States. Not until 1968 was it suspected that both hunger and malnutrition were much more common than had been assumed. In that year, *Hunger U.S.A.*, published by the Citizens' Board of Inquiry into Hunger and Malnutrition, provided evidence that not all Americans were benefitting from being citizens of a land of plenty. Compared to many other parts of the world, the United States can still be said to be relatively free of nutritional deficiencies; indeed, overnutrition is a more common problem than is undernutrition. Nevertheless, the existence of hunger or nutritional deficiency in even one person cannot be justified or accepted with complacency.

Studies of food consumption have long been conducted, primarily by the U.S. Department of Agriculture. In these studies, diets are rated as follows:

"good": provide recommended intakes of all nutrients
"fair": provide more than two-thirds, but less than 100 percent, of the recommended intake of one or more nutrients
"poor": provide less than two-thirds of the recommended intake of one or more nutrients

In the 1965 survey, for example, approximately one-half of the household's diets were rated "good," almost one-third were rated "fair," and approximately one-fifth were judged "poor."

However, these studies were studies of food intake only, and in themselves did not provide objective or comprehensive information on nutritional status. The value of publications such as *Hunger U.S.A.* was that they publicized the existence of previously unsuspected problems, particularly among the poor. They were intended to arouse emotion and lead to action, and they accomplished this purpose admirably, but they did not provide the carefully documented evidence demanded, of a rigorous scientific study.

For this reason, the U.S. Public Health Service was authorized to conduct the first comprehensive study of the nutritional status of Americans, beginning in 1968. This study, the *National Nutrition Survey,* was designed to document the existence of malnutrition among people of low-income areas, because food-consumption surveys have repeatedly shown that as incomes decrease, diets generally become less likely to provide recommended intakes of essential nutrients. Because it would be virtually impossible to study all of the low-income people in the United States, a random sample of more than 70,000 individuals was selected from ten states: Washington, California, Texas, Louisiana, South Carolina, Kentucky, West Virginia, Michigan, Massachusetts, and New York (including a separate survey of New York City). Most of the families finally selected had incomes below $3000 per year; however, a few middle- and upper-income families were included because they lived within low-income areas. For this and other reasons, it must be recognized that the population studied in the *National Nutrition Survey* was not representative of the entire population of the United States, nor even of the states within which samples were drawn.

Approximately 40,000 of the subjects participated in a clinical evaluation, which included a physical examination, anthropometric measurements, x-ray examination of the wrist, dental examination, and collection of blood for biochemical analysis. Subgroups were then selected for more detailed dietary and biochemical evaluation, with heavy representation of high-risk populations such as infants and young children, adolescents, pregnant or lactating women, and those over sixty years of age.

The main findings of this comprehensive study of nutritional status can be summarized as follows:

1. A significant proportion of the population surveyed was malnourished or at high risk of developing nutritional problems. However, different segments of the population varied with respect to the severity of malnutrition and in regard to the specific nutrients involved. A striking example is the prevalence of low vitamin A levels in the serum; low levels were much more common among the Mexican-Americans than among the Puerto Ricans in the study. These findings show that the kinds and degrees of malnutrition vary from one locality to another, and that the situation found in one local situation cannot be assumed to exist among the poor elsewhere.

2. Although generalizations may be misleading, a few clear-cut ones emerged. Malnutrition was found most commonly among blacks, less commonly among Spanish-Americans, and least commonly among whites. In general there was increasing evidence of malnutrition as income level decreased. However, comparison of individuals of similar income level and ethnic background but living in different states showed that income is not the only determinant of nutritional status; factors such as social and cultural differences are also important.

3. Of all age groups studied, individuals between the ages of 10 and 16 were most likely to be malnourished, and males in this age group were more likely to have unsatisfactory nutritional status than females were.

4. There was a positive relationship between nutritional status and the level of educational attainment. Whether this indicates a specific effect of education is not known, since the number of years of school completed is associated with income level and other factors affecting nutritional status.

5. School lunches contributed a significant proportion of the total nutrient intake of children, particularly among black children.

6. Evidence was found of retarded growth and development in children and adolescents. However, black children were taller than white children and were more advanced in bone and tooth development, which indicates that inherited racial differences affect growth and development and may even offset some of the detrimental effects of malnutrition.

7. Obesity was most prevalent in adult women, particularly black women. Among males, obesity was more common in whites than in blacks.

8. With regard to specific nutrients, the prevalence of malnutrition ranged from surprisingly high to extremely low:

Iron. Iron deficiency anemia was the only nutrient deficiency disease found in large numbers of individuals throughout all segments of the sample population.

Protein. Low serum albumin levels, suggesting marginal protein nutriture, were found in a relatively large proportion of pregnant and lactating women, but not in others.

FIGURE 10–3
Donated food used to help people improve their nutritional status. (USDA photo.)

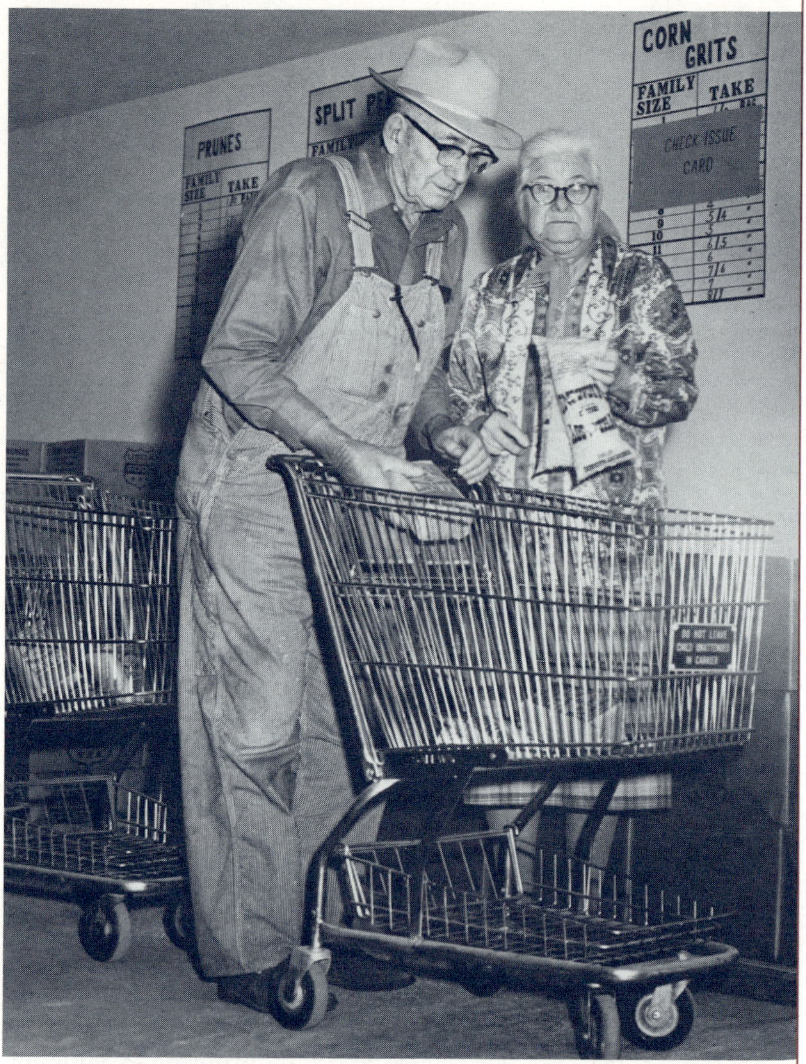

Vitamin A. Young people in all subgroups had a high prevalence of low vitamin A levels, based on biochemical measurements; Mexican-Americans in Texas had a particular problem with regard to this vitamin. However, clinical evidence of deficiency, such as skin or eye changes, was lacking.

Vitamin C. Nutritional status with respect to vitamin C was not a major problem among any of the groups surveyed. In general, males had a greater prevalence of low serum levels of vitamin C than females did, and the prevalence of unsatisfactory status increased with age.

Riboflavin. As evaluated from urinary excretion studies, riboflavin status was poorest among blacks and among young people of all ethnic groups.

Thiamin. On the basis of urinary excretion data, nutritional status with respect to thiamin did not appear to be a problem among any group.

Iodine. Clinically, goiter was found to be more prevalent than had been anticipated. However, no relationship was found between the prevalence of goiter and nutritional status with respect to iodine, suggesting that the goiter was caused by factors other than nutrition.

It must be emphasized that, although the *National Nutrition Survey* was the most nearly complete survey of its kind ever accomplished in the United States, it was limited both as to the size of the population surveyed and as to the number of nutrients studied. Biochemical methods have not yet even been developed to monitor the status of people with respect to most of the essential nutrients. Therefore, the *National Nutrition Survey* should be regarded as an important step in the continuing close observation of the American population, rather than as the final answer regarding nutritional status in Americans.

PROGRAMS TO IMPROVE NUTRITION IN THE UNITED STATES

The occasional food basket donated to a needy family obviously cannot accomplish the purpose of alleviating hunger and malnutrition in a nation. Large-scale programs, many of which are authorized through laws and financed by government funds, are necessary. Some of the more important of these are the following:

Donated food program. The Surplus Food Program, started in the 1930s, was the first government food program. Originally, a few commodities, or staple foods, were distributed to needy people; later, the program was expanded to include over twenty types of foods, not all of which were available in surplus (Figure 10–3).

Food stamp program. In the 1960s, this program was initiated in order to provide buying power. Recipients purchase the stamps at a price dependent upon their ability to pay, and then use the stamps to purchase food. The federal government pays the difference between the value of the stamps and the money paid for the stamps. In effect, therefore, people use their limited funds to purchase stamps which they then spend for more food than they could otherwise afford.

School feeding programs. Under the National School Lunch Program, free or reduced-cost lunches are available to children who cannot afford to pay the regular price. The same act that regulates the school lunch program also provides support for the Special Milk Program, which makes milk available at low cost to children in various organized groups, including schools. The Child Nutrition Act provided funds for purchasing equipment needed by schools wishing to participate in the School Lunch Program, and authorized the use of federal funds for a School Breakfast Program as well.

Head start. The main purpose of this program is to provide im-

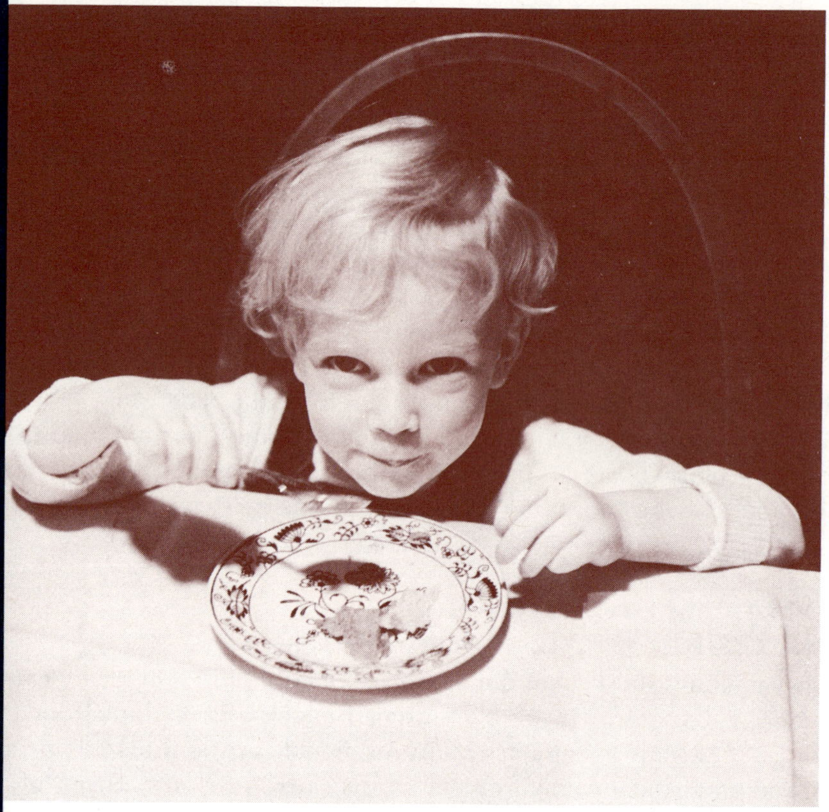

FIGURE 10–4
Food as well as education is an important component of many programs for young children. (Photo by Donald R. Depew, courtesy of DHEW.)

proved conditions for intellectual and social development of preschool children from disadvantaged families. As a part of this program, however, improved nutrition is provided, both by providing food and through the educational component of the program (Figure 10–4).

Expanded nutrition program. Nutrition aides, trained through the Extension Service of the U. S. Department of Agriculture, work to provide low-income homemakers with the knowledge and skills required to utilize their available food resources to best advantage. In addition, funds are allocated to support the efforts of inner city professionals who incorporate nutrition education into their work with young people.

Medicare. Standards for nutrition are included in the requirements for institutions such as hospitals and nursing homes in which substantial numbers of elderly people live. Nutritional assistance is not, however, provided for the majority of older people who live in their own homes or in the homes of others.

These programs, along with many others, seek to alleviate hunger and malnutrition in two main ways: by making more food available, and by educating people as to the best use of available food. Support of this type of program, however, depends upon the nonhungry and the well nourished. It is unfortunate that many tend to believe that those who are poor or hungry are less deserving than others, that poverty is usually the result of laziness and shortsightedness, and that "those who do not work do not eat." Perhaps one of the greatest needs for education, then, is not among those who need the programs, but among those who are fortunate enough not to need them.

HUNGER AND MALNUTRITION IN THE DEVELOPING COUNTRIES

Of our 3.5 billion, a billion are hungry or *dangerously* undernourished, or both; while in the affluent food-rich societies, many are more concerned with reducing their own weight than reducing the weight of hunger that presses on the great majority.

–Speech delivered by the Rt. Hon. Lester B. Pearson, former Prime Minister of Canada, Second World Food Congress, The Hague, The Netherlands, 1970.

What, then, does the world look like in 1970? On balance, it is not a very pretty picture . . . And much of this is due to the fact that man lives on one planet, but in two worlds. . . . There is a world of luxury foods, and another where food is the only luxury known.

–Keynote address delivered by A. H. Boerma, Director-General of the Food and Agriculture Organization, Second World Food Congress, The Hague, The Netherlands, 1970.

The "two worlds" in which people live are shown in Figure 10–5. In the area known as the developed countries are found one-third of the world's people, among whom hunger exists mostly in isolated pockets, and where overnutrition is more common than undernutrition. In the other, which includes the developing countries, are found two-thirds of the world's people; also found here are crushing problems of poverty, overpopulation, illiteracy, and unemployment, as well as hunger and malnutrition.

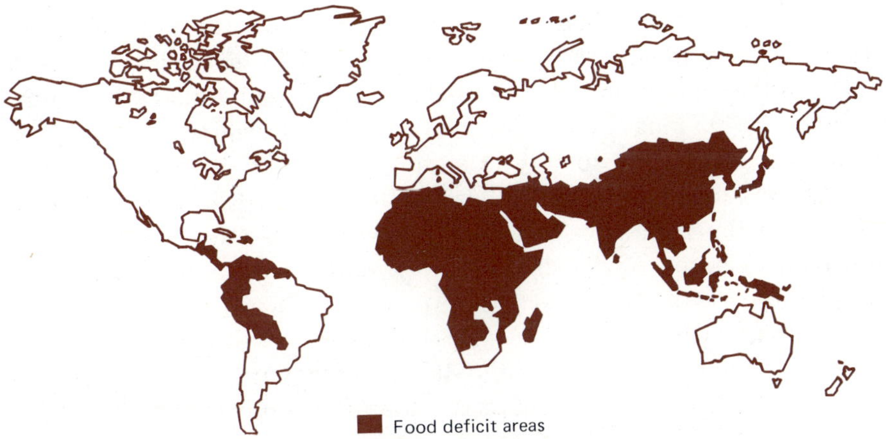

FIGURE 10–5. The "Two Worlds" in which humanity lives.

The nutrition problems of the developing countries are so well known that there is little need to document further evidence. It is estimated that *between one-half and two-thirds* of the world's people suffer from hunger or from some type of undernutrition; that there are in the world *approximately 1 billion* nutritionally deprived children below the age of 14; that in India alone some *10,000* children become blind each year because of vitamin A deficiency; and that mortality of infants and children in the developing countries is such that the average life span in these countries is *no more than forty years.* Food balance sheets, diet surveys, clinical examinations, information from vital statistics, laboratory tests, and other methods have all been used to assess nutritional adequacy among people of the developing countries. Generally, these studies are done by people from outside the area being studied. Surveys in other countries are more difficult to do than surveys in one's own country because of various factors: the language barrier, antagonism toward foreigners, lack of qualified technical personnel, inadequate laboratory facilities, and religious beliefs or cultural mores which may interfere with necessary procedures—such as the taking of blood samples or the examination of females. Despite these difficulties, enough nutrition surveys have been done to support the conclusion that the majority of the world's people today still live in the fear of hunger and malnutrition which has existed since the human species evolved, and from which we of the developed countries have been freed only in recent centuries.

More important than the presentation of statistics on world nutrition problems is the examination of two related subjects. One is the question of why large numbers of people are hungry and malnourished; the other is concerned with the organized efforts to improve nutrition.

The roots of hunger and malnutrition in developing countries

The causes of nutritional problems are multiple and intertwined, but identification and understanding of them is necessary in seeking solutions. Some of the most important are the following:

Poverty. In some of the developing countries, the annual income per person is typically *10 percent or less* of the average per capita income in the United States. The effect upon the individual's food buying power is obvious. Equally important is the effect of national poverty on the ability of a society to supply the roads, schools, sanitation systems, medical centers, and other facilities needed for activities such as food distribution, education of people regarding nutrition, and treatment or prevention of diseases which interact with and contribute to malnutrition.

Overpopulation. The rate of population growth is so much more rapid in the developing than in the developed countries that it has been estimated that by the year 2000, more than three-fourths of the world's population will live in the developing countries. Thus, although total food production increased during the 1960s, the amount of food available *per person* increased only slightly or not at all in Latin America and the Far East, and actually declined in Africa.

Increasing urbanization. Malnutrition has long existed among the rural people who constitute the majority of the populations of the developing countries. However, even more extreme deprivations may await those who, in increasing numbers, move to urban areas only to find unemployment, slum dwellings, and lack of opportunity to raise food or forage for food as they did previously.

Antiquated agricultural methods. The tools and methods used to produce food in parts of the world are typical, not of the nineteenth-century Western world, but more of the fifteenth century, or even earlier. Only primitive methods of plowing and irrigation are used in some areas, and food production may rely on human labor rather than on machines or even on animals. As a result, much of the energy derived from today's food is used in an attempt to wrest tomorrow's food from the soil. The land may be farmed by those who do not own it, as in the feudal system of earlier Europe; under these conditions rural people have little incentive (or may not even have the right) to change their methods of food production. Alternatively, land may have been divided and subdivided into small portions within a family, so that modern mechanized agriculture would be difficult to introduce. The soil may be unproductive for a variety of reasons: underuse of fertilizers, soil erosion, lack of water, or overgrazing by cattle—which may be kept primarily for prestige value, or which are protected as sacred.

Lack of education. From the viewpoint of long-range programs, lack of education is one of the most serious barriers to improving the nutrition of a society. Illiteracy makes it extremely difficult to teach better methods of food production and utilization, and uneducated people are apt to have little awareness of the relationship of nutrition to health, or of the benefits of limiting family size so as to have a smaller number of better-fed, healthier children. Uneducated people also commonly accept without question superstitions and taboos that contribute to malnutrition, such as the belief that numerous foods must be avoided by pregnant women in order to protect the fetus, or that diseases can be driven away by starving the patient.

Widespread health problems. Although many of the diseases of tropical countries are parasitic and infectious rather than nutritional in origin, the decreased physical vigor of a malnourished community can lead to continued low ability to produce food. The end result can be a vicious circle of low food production, malnutrition, decreased susceptibility to diseases in general, and continued low productivity.

Programs to improve nutrition in developing countries

None of the problems of the developing countries can be considered in isolation. Hence programs which improve the situation with respect to

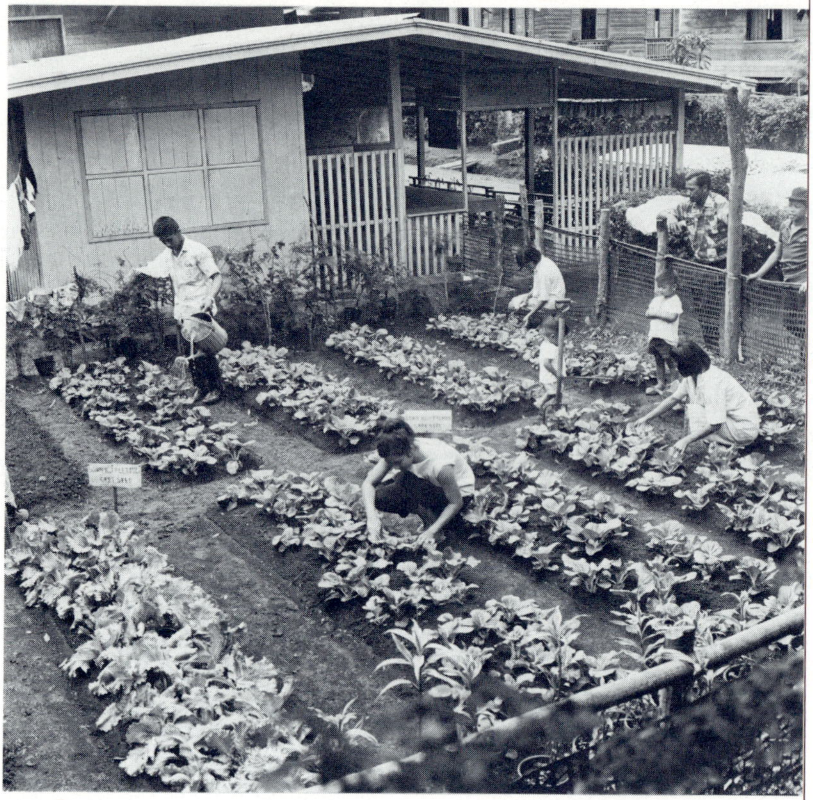

FIGURE 10–6
A CARE-sponsored program in the Philippines; seeds and hand tools are donated, with the recipients providing self-help in the form of labor. (CARE photo.)

one area will almost inevitably have implications for others. Programs may therefore be involved in a broad spectrum of services such as educational, medical, social, and economic, as well as those related specifically to nutritional improvement.

Nongovernmental agencies such as the Ford Foundation and Rockefeller Foundation have funded research on the development of new food mixtures and new strains of plants which provide better nutrition than do the conventional foods available in some of the developing countries. Some of these will be discussed in later chapters.

Church groups provide direct aid by distributing food to those living in the areas in which the churches work. In addition, some provide more long-term assistance by conducting educational programs on subjects ranging from improved agricultural methods to family planning. Unfortunately, some churches place the principal emphasis upon gaining converts rather than meeting the needs of the general population, and in the process may create social problems as serious as those already existing.

Voluntary agencies in the United States and other developed countries provide assistance in the form of vast feeding and self-help projects within the developing countries. One of the best known is CARE

(Cooperative for American Relief Everywhere). This organization obtains funds and materials from various sources: donations of money from private citizens, contributions of foods from the United States Government, and equipment or funds from industries and business. The governments of recipient countries provide transport and warehousing, and the individuals who finally receive help may contribute their own labor to the projects financed by CARE (Figure 10–6). By sharing costs, the recipients help to make the project their own accomplishment, rather than a form of charity which could stifle their dignity and self-determination.

However, as important as the work of voluntary groups is, the scope of the world problem is too great for them to solve alone. For this reason, a number of organizations within the United Nations are involved in food and nutrition programs in various ways.

The United Nations International Children's Emergency Fund (UNICEF) was originally formed to provide emergency aid to children in countries devastated by World War II. Since 1950, the programs have been broadened to provide less direct but longer-range aid to children of the developing countries. Funds for UNICEF's work, provided voluntarily through the governments of about one hundred nations, support a variety of programs related to the welfare of children. These include maternal and child health clinics, school health programs, disease control centers, and education programs for the training of doctors, midwives, nurses, teachers, and others needed to insure the health of children. Assistance to family planning programs, included as part of maternal and child health services since the late 1960s, may at first sight seem to be far removed from the original purpose of UNICEF, but is ultimately a more effective step toward child welfare than are stopgap measures whereby emergency aid is given to ever increasing numbers of undernourished children.

Another specialized United Nations Agency, the World Health Organization (WHO), provides health assistance in many forms to people of all ages. The training of personnel in the health professions, the improvement of environmental sanitation, and the control of major diseases are important parts of the mandate of WHO. To some extent, WHO is directly involved in nutrition programs, many of which are conducted in cooperation with other United Nations agencies such as UNICEF. To a much larger extent, WHO contributes indirectly to nutritional improvement through improving the general health of populations. Healthier people are more effective workers and thus produce more food; control of infectious diseases prevents the synergistic effect seen when malnutrition and infection together produce a more serious illness than malnutrition alone; and educational programs stress improved nutrition as an important part of total human health.

The Food and Agriculture Organization (FAO) is a United Nations agency with several main objectives. One is to assist member nations to increase food production through such means as irrigation projects, programs to provide agricultural machinery, and technical assistance in production of domestic animals and crops. Another important function is to obtain information on the food supplies of nations as well as on their particular agricultural problems. This information is necessary to enable the development of long-range plans for production of food in order to help nations raise their general standard of living as well as improve the nutrition of their people.

In summary, programs to combat hunger and malnutrition in developing countries are at present aimed at making nations self-sufficient rather than merely providing temporary assistance in the form of food. Family planning programs have been initiated in a number of areas with the goal of increasing the availability of food per person, because rapid population growth offsets gains in food production. Population planning, as distinct from individual family planning, will probably be necessary eventually in order to bring the reproductive behavior of people into accord with the social and economic needs of nations. Because attitudes toward reproduction change very slowly, results should not be expected soon, and the realistic goal for at least the next decade is to intensify efforts to increase food production and improve the general standard of living of people throughout the world. However, the possibility that increased food and other resources will eventually improve the *quality* of life, rather than being used largely to support mere existence for ever larger *numbers* of people, may be regarded at least with guarded optimism.

SUGGESTED READINGS

Clark, F. "Recent Food Consumption Surveys and Their Uses." Federation Proceedings 33 (1974):2270.

"Ten-State Nutrition Survey, 1968–1970 (highlights)." Atlanta: U. S. Dept. of HEW, Center for Disease Control, DHEW Publ. No. (HSM)72–8134.

Elwood, P. C. "Evaluation of the Clinical Importance of Anemia." *American Journal of Clinical Nutrition* 26 (1973):958.

Garn, S. M., S. T. Sandusky, J. M. Nagy, and M. B. McCann. "Advanced Skeletal Development in Low-income Negro Children." *Journal of Pediatrics* 80 (1972):965.

Hiemstra, S. J. "Nutritional Standards in School Food Service." *Journal of School Health* 42 (1972):317.

Krehl, W. A. "The Evaluation of Nutritional Status." *Medical Clinics of North America* 48 (1964):1129.

Leverton, R. M. "The Paradox of Teen-Age Nutrition." *Journal of American Dietetic Association* 53 (1968):13.

Lewis, I. J. "National Nutrition Survey: Viewpoint of a Public Administrator." *American Journal of Clinical Nutrition* 25 (1972):956.

Lowe, C. U. "National Nutrition Survey: Viewpoint of a Nutritionist." *American Journal of Clinical Nutrition* 25 (1972):964.

Perryman, J. N. "The School Administrator and the Food Service Program." National Education Association, Washington, D.C., 1972.

Sauberlich, H. E., R. P. Dowdy, and J. H. Skala. "Laboratory Tests for the Assessment of Nutritional Status." Cleveland: CRC Press, Inc., 1974.

11

pathways of change: metabolism and related life processes

Biochemical nutrition is really a tautological term, since all nutrition is essentially biochemical and all biochemistry in living matter is dependent on nutrition.

–Peter Hahn, "Nutrition and Development," M. Winick, ed., New York: Wiley, 1972.

The conversion of food into life can be explained in terms of two types of biochemicals: those which serve as nutrients and those which determine how nutrients are utilized within the living organism. A discussion at the molecular level can interpret nutrition more precisely than is possible at the level of populations, whole organisms, or cells. This chapter is therefore necessarily presented in the language of chemistry. However, the discussion has been simplified in two major ways:

First, words rather than chemical formulas have been used in most cases. A common reaction to a chart covered with chemical structures is to turn the page—a response which this discussion is not intended to provoke.

Second, many details have been omitted so that the most important points may stand out more clearly. Thus an entire pathway or process may be represented by words indicating the starting materials and the final products, with most or all of the intermediates omitted.

It will not be possible to describe in detail the processes whereby nonliving atoms and molecules from the environment are transformed into *protoplasm,* of which life is made. The main outlines of these processes, however, can provide some insight into the inner world wherein the dynamic processes of nutrition ultimately occur.

THE CHEMICAL COMPOSITION OF LIFE: THE CONSUMER AND THE CONSUMED

The chemical elements which make up all living matter are basically much the same. However, different kinds of organisms, as well as different cell types within the same kind of organism, differ from one another in several important respects: the structures of the molecules into which the elements are built, the relative quantities of various chemical substances present, and the functions which the materials perform in living things.

Structure and function are intimately linked. Thus the proteins known as *keratins,* found in large amounts in such structures as skin, hair, hoofs, nails, and quills, have a structure that makes them highly insoluble. This is an obvious advantage, considering the consequences of being caught in the rain with soluble skin and hair. By contrast, many of the proteins of the blood, liver, brain, and other internal parts must move about in the cells or body fluids in order to perform their roles. Their chemical structures are such that they dissolve readily in water, thereby enabling them to travel freely.

In some cases, the chemical composition of an organism is quite similar to the composition of what it consumes, as when an animal lives by preying on closely related species. Cannibalism, the eating of other members of the same species, is the closest an organism can come to having a diet identical to its own composition, although of course no species could survive if its members lived exclusively by eating each other. At any rate, for most forms of life there are vast differences between the organism and what it consumes. Plant-eating animals must produce their own tissues from the plants they eat, and plants must grow by using the very simple materials they absorb from the soil and air. People eat an incredible variety of foods, and the substances that function effectively in the organisms from which these foods are derived are far from identical to those necessary for the functioning of the human organism. In fact, many of the components of foods would be extremely detrimental if they were somehow incorporated unaltered into human cells.

The expression, "You are what you eat," therefore cannot be literally true. You are the end result, not only of the materials you derive from the environment, but also of what your body does with these materials. The alteration of food substances into human life is accomplished by three major interrelated processes: digestion, metabolism, and excretion. Each of these processes involves a large number of chemical reactions, with each reaction catalyzed by a specific enzyme. Therefore, a consideration of enzymes is a reasonable point to begin the study of how nutrients are transformed into life.

ENZYMES: BIOLOGICAL ACCELERATORS

Any chemical reaction that occurs in living material can also occur in nonliving material. Therefore, an outstanding characteristic of biochemical systems is not the nature or type of reactions, but their extremely rapid rate under the conditions found within the body. This rapidity is made possible through the intervention of catalysts known as *enzymes*, which are found in all plants and animals. Although all enzymes are proteins, the thousands of different enzymes found in a human differ from the thousands of different enzymes found, say, in a fish, a bird, or a rose bush. These differences are, of course, the result of the genetic differences that make each species unique, and which enable each species to produce the kinds and amounts of enzymes appropriate to its own particular needs. Within a given organism, also, different types of cells have unique enzyme patterns, depending upon the cells' particular functions. However, *all* enzymes have the following characteristics in common:

1. They are proteins, and are therefore sensitive to heat, acids, and other factors which in general alter proteins.

2. They are specific in action, catalyzing reactions involving only one substance or at most a small group of substances which are referred to as the *substrates.*

3. They act by combining with one or more substrates to form an enzyme-substrate complex. The substrates thus bound are less stable

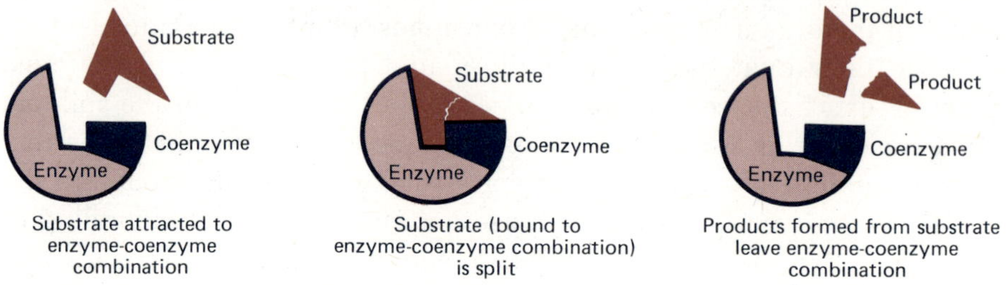

FIGURE 11–1. An enzyme in action. Enzymes may catalyze the breakdown of substances into smaller products, as in this example, or may combine two or more substrates to form larger products.

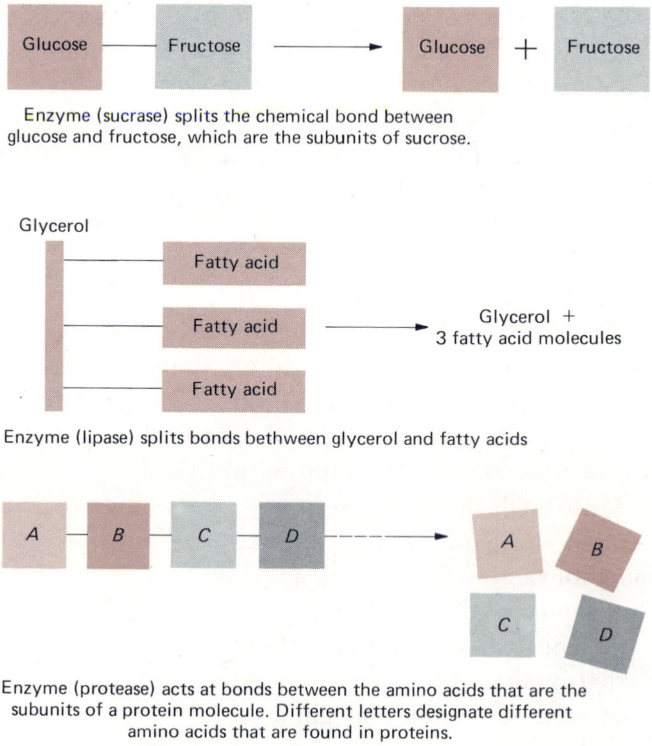

FIGURE 11–2. Action of sucrase, a lipase, and a protease.

than they are in the unbound state, and therefore readily change to one or more new substances, called the *products.* The products then leave the enzyme, which itself remains unchanged and available for recombination with another substrate molecule (Figure 11–1). Thus the same enzyme molecule may be *reused* thousands or millions of times before it is broken down, as all cell constituents ultimately must be.

Some but not all enzymes have the following additional characteristics:

1. Many are named according to their substrates, with the suffix *ase* added. For example, *sucrase* is a digestive enzyme which splits the disaccharide sucrose, and *proteases* are enzymes which liberate amino acids by splitting the bonds in protein molecules (Figure 11–2).

2. They may contain nonprotein substances as parts of their structure. The nonprotein portion, called a *coenzyme* or *cofactor,* may be a mineral or a compound produced in the cells from a vitamin or some other compound.

Homeostasis, the maintenance of an internal environment compatible with normal life processes, is accomplished by regulating the amounts of substrates, cofactors, hormones, and other biochemicals necessary for the organism's functions, and this regulation is possible largely through the action of enzymes. In turn, however, the substrates, cofactors, hormones, and other biochemicals modify the rates of many enzymatic reactions. Nature thus operates by an elaborate system of checks and balances. Failure at any point in the system can lead to impaired functioning, which we call disease. Indeed, all diseases and deaths must ultimately be explained on the basis of loss of control over one or more biochemical reactions.

Some aspects of functioning, such as the structures of the protein portions of enzyme molecules, are ultimately controlled by the structures of the internal factors, the genes. Upon areas such as these, nutritional intake can have no effect. However, other aspects of metabolism, such as the amounts of substrates and coenzymes available, can be profoundly influenced by diet.

DIGESTION

Properly speaking, digestion occurs *outside* the body, rather than inside it (Figure 11–3). Although the cellular walls of the digestive organs are properly considered part of the body, it is in the *lumen,* or inner open space, that food is digested. The lumen of the digestive tract, which is actually a hollow tube continuous with the environment, is not really part of the body at all. Although this may seem to be a minor point, it is very important. Nutrients cannot be utilized by cells until after they are absorbed from the digestive tract into the body itself. Of the six nutrient classes, only water, vitamins, and mineral elements can be absorbed in the forms in which they ordinarily occur in foods; other

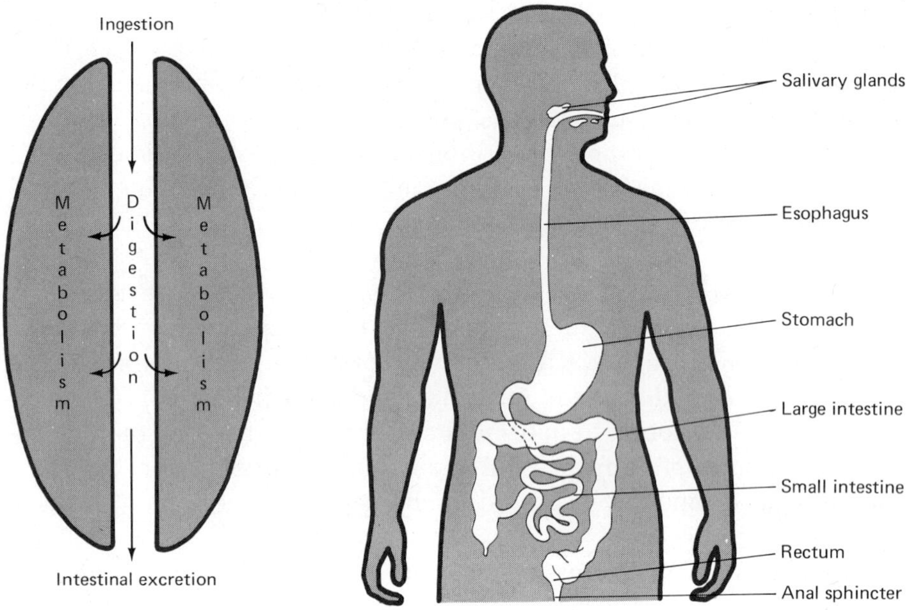

FIGURE 11–3. The human digestive system; note that the space within the digestive tract is outside the body.

nutrients must first be altered by digestion. Impaired digestion and absorption can therefore result in severe malnutrition even though the diet contains the kinds and amounts of nutrients ideal for the normal individual.

The over-all result of digestion is that large particles are made small enough to be absorbed across the walls of the digestive tract into the body (Figure 11–4). Digestion is accomplished in two major ways. *Mechanical* processes, performed by muscles, reduce the size of large pieces of food to smaller bits, which, however, are still much too large to be absorbed. It is through *chemical* processes, catalyzed by enzymes, that individual nutrient molecules are reduced in size until the products are small enough to be absorbed.

What happens in the various parts of the digestive systems is as follows:

In the mouth, food is mechanically ground into smaller pieces by the teeth, and mixed with saliva which moistens and lubricates it. *Amylase,* a starch-digesting enzyme, is present in saliva, but actually causes little chemical change in starch because food ordinarily remains in the mouth for only a short time. Therefore, changes in the mouth are almost entirely of the mechanical rather than of the chemical type.

Food passes along the esophagus so rapidly that no digestion of either type occurs here. It is therefore in the stomach that enzymatic digestion begins to a significant degree. Gastric juice secreted by the stomach contains proteases which begin to split proteins into smaller amino acid chains known as *peptides.* Fat-digesting enzymes called *lipases* also begin to work here. Carbohydrate digestion, however, does not occur to any great extent in the stomach, because cells lining the stomach pour out *hydrochloric acid*. This acid inhibits the action of the carbohydrate-splitting amylase swallowed along with food, although it stimulates the activity of proteases secreted by the stomach.

In addition to performing chemical digestion, the stomach mechanically mixes its contents through vigorous churning motions of the muscular walls. During a period that ordinarily lasts several hours, the partially digested mass gradually leaves the stomach and enters the small intestine.

It is *in the small intestine* that the greatest portion of digestion really occurs. Into the small intestine flow three kinds of digestive fluids:

1. The pancreas secretes a fluid important in the digestion of all three classes of energy nutrients: present are several proteases, a fat-splitting enzyme, and a number of carbohydrate-digesting enzymes. In addition, pancreatic juice contains bicarbonate, which neutralizes the hydrochloric acid entering the intestine together with the stomach's contents. This creates a nonacidic environment, ideal for the work of the enzymes that catalyze the remainder of the digestive process.

2. Intestinal juice, produced by cells lining the intestine itself, contains a number of carbohydratases that split disaccharides to monosaccharides. Sucrase splits sucrose to glucose and fructose; maltase splits maltose into two glucose units; and lactase splits lactose into glucose and galactose. The intestinal juice also contains lipases, which remove fatty acids from fat molecules, and enzymes which complete the digestion of proteins by liberating amino acids from peptides formed earlier in the stomach.

3. Bile, a fluid produced by the liver and stored in the gallbladder, is ejected into the intestine when food is present. However, unlike the other two digestive fluids, bile does not contain digestive enzymes; its chief contribution to digestion is its action as a detergent. Components known as *bile salts* emulsify fats, breaking large fat droplets into smaller droplets. These can then be attacked by lipases in the pancreatic juice and intestinal juice.

After passing along the length of the small intestine, material that has resisted digestion enters the large intestine or colon. Because no digestive enzymes are produced in this part of the tract, anything not digested previously will pass along the colon without further alteration. The principal change occurring in the large intestine is absorption into the blood stream of additional amounts of water and dissolved salts (minerals). Thus the liquified mass which enters the colon is converted into more solid material, which is eventually excreted as the feces.

Approximately two-thirds of the remnants excreted as feces consists of water; most of the remaining one-third consists of all of the cellulose which was eaten, plus enormous numbers of bacteria. Ordinarily, these intestinal bacteria are harmless or even friendly, producing substances such as vitamin K, which can be absorbed and utilized by the body. Only minute amounts of unabsorbed minerals and vitamins are excreted in the feces, because these are present in foods in relatively small amounts. Also, because the energy nutrients in foods are ordinarily digested and absorbed almost 100 percent efficiently, very little of these remain to be excreted in the intestinal waste of normal people.

Regulation of digestion

At the very least, secretion of digestive fluids into an empty tract would be wasteful; at worst, the enzymes in the juices might start to nibble away at the digestive tract itself, if food were not present. Therefore, organisms have evolved mechanisms for insuring that large amounts of the various juices are secreted into the digestive tract only when it contains food, so that the presence of enzymes and substrates is co-

FIGURE 11–4. Change and nonchange in digestion. Nutrients themselves or products of nutrient digestion are absorbed into the bloodstream if they are water-soluble, and into the lymph stream if they are fat-soluble.

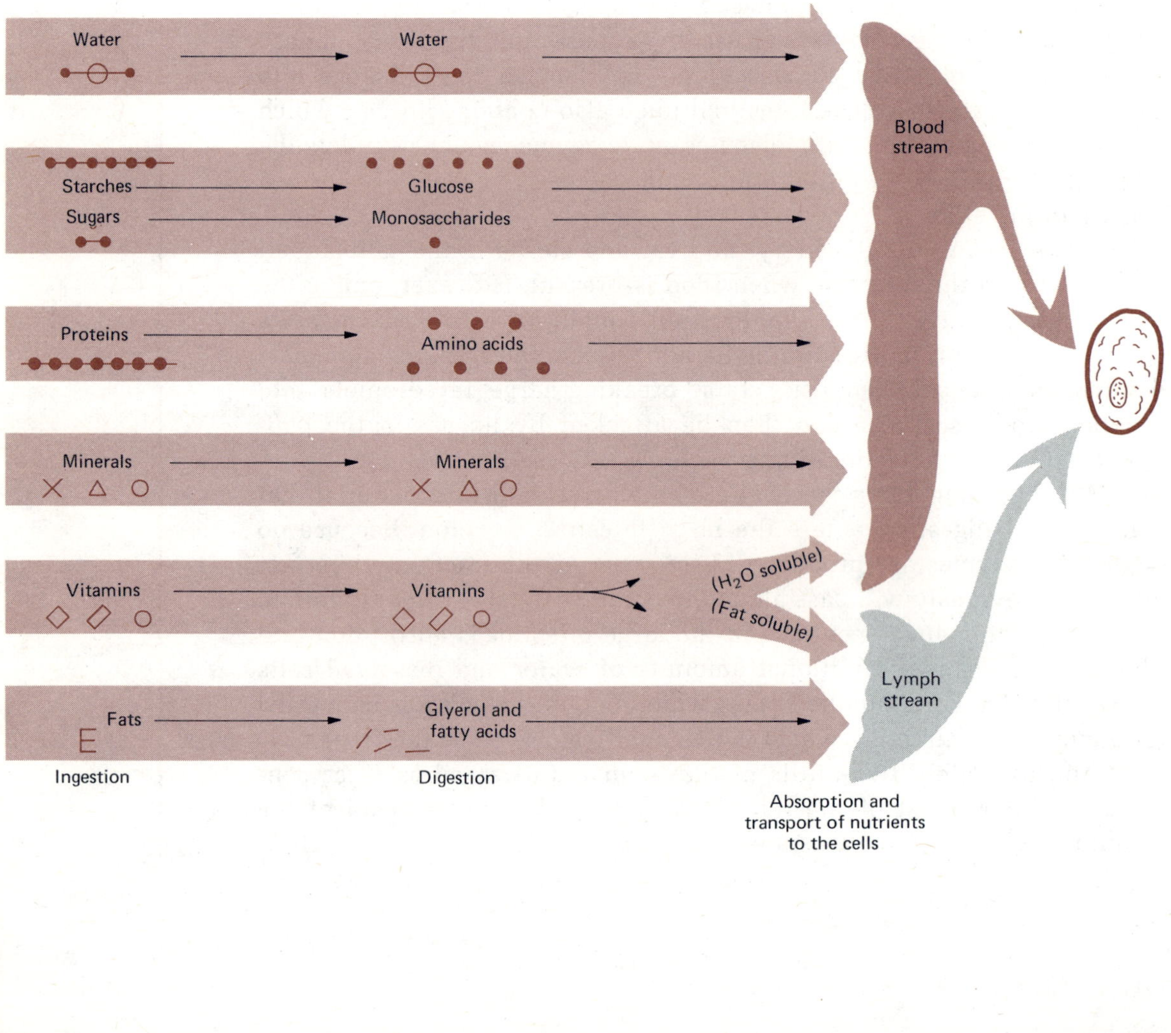

ordinated. This control is achieved by both of the organ systems specialized for regulation and integration: the nervous system and the endocrine system.

In the mouth, saliva is secreted in response to chemicals which stimulate *nerves;* an acid such as vinegar, for example, causes an immediate increase in salivation. Mechanical nerve stimulation, which occurs when an object is present in the mouth, can also simulate saliva flow; in fact, hikers often carry small stones in their mouths to stimulate saliva secretion and thereby relieve the thirst felt when the mouth is dry. Normally, of course, it is food of some sort which acts as the mechanical stimulus. In addition, purely psychic influences—the sight of, or even the thought of, food—can, through neural stimulation, induce salivation in anticipation of food.

In the stomach and intestine, *hormones* largely regulate the secretion of digestive juices. The hormones are not secreted into the lumen of the digestive system as digestive enzymes are; rather they enter the blood stream, which carries them to their distant target organs. Six different hormones have been identified as factors in regulating secre-

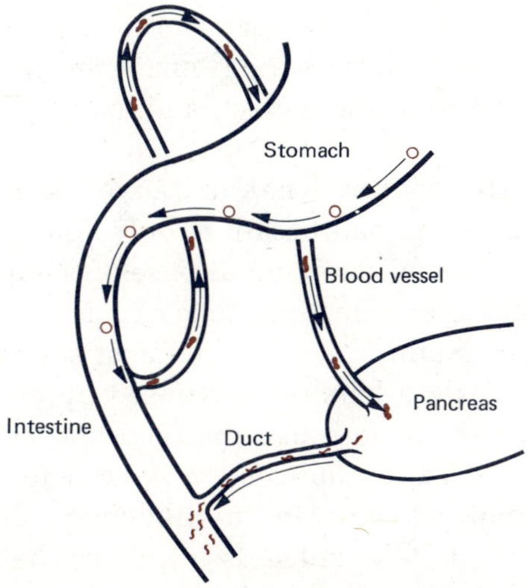

FIGURE 11–5. Control of pancreatic juice secretion by the hormone secretin. Hydrochloric acid (white dots) from the stomach stimulates intestinal cells to produce secretin (black marks). Secretin enters the bloodstream, which carries it to the pancreas. In response, the pancreas pours its digestive juice (black curls) into the intestine. Enzymes in the pancreatic juice digest nutrients; bicarbonate in the juice creates a favorable environment for the action of the enzymes.

tion of the various digestive juices. Figure 11–5 explains how the secretion of one type of digestive juice is regulated by one particular hormone, *secretin.*

In addition to regulation by hormones, modification by nerves affects secretion in the stomach and intestine. Purely psychic factors, as well as the presence of food in the digestive tract, can stimulate nerves; fear and anger, for example, can inhibit secretion of gastric juice by the stomach and thereby interfere with digestions. Mechanical digestion—the moving and churning of food by *peristalsis,* or the coordinated action of muscles in the digestive tract—can also be altered by nerve activity; strong emotions can retard the movements of the digestive organs, or, conversely, may sometimes speed them up so that much of the food is hurried along the digestive tract too rapidly for digestion and absorption to be completed. Thus nutritional status can be altered by the state of mind as well as by the quality of the diet.

Nutrition-related digestive system disorders

People who would never consider trying to treat their own disorders of the heart, kidneys, or other organs may nevertheless believe that "do it yourself" medicine is good enough for the digestive system. In this belief, they are encouraged by producers of remedies for a variety of real or imagined disorders. Of course it is not necessary to consult a physician for each temporary digestive problem, some of which are merely nuisances or social disadvantages rather than medical matters. However, judging from the number of products sold for the treatment of various parts of the digestive system, many people need to know more than they do about the subject, and may find the following brief discussion helpful.

Bad breath. No matter what the advertisements of toothpastes and mouthwashes imply, bad breath is only a symptom, not a disease. It can be caused by heavy smoking; disease of the tonsils, nose, sinuses, lungs, liver, stomach, or intestine; foods such as garlic, onions, or alcoholic beverages; or other factors. The most common cause, however, is food particles that are being decomposed by bacteria in the mouth. The obvious treatment is to brush the food particles off the teeth.

Indigestion. The term *indigestion* is used for a variety of conditions: nausea, vomiting, pain in the abdomen, diarrhea, and so on. Although many people take antacids to relieve the "acid stomach" believed to cause these symptoms, the stomach is normally acid and it would be undesirable to change this condition, even if it were possible. However, frequent indigestion, or any severe abdominal pain, may represent a serious condition, the cause of which a physician should determine.

Vomiting. Because vomiting is a way of ridding the stomach of its contents, people commonly assume that the cause invariably "must be something I ate" (or drank). Actually, vomiting is controlled by a part of the brain, and can therefore be induced by any factor that can affect that organ: drugs, motion, unpleasant odors, or even strong emotions. The most important nutritional implication of vomiting is the loss of fluid, which can rapidly lead to dehydration. Although this is especially serious in infants and young children, persistent vomiting in any individual requires prompt medical attention. Popular home remedies, such as dilute salt solutions, may actually do more harm than good.

Ulcers. An ulcer, or open sore, in the stomach or intestine can cause extreme pain, and if the ulcer bleeds the blood loss can result in severe anemia. The pain can often be relieved temporarily either by taking antacids or by eating, but this merely covers up a symptom. Although foods do not cause an ulcer, certain foods may aggravate it. Diet is therefore part of the treatment, but the patient should always be under the care of a physician. Self-treatment with special diets (all milk, strained baby foods, and similar regimens) is definitely not recommended.

Gallbladder disease. Gallbladder disease is most commonly caused by the presence of gallstones, solid concretions which form in the gallbladder. The victim is most often an obese woman of middle age or older. Because secretion of bile into the intestine is decreased, fat digestion is impaired when the gallbladder is diseased. However, the number of people who claim that they find fats indigestible because of their "gallbladder condition" is surely much larger than the number who actually have a diseased gallbladder. Obviously, diagnosis by a physician is indicated.

Irritable colon. One whose colon is irritable and subject to painful spasms is said, quite incorrectly, to suffer from *colitis*. Properly, colitis means inflammation of the colon, and victims of so-called "colitis" do not have any such problem. The colon itself is normal, and it is only the nervous impulses to the colon that are abnormal. (However, this may be no more comforting than a dentist's finding that the teeth are fine, and it is *only* the gums that are diseased.) An irritable colon is sometimes considered a prestigious condition, affecting as it often does those who are sensitive and highly emotional. Unfortunately the symptoms—passage of gas and mucus from the rectum—are hardly compatible with a self-image of delicacy. Avoiding foods that the particular individual finds to be gas-forming can help.

Constipation. Judging from the number of laxatives sold for regulating the colon, many people have peculiar ideas regarding constipation. This is particularly true for older people, perhaps because of the intense preoccupation with this subject a generation or two ago; "irregularity" was believed to be a very serious matter, leading to a toxic state as the result of absorption of "necrones" formed by intestinal bacteria. In fact, these postulated toxic materials do not exist; the uncomfortable feelings caused by constipation are merely the result of distention of the colon by the hard, dry, retained stools. Nevertheless, self-medication with laxatives is very common, apparently based on the belief that a daily "cleaning out" is beneficial or even necessary to health.

If constipation is a problem, it can often be relieved by increasing the cellulose intake by eating more fruits, vegetables, and whole grain breads and cereals. In fact, today's breakfast cereals are an outgrowth of the bran-containing products originally developed to prevent and treat constipation. A few foods, most notably prunes and prune juice, have a marked laxative effect over and above that due to their cellulose content. Contrary to popular opinion, however, drinking copious amounts of water has no effect on the colon contents, because the extra water is absorbed before reaching the large intestine.

It is only fair to those who suffer from *spastic* constipation, as opposed to the *atonic* type which is much more common, to mention that the increased cellulose intake recommended for common constipation would make the other type worse. Again, medical advice is indicated.

ABSORPTION

In absorption, nutrients move from the external environment (the intestinal lumen) to the internal environment (the organism proper). To do this, nutrients must gain entry into one of the cells lining the digestive tract, move across the cell, and finally exit from the cell on the opposite side from which it entered.

The structure of the small intestine is uniquely suited to absorption. Tiny finger-like projections called *villi,* found all along the lining, increase the absorption area of the intestine tremendously (Figure 11–6).

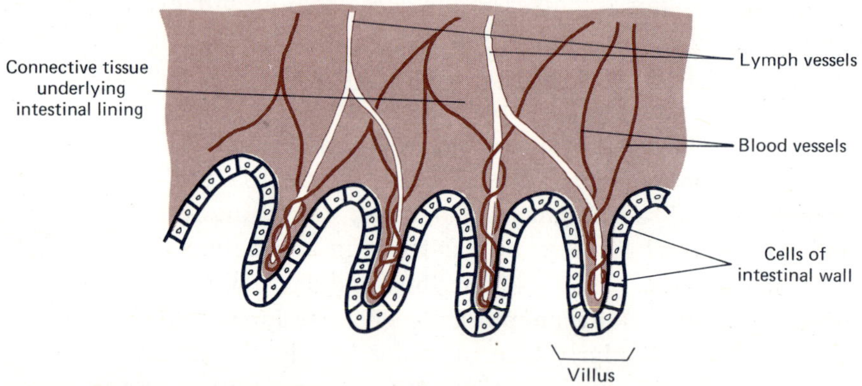

FIGURE 11–6. Villi of the digestive tract.

As a result of this folding and pocketing, as much as 300 square yards of surface area is made available across which absorption may occur. Each villus contains extremely small vessels of the blood and lymph systems, which pick up absorbed nutrients and transport them to the cells of the body. In general, water-soluble substances such as simple sugars, amino acids, and minerals enter the blood vessels, and fat-soluble substances enter the lymph vessels. Exactly how nutrients manage to penetrate the barriers they must cross is not completely understood. However, several general mechanisms are known to operate (Figure 11–7).

For some nutrients, absorption is by *diffusion,* just as sugar molecules added to a cup of coffee eventually mix or diffuse with the liquid, even without stirring. This is because substances naturally tend to travel from an area of high concentration to an area of lower concentration. Relatively small substances—water, certain minerals, and alcohol—appear to be absorbed in this manner. It is postulated that they pass through tiny holes or pores in the cell walls, although no pores have ever actually been seen in cells, even with the most powerful microscopes.

For other nutrients, specific *carriers* transport them across the intestinal wall, linking to the nutrient at one side and releasing them at the other. The use of carriers facilitates absorption of many water-soluble nutrients that could not otherwise readily penetrate the lipid-containing walls of the cells lining the intestine.

A third means of absorption is by *active transport,* in which a nutrient travels to an area of *greater* concentration rather than to an area of lower concentration. Because this is opposite to the way materials flow spontaneously, energy is required, just as it is for pumping water upward against the force of gravity. Glucose is an example of a nutrient that is actively transported across the intestinal wall: even after the concentration in the blood stream exceeds that in the digestive tract, active transport allows still more glucose to be absorbed. As a result, nutrients are absorbed that would otherwise remain in the intestinal lumen and eventually be wasted by excretion.

METABOLISM

Metabolism differs from digestion in a number of important ways, some of which are shown in Table 11–1. Additional points include the following:

Metabolism is a universal characteristic of life, whereas digestion does not occur in all organisms. Green plants (with a few exceptions such as the Venus Fly Trap) and microorganisms that subsist on simple materials from their environments have no need for digestion.

Metabolism includes two types of reactions, *anabolic* and *catabolic,* which occur simultaneously and continuously. Anabolic reactions, which in general require energy, result in products that are larger than the beginning materials, as in the synthesis of a protein molecule from amino acids, or of a glycogen molecule from glucose. Catabolic reactions, in which energy is released, result in a "breaking-down" (Figure 11–8).

Cessation of metabolism would result in almost immediate death,

TABLE 11–1
Digestion and metabolism compared

	Digestion	Metabolism
Classes of nutrients altered	All except water, vitamins, minerals	All
Site	*Outside* the body proper	*Inside* the body proper
End result	To prepare nutrients for absorption	Twofold: (1) to provide energy for energy-requiring processes (2) to transform nutrients into cellular material
Means	Physical (mechanical) and chemical (enzymatic)	Chemical (enzymatic) only
Effect on size of substances	Nutrients converted to smaller substances	Nutrients converted to larger or to smaller substances
Energy changes	No useful energy changes	Energy released when certain organic compounds are split; energy utilized when nutrients are changed to larger substances
End products	Substances small enough to be absorbed	Substances that (1) become part of body structure, or (2) are discharged into the environment

whereas organisms may survive for long periods of time without digestion. In organisms such as humans, who eat at relatively short intervals, digestion normally proceeds continuously, but it need not necessarily do so.

Metabolism consists of a much larger number of chemical reactions than does digestion. A complete discussion of metabolism would require many pages of *metabolic maps*. These maps, which are diagrams depicting the detailed chemical reactions in which nutrients participate,

FIGURE 11–7. Absorption of nutrients: (a) Simple diffusion, (b) Carrier-mediated absorption, and (c) Active transport (an energy-requiring process).

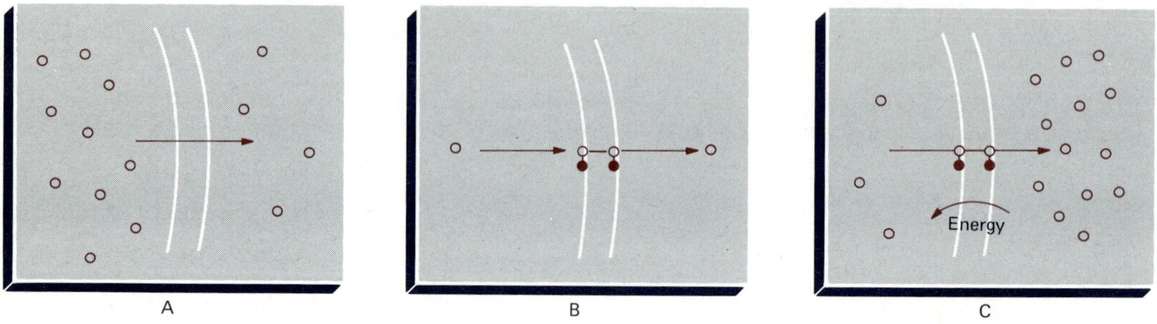

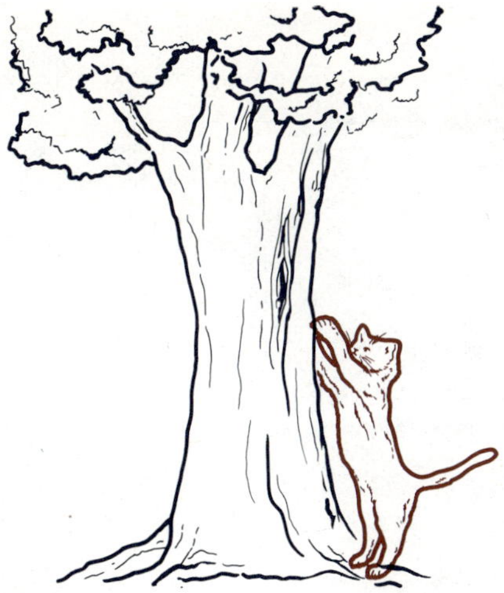

FIGURE 11–8. CATabolism: an energy-releasing process of *breakdown*. This memory device is familiar to any owner of a CAT that works at the breakdown of tree bark, furniture upholstery, and the like.

are commonly large enough to cover a sizable portion of an entire wall. Fitting them into a few book pages, or into the mind of anyone but a biochemist, is nearly impossible.

The reactions that make up metabolism

By convention, reactions are represented by drawing arrows between the substrate and the product. In metabolic reactions, the arrows may be drawn in three different ways:

In a *completely reversible* reaction, the same enzyme which catalyzes the conversion of one substance to another also catalyzes the opposite reaction, as in

$$\text{Substance A} \longleftrightarrow \text{Substance B}$$

The double-pointed arrow indicates that this reaction is completely reversible, and whether A is a starting material or a product depends on the observer's point of view.

In a *completely irreversible* reaction, starting materials can be converted to products, but the products cannot then be reconverted to the original materials. This type of reaction is designated by a single-ended arrow, as:

$$\text{Substance A} \longrightarrow \text{Substance B}$$

Many biochemical reactions are intermediate between the above two extremes. The process is reversible, but catalyzed by different enzymes in the two different directions, as in the following example:

$$\text{Substance A} \underset{\text{enzyme \#1}}{\overset{\text{enzyme \#2}}{\rightleftarrows}} \text{Substance B}$$

FIGURE 11–9

Energy is released when foods are burned, although the forms of energy (heat and light in this case) may not be forms useful in the body.

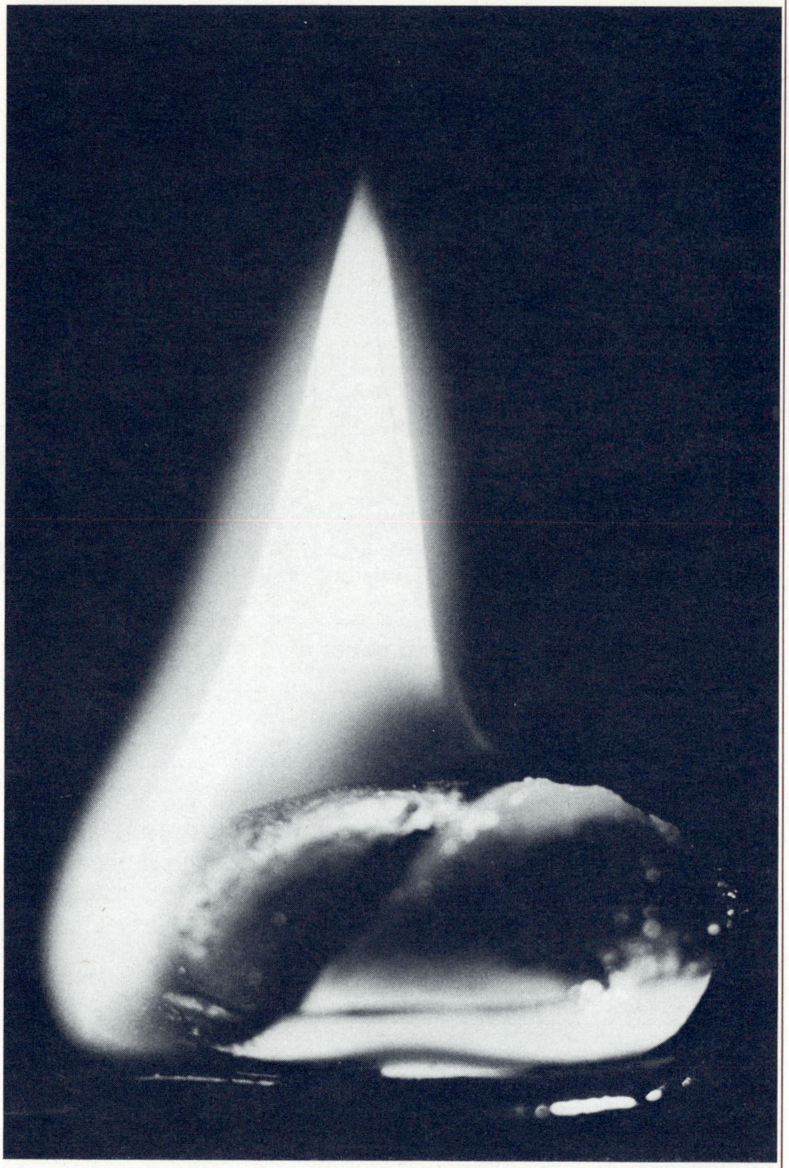

At first glance, this may seem an inefficient system in that the cell must produce two *different* enzymes rather than the single enzyme used in a completely reversible reaction. However, consider the advantage of separate exits and entrances in a building. Although they are "inefficient" in that they require the installation of more doors, they allow for rapid regulation of the population inside the building. The population can be increased rapidly because entrances are not blocked by those who are trying to leave, or it can be decreased rapidly because those who are leaving are not impeded by incoming people. Also, if the entrance doors are locked while the exits are left open, the building will gradually empty.

In a similar manner, a cell can control the "population" of a given type of molecule in the cell. By stimulating the enzyme which catalyzes the conversion of Substance A to Substance B, the amount of Substance B can be increased; by stimulating the enzyme which catalyzes the opposite reaction, the amount of Substance A can be increased. This type of control could never be achieved if a single enzyme catalyzed the reaction in both directions, because stimulation of the enzyme would increase the rate of the reaction in both directions, and the net result would be nil.

Biological oxidation and oxidative phosphorylation

These processes are not nearly as formidable as their names might suggest. In fact, the main features are relatively simple.

Materials, including food, can be burned in the presence of oxygen, and the uncontrolled release of energy in the form of heat and light is readily observed (Figure 11–9). However, this type of oxidation would be not only useless, but very detrimental to cells. *Oxidation*, in biology, does not involve direct combination of a substance with oxygen, as burning does. Rather it consists of the *removal of electrons from a compound*. Hydrogen atoms, each with an extra electron attached, are passed along a line of carriers. Ultimately the hydrogen combines with oxygen, forming water. Biological oxidation therefore refers to the *transport of electrons from organic substances to oxygen* with the electrons attached to hydrogen atoms rather than floating around free. By this means, about half of the energy from nutrients is trapped or harnessed in the form of the special chemical adenosine triphosphate (ATP). The energy of ATP can then be used to power the *endergonic*, or energy-requiring, processes of the cell. That portion of energy *not* harnessed in ATP is released as heat, which is lost continuously from the body.

Oxidative phosphorylation means that phosphate is added to *adenosine diphosphate*, or ADP; as electrons flow toward oxygen, energy is released and used for the phosphorylation of ADP to form ATP (Figure 11–10).

The principal features of nutrient metabolism can now be examined. Although each nutrient class will be discussed separately, it is important to keep in mind that the metabolism of each nutrient is intimately linked to that of others. Many of these interrelationships will emerge as the discussion progresses.

The metabolism of carbohydrates

To a very large degree, the metabolism of carbohydrates is the metabolism of glucose, either "free" or present as parts of large carbohydrate molecules. Some of the glucose available to cells is not immedi-

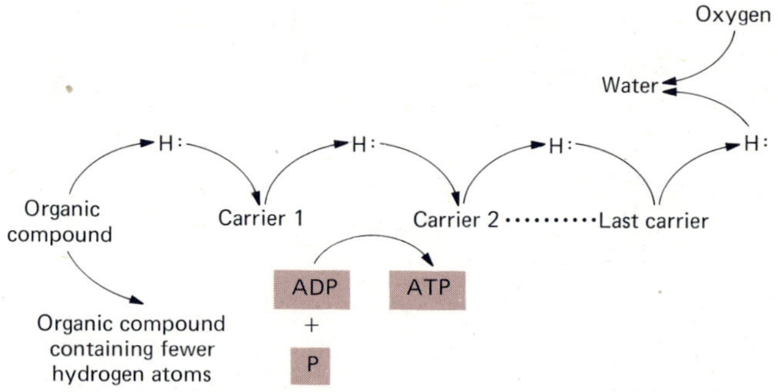

FIGURE 11–10. Biological oxidation (transfer of electrons from organic compounds to oxygen) and oxidative phosphorylation (ATP formation using energy released when electrons move toward oxygen). The electrons are attached to hydrogen atoms, which eventually combine with oxygen to form water molecules.

ately oxidized. It may be converted to other monosaccharides, such as the 5-carbon sugars found as parts of DNA and RNA molecules. Similarly, lactose, secreted in milk, need not be present in the diet of a lactating woman because cells are able to convert glucose to galactose; the galactose can then be linked to glucose molecules to yield lactose as needed. Glucose is also a starting material from which cells produce the nonnitrogen part of nonessential amino acids. Finally, glucose in excess of immediate needs is converted to the storage form of carbohydrate, glycogen, until the capacity of the body to store glycogen is reached. Any further excess is converted to fat and stored in that form. These various fates are summarized in Figure 11–11.

Most glucose, however, is oxidized to yield energy. As a matter of fact, 38 molecules of ATP (as well as a considerable amount of heat) are produced as the result of oxidizing a single glucose molecule. The over-all reaction can therefore be represented as shown in Figure 11–12. Now it is fairly obvious that the over-all process of glucose oxidation cannot be accomplished in a single chemical reaction, for fully *83 particles of matter* participate as substrates. Imagine trying to crowd all of those substances on a single enzyme molecule at the same time. Thus glucose must be oxidized in a stepwise fashion, and the individual steps make up two of the most famous of all known metabolic pathways: *glycolysis and the citric acid cycle.*

Glycolysis

Glycolysis—the word literally means *sugar breaking*—is a process in which each molecule of glucose is eventually split into *two* molecules of the 3-carbon compound, *pyruvic acid* (Figure 11–11).

Actually, glycolysis consists of 10 distinct chemical reactions, each catalyzed by a different enzyme. The resulting 2 molecules of pyruvic acid contain altogether only 8 of the 12 hydrogen atoms originally present in the glucose molecule; the 4 "missing" hydrogen atoms have been

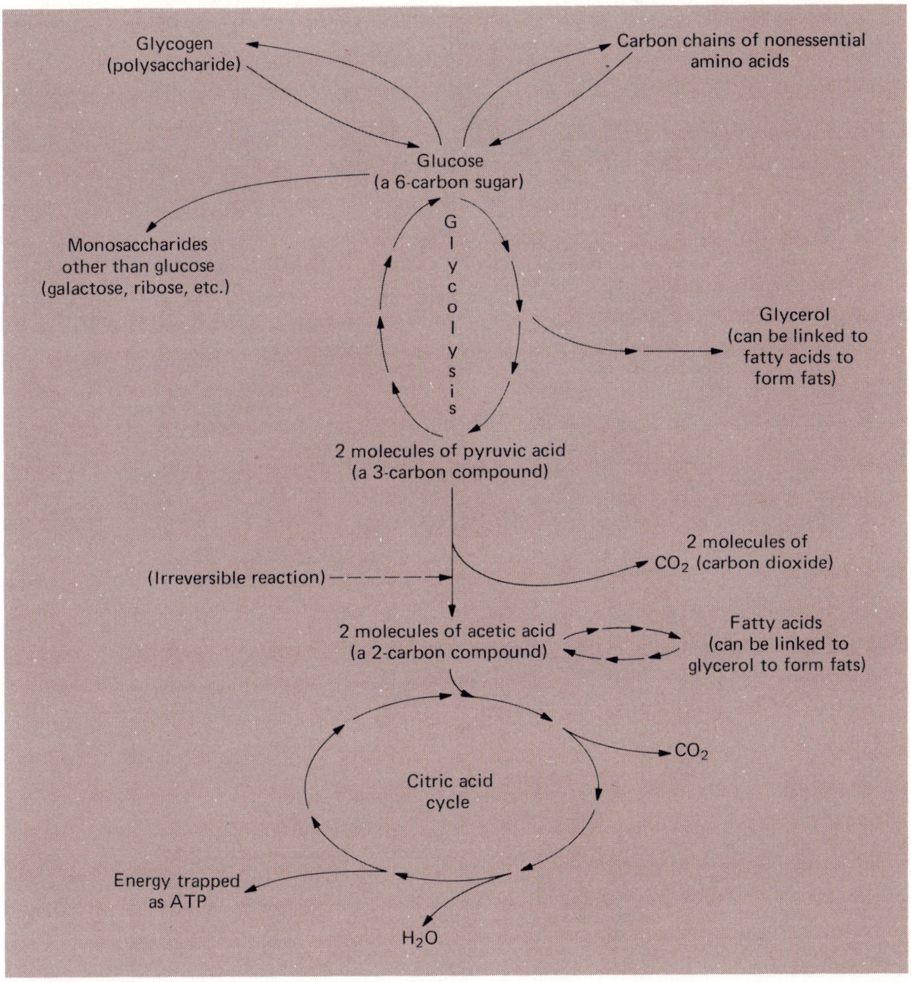

FIGURE 11–11. Various fates of glucose. Note that the conversion of pyruvic acid to acetic acid is an irreversible step. Acetic acid therefore cannot be used to produce glucose in the body.

transferred along a chain of carriers and eventually accepted by oxygen. In this manner, some of the energy available from glucose has been released.

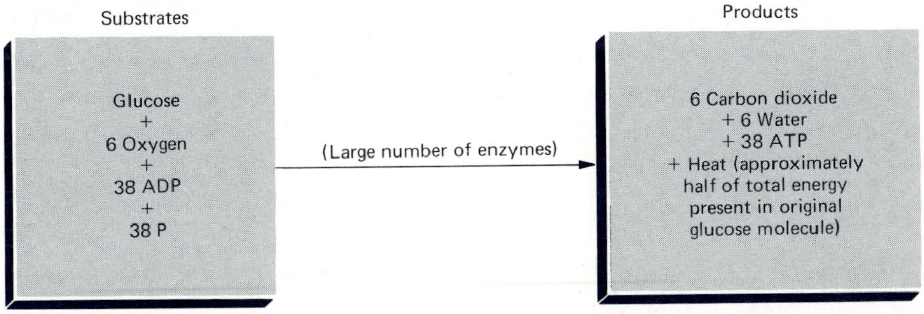

FIGURE 11–12. The overall result of the complete breakdown of glucose.

There is, however, still a great deal of hydrogen remaining in the pyruvic acid molecules. In order to release more energy, therefore, pyruvic acid is converted to *acetic acid*, the familiar acid found in vinegar. In the process, carbon dioxide is liberated (Figure 11–11). This carbon dioxide is then excreted by the lungs.

The citric acid cycle

Acetic acid enters a remarkable reaction sequence which ultimately accounts for the catabolism of all classes of energy nutrients. These reactions are collectively known as the *citric acid cycle*, or *Krebs cycle*. Although the cycle actually consists of ten separate reactions, it may be represented as:

$$\underset{\text{acetic acid}}{CH_3\text{—}COOH} + \underset{\text{oxygen}}{2O_2} \longrightarrow \underset{\text{carbon dioxide}}{2CO_2} + \underset{\text{water}}{2H_2O}$$

Figure 11–13 shows the main features of the citric acid cycle as well as its relationship to glycolysis. In the first step, acetic acid com-

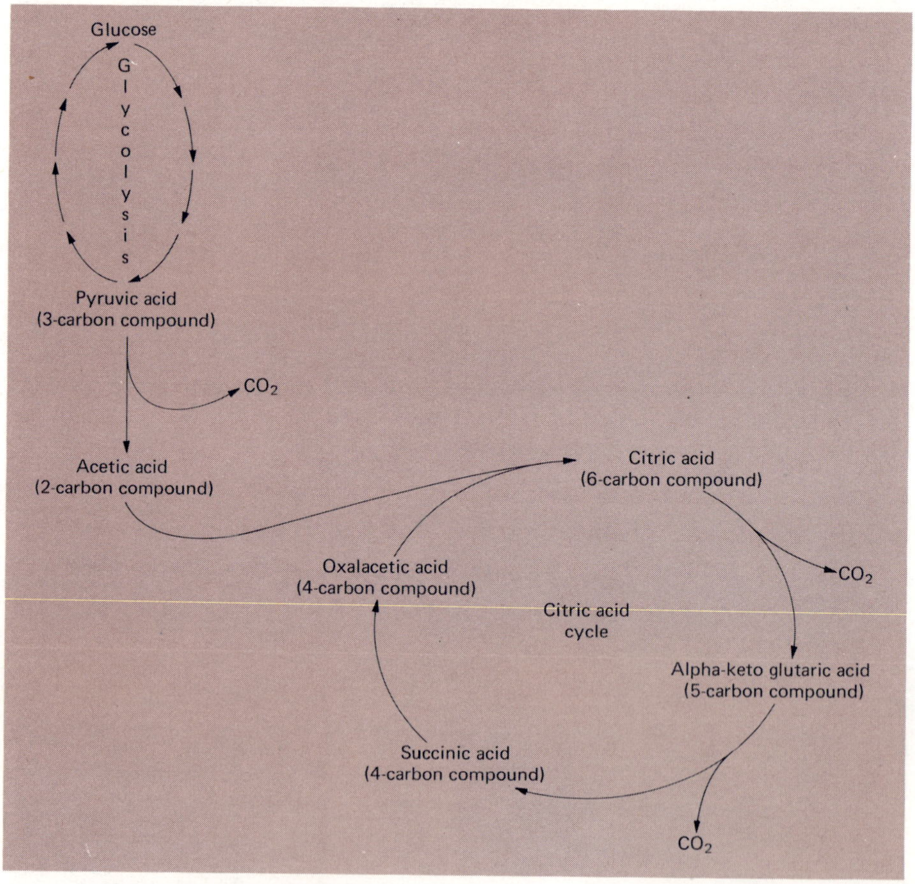

FIGURE 11–13. The main features of the citric acid cycle, and the relationship of this cycle to glycolysis.

bines with a 4-carbon compound to yield citric acid (hence the name of the cycle). Citric acid is then converted to the next compound of the cycle, and so on, until the original 4-carbon compound is regenerated, ready to accept another acetic acid molecule.

A nose count of atoms shows that, as the result of each turn of the cycle, four hydrogen atoms are transferred from acetic acid to oxygen. Because this is the principal means whereby useful energy becomes available to the cell, and because 2 acetic acid molecules are derived from each glucose molecule, it is obvious that much more energy is obtained from the final breakdown of glucose in the citric acid cycle than from glycolysis alone.

The metabolism of fats

Because fats consist of two different types of subunit, each of these must be considered separately. However, of the 50 or so carbon atoms present in a typical fat, only 3 are in the glycerol subunit, with all the rest in the 3 fatty acid subunits.

Each of the fatty acids is broken down in a stepwise manner to form the 2-carbon compound, acetic acid (Figure 11–14). Thus a fatty

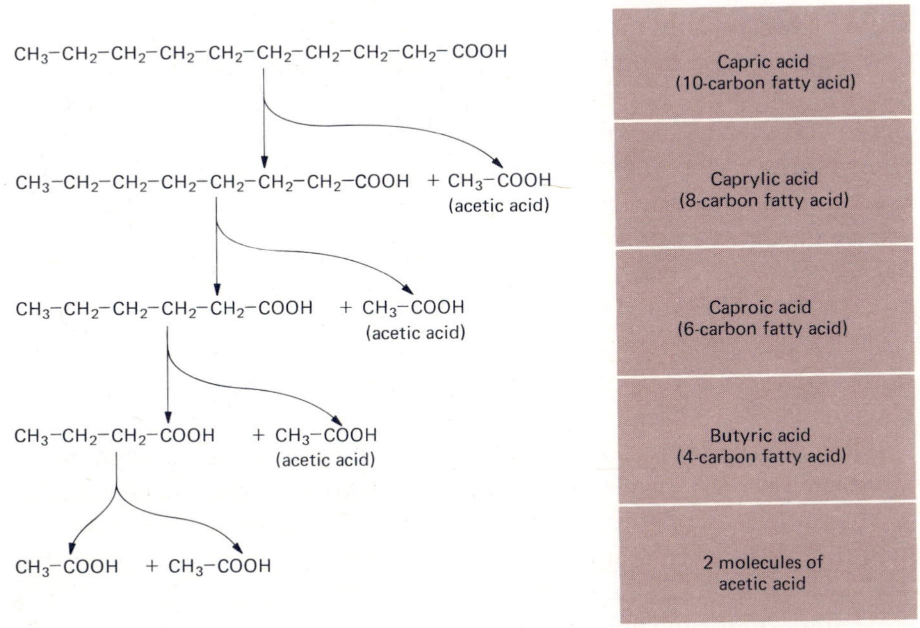

FIGURE 11–14. The breakdown of a fatty acid to acetic acid molecules.

acid containing 18 carbons would yield 9 molecules of acetic acid, one containing 14 carbon atoms would yield 7 acetic acid molecules, and so on. The acetic acid can then be completely oxidized via the citric acid cycle, just as the acetic acid derived from glucose can be. Alternatively, acetic acid can be used to resynthesize fatty acids, essentially by reversing the pathway whereby fatty acids were broken down to acetic acid.

Acetic acid is also important in the synthesis of the group of lipids known as *steroids*. Among the steroids important in nutrition are cholesterol, bile salts, vitamin D, and steroid hormones. Because they can be produced in the body, none of these is essential in the diet. The exception is vitamin D, and even this can be synthesized in sufficient amounts upon adequate exposure of the skin to the radiation of the sun.

If the supply of acetic acid is unusually great, it may be converted to compounds known as *ketone bodies*. These should not be confused with the *phenylketones* formed in the genetic disease phenylketonuria (PKU). Ketone bodies are 3-carbon or 4-carbon compounds that accumulate when fatty acid breakdown is unusually rapid; *acetone*, which is a ketone body, can easily be detected on the breath of a person whose ketone body production is abnormally high.

One option which is *not* open to acetic acid is its conversion to pyruvic acid and hence to glucose. The reason this is impossible is because the conversion of pyruvic acid to acetic acid is irreversible. Hence, although glucose is freely converted to fatty acids, fatty acids cannot in turn be converted to glucose.

The second subunit of fats, the glycerol molecule, can be converted to a 3-carbon compound, which is an intermediate in glycolysis. From there, it can by a reversal of *glycolysis* be used to produce glucose. However, the amount of glucose synthesized in this manner is trivial compared to the total amount of glucose needed by the cells for normal functioning. For all practical purposes, therefore, fat is not a significant source of glucose in the body.

The metabolism of amino acids and proteins

Amino acids are the protein subunits that are delivered to the cells by the blood, and it is therefore the metabolism of these which will be considered. Each different amino acid is metabolized somewhat differently than other amino acids are, but the general features common to all are shown in Figure 11–15. Amino acids are of course necessary for production of cell proteins. In addition, amino acids are converted to nonprotein nitrogen-containing compounds: nucleic acids (DNA and RNA), the hormones adrenaline and thyroxine, and a large number of other important biochemicals. The amino acids not used for synthesis of nitrogen-containing compounds are *deaminated* and subsequently oxidized as energy sources. Deamination is the stripping off of the amino group (the nitrogen-containing part) from the rest of the molecule (the carbon-hydrogen-oxygen part, or *carbon chain* of the amino acid).

The nitrogen-containing part removed is, for a brief instant, in the form of ammonia. Because ammonia is highly toxic to cells, it must be

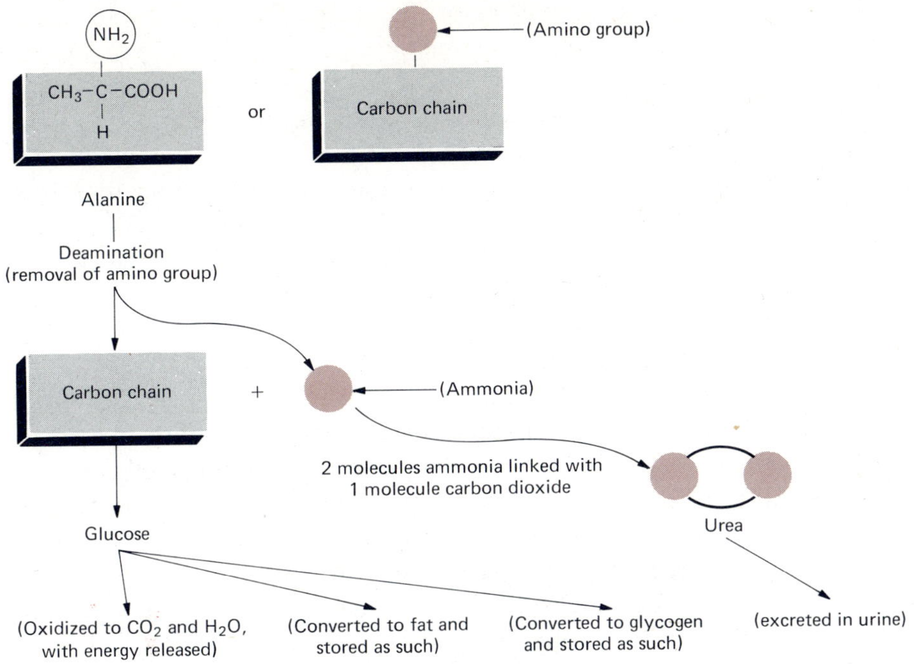

FIGURE 11–15. The breakdown of an amino acid.

converted immediately to a less toxic form. In human cells, this is accomplished by changing ammonia into *urea,* a relatively innocuous substance.

The remaining portion of the amino acid, the carbon-hydrogen-oxygen part, can enter a variety of pathways, depending upon which amino acid is being discussed. Some molecules can be converted to intermediates of glycolysis, and hence to glucose. This process is known as *gluconeogenesis* (neo = new; genesis = formation), the formation of glucose from noncarbohydrates. This is an important role of amino acids, because glucose cannot, as has been seen, be formed to any significant degree from fats. A few amino acids, however, are converted more or less directly to acetic acid, and therefore cannot be used for production of glucose.

The principal features of energy-nutrient metabolism are summarized in Figure 11–16, which shows some of the interrelationships of various nutrient classes.

The metabolism of vitamins

As a general rule, a vitamin in itself is useless to the cell. It is active only after it has been incorporated into the structure of a coenzyme, which is then used to complete the structure of one or more enzymes. Thus, although vitamins are not broken down to provide energy, they are necessary for the activity of many enzymes that oxidize the fats, carbohydrates, and amino acids which yield energy. None of the metabolic pathways, such as glycolysis or the citric acid cycle, can proceed normally without coenzymes, of which various vitamins form important parts.

Each specific vitamin is used for producing one or more specific coenzymes, and one vitamin cannot substitute for another in this regard. Discussion of the metabolism of individual vitamins therefore involves more detail than does a general outline of energy-nutrient metabolism. However, the details are fortunately not necessary to a basic understanding of metabolism.

The metabolism of minerals

Minerals perform two important general roles in the body; as structural components and as necessary parts of biological regulators such as enzyme systems. The metabolism of a mineral includes all changes which result in the use of a mineral for either of these two general functions. A calcium ion, for example, can become part of the structure of a bone or tooth, or may be used to activate an enzyme involved in blood clotting or muscle contraction. Because the unique roles of individual minerals vary so much, generalizations are difficult. Their specific aspects will be discussed as individual minerals are considered in Chapter 16.

FIGURE 11–16. The overall picture of energy nutrient metabolism.

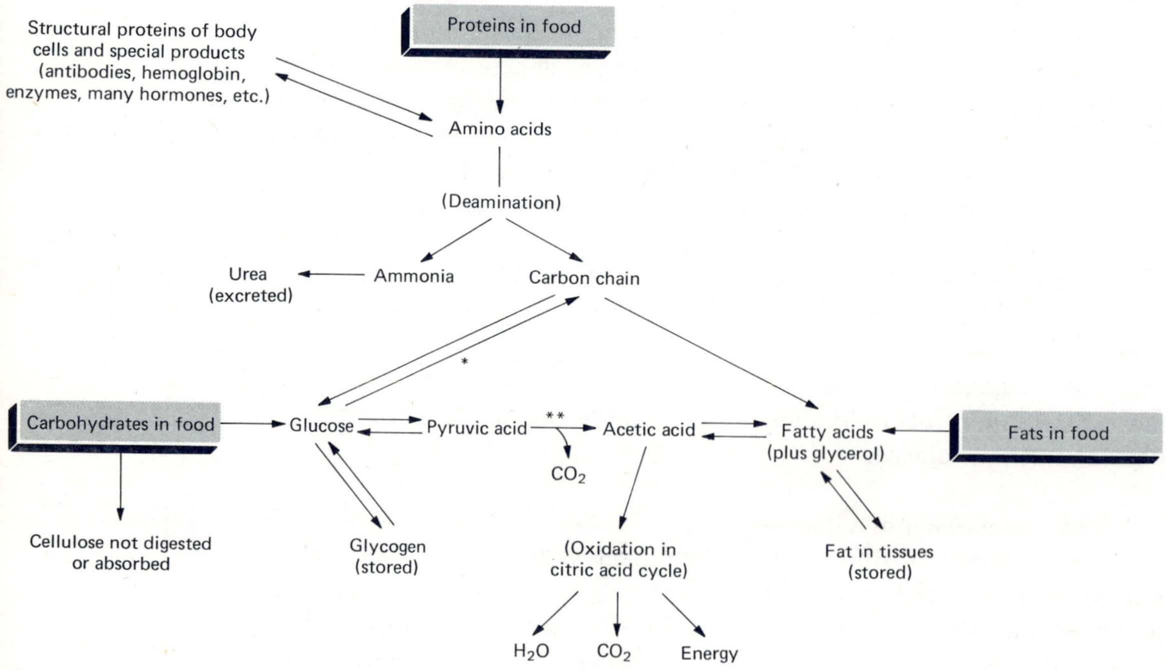

*Glucose can be used for sythesis of *nonessential* amino acids.
**Irreversible reaction.

The metabolism of water

Of the huge number of water molecules which enter and leave the body each day, the vast majority undergo no chemical changes during their journey through the system. However, some water molecules enter into important chemical changes, known as *hydrolysis* reactions. When a molecule such as a fat, a protein, or a polysaccharide is split into smaller units, water molecules enter into the reactions by splitting and becoming parts of each of the resulting products. Thus water is to some extent consumed in biochemical reactions, as it is formed when hydrogen removed from energy nutrients is donated to oxygen from the air.

Regulation of metabolism by nutrients

The ultimate control of enzymes, and hence of the basic pattern of metabolism, resides in the genes. However, metabolism can be modified by a variety of factors such as hormones, nerve activity, drugs, and nutrients. The following discussion covers some of the ways in which diet exerts effects upon metabolism.

A relatively recent area of study is that of the effects of diet on adaptive enzymes—those which change in activity in response to altered conditions in the body. Enzyme activity can be changed by increasing or decreasing the number of enzyme molecules produced in the cells; this alters the *degree* to which the enzyme operates, although the *kind* of reaction catalyzed is unaffected. The ability of enzymes to change in response to dietary changes appears to be important to survival in that it allows the organism to adapt to nutrient intakes much lower or much higher than that available under ideal conditions.

Variations in protein intake, for example, have pronounced effects upon the levels of certain enzymes involved in protein metabolism. When protein intake is very low, the activities of enzymes involved in amino acid breakdown are decreased, helping to insure that cells use the limited supply of amino acids for protein synthesis rather than for fuel. When protein intake is high, such extreme frugality is of course unnecessary.

An entirely different situation is seen in starvation, when *all* energy nutrients, not just proteins specifically, are lacking. Glucose, which is specifically needed as an energy source by the brain and nerves, cannot be produced in significant amounts from fats stored in the body. Amino acids must therefore be deaminated so that the nonnitrogen-containing part can be converted to glucose. Here is seen a definite hierarchy of priorities: providing glucose to the brain takes precedence over protein synthesis to maintain the body as a whole, for if the brain is starved the whole organism will die. Proteins of the heart, kidneys, liver—all organs, in fact—are sacrificed in the service of the brain.

Fat metabolism responds dramatically to a number of dietary changes, including the frequency of eating. Animal experiments have studied the effects of meal-feeding versus the rat's normal pattern of nibbling frequently throughout the day and night. In rats given access to food only at specified times, there is an increase in enzymes involved in fat synthesis, apparently caused by the sudden increase of large amounts of substrates available in infrequent bursts.

Fat metabolism also responds to the ratio of fat and carbohydrate in the diet. On diets high in carbohydrate, there is an increase in the activity of enzymes involved in fat synthesis; this enhances the conversion of excess carbohydrate to fat. Conversely, as the fat content of diets increases, the fat-synthesizing capacity of the cells decreases via decreased activity of enzymes which catalyze fat synthesis. In this way cells avoid the wasteful activity of producing large amounts of enzymes that, for the time being, are not needed. It should be recognized, however, that these changes in enzyme activity cannot in themselves bring about a gain or loss of body fat. A supply of energy nutrients in excess of the body's needs is always necessary in order to gain body fat, because the enzymes can of course act only in the presence of substrates to act upon.

EXCRETION OF THE END PRODUCTS OF METABOLISM

So far, so good. Nutrients have been ingested, digested, absorbed, carried via the blood and lymph to the cells, and finally altered in a variety of ways by means of the various metabolic pathways. As the end result of all of these processes, some nutrients have been utilized as building materials, becoming a more or less permanent part of the physical structure of the body. Other nutrients have been oxidized, thereby releasing energy, either to support the cells' activities or uselessly as heat. Still others have participated in regulatory roles in various types of reactions.

Because the kinds and amounts of nutrients entering the organism can never be exactly what the body needs, some unusable materials are inevitably left over. Also, as a glance back at the figures representing metabolism will show, the cells themselves have produced substances that must now be eliminated. These include carbon dioxide, urea, and water formed from the oxidation of energy nutrients. Heat energy, although not a substance, cannot be used to perform work by cells and is therefore also considered an end product of metabolism. In order to keep all body components at tolerable levels, the body has developed specialized organs for excretion. These organs maintain homeostasis by discharging useless materials and energy in the form of heat from the body back into the external environment from which, in different forms, they originally came, The lungs, kidneys, and skin are the organs responsible for excreting metabolic end products.

The lungs. Carbon dioxide is excreted almost exclusively via the lungs; water vapor and heat energy are also excreted to some extent via these organs, as can be seen by exhaling into surrounding cold air. All of these end products flow from the bloodstream into the lung spaces as a result of concentration differences; because their concentration is greater inside the body than in the air inside the lungs, they move spontaneously out of the body.

The kidneys. Although the excretion of various substances by the kidneys is very complex, the main points are rather easily grasped. Essentially, the kidneys act as filters to clear the blood of unwanted materials. This process can be compared to the familiar process of cleaning out a cluttered closet (Figure 11–17).

In the first step, everything is removed except for those items that cannot be removed. Blood cells and protein molecules, for example, are too large to pass the barrier between the blood and the inside of the *nephron* or basic kidney unit, just as items such as built-in shelves and clothes rods are not easily removed from a closet. No further selection occurs at this point, everything being moved out of the blood (or the closet) except for things which cannot be removed.

In the second step, definite decisions and selections are made. The kidney retains those materials which are useless or perhaps even harmful and which the body must therefore eliminate: urea, excess minerals and vitamins, and similar substances. Other materials, however—glucose, large amounts of water, amino acids, and similar materials which can be of use to the body—are put back into the blood, to be recirculated to the body cells. This is similar to deciding which items are worth putting back into the closet and saving.

The final part of the process is the elimination of those things that have *not* been chosen to be retained. These flow down a series of ever enlarging and merging channels in the kidneys until they reach the ureters. Along these tubes the liquid, now known as urine, flows to the bladder, where it is stored until urination occurs. This can be compared to the final disposition of items originally taken from the closet; what is no longer necessary or useful is eliminated (given away, sold at a rummage sale, or otherwise disposed of).

The complexity of kidney function is therefore actually very efficient. Substances that are unnecessary or detrimental are discharged from the body; substances that the body can use are conserved in order to avoid wasteful losses. Consider the example of water conservation. In an adult, up to 200 quarts of water may be removed from the blood by the kidneys each day. Of this, some 99 percent is reabsorbed into the blood because of the action of antidiuretic hormone, and only about 1 to 2 quarts eventually leave the body in the urine. Imagine the problems that would result if the kidneys were incapable of reabsorbing water. One's life would literally center on two major activities: urinating and drinking copious amounts of water to replace that lost in the urine.

There is, however, a minimum amount of water which must be lost daily in the urine in order to eliminate waste products. This minimum, known as the *obligatory loss,* is estimated at somewhere between 1½ and 2 cups. If fluid intake is so low that this amount is not available for urine formation, metabolic waste products can accumulate in the body until they reach toxic concentrations. This forces the kidneys to obtain water necessary for urine formation by excreting water that would otherwise be reabsorbed into the blood. If this continues long enough, the body content of water is decreased until the individual becomes dehydrated.

The maximum amount of water that can be excreted daily in urine is extremely great in most healthy individuals, although intakes far above needs can rarely result in a dilution of body fluids, a very serious condition known as *water intoxication.* Although the sense of thirst generally insures that water intake matches the needs of the body, numerous mental and physical disorders can interfere with this normal control.

The skin. The advantage of water loss via the skin is not primarily to eliminate excess water, for the kidneys could do this without assistance from other organs. Rather, sweating is the principal means whereby the body excretes heat energy in order to keep its internal temperature under control. Some 1½ to 3 cups of water are evaporated from the surface of the skin daily, exerting a considerable cooling effect. The importance of this can be shown by a very rough calculation of the

FIGURE 11–17. A simplified version of kidney function.

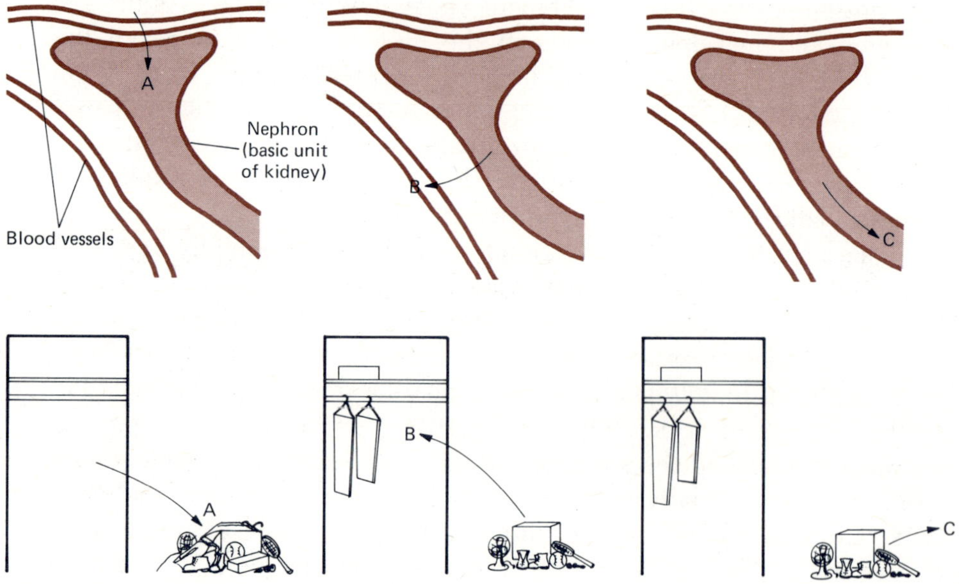

Step A—Everything removable is removed (from the blood or from the closet).

Step B—Useful materials are retained by putting them back (into the blood or into the closet).

Step C—Useless materials are discarded.

effects of daily heat production on body temperature if heat were not continuously eliminated. As an example, consider an average adult male weighing 70 kilograms (approximately 154 pounds) and utilizing the number of calories recommended by the RDA. Each day, this individual produces an amount of heat that would increase his body temperature by about 40° Centigrade (some 70° Fahrenheit) if all of this heat remained in the body.

During exercise, when energy nutrients are oxidized at a very rapid rate to support muscular activity, the amount of heat produced is correspondingly increased. In response to the greater need to eliminate heat, as much as six quarts of sweat may be lost per hour. Under ordinary conditions, however, exercise this intense cannot continue for long.

In addition to water, various minerals as well as small amounts of urea are lost coincidentally in the sweat; in fact, sodium and chloride are lost to such an extent that sweat has a noticeably salty taste. The amounts of other minerals in sweat are generally quite small, however, so that very sensitive analytical methods may be required to detect some of them. Increased sweating does not occur in order to compensate for excess intakes of water or minerals. Rather, excess intakes of these result in greater volumes of urine. Any physiologist can verify this. So, for that matter, can any beer drinker.

SUGGESTED READINGS

Donaldson, R. M. "The Muddle of Diets for Gastrointestinal Disorders." *Journal of the American Medical Association* 225 (1973):1243.

Guyton, A. C. *Function of the Human Body,* fourth edition. Philadelphia: Saunders, 1974.

Haenal, H. "Human Normal and Abnormal Gastrointestinal Flora." *American Journal of Clinical Nutrition* 23 (1970):1433.

McGilvery, R. W. Biochemical Concepts. Philadelphia: Saunders, 1975.

12

energy and weight control

Among the majority of the people of the world, the most serious nutritional problem is not a deficiency of any specific nutrient, but sheer lack of an adequate energy supply. When diets fail to provide enough energy to meet needs, people are forced to consume the materials of their own bodies for fuel. During prolonged undernutrition, not only are the stores of carbohydrate and fat exhausted, but cells of various organs are sacrificed in order to use their proteins as fuel. Finally, when no more energy can be obtained from these sources, life flickers and dies, as does the light of a candle when the wax has been consumed.

By contrast, people in the developed countries are more concerned with excess energy than with any other aspect of nutrition; obesity, the result of calorie excess, is the most common form of malnutrition seen in countries such as the United States.

ENERGY: WHAT IT IS AND IS NOT

Energy is the capacity to do work. It is *not* a feeling of vigor, enthusiasm, or "pep" as the term is popularly used. Overweight people may feel, or say, that they "lack energy," meaning that they have no particular desire for activity or accomplishment; but in the physical sense of the word they are actually overloaded with stored energy in the form of fat. Undernourished people can also feel fatigued, but having no energy is literally impossible, because an organism that has no energy ceases to be a living system.

The term *work* includes all changes that the body accomplishes. Some forms of work are obvious: moving furniture, walking, climbing stairs, cleaning windows. However, activities such as dancing, playing tennis, and swimming are also considered forms of work, because the physiologist's definition of work does not depend in any way upon whether the activity is pleasurable or odious.

Work that is not outwardly obvious is also continuously being performed by the body. Just lying quietly and continuing to live requires that the internal organs expend energy in performing their various functions. Thus, although we are seldom aware of these continuous internal activities, they all constitute work which is vital to our continued existence.

Measuring energy: calories and kilojoules

The basic unit of energy used in the science of nutrition is the *Calorie*. Whenever the energy value of a food is specified, it should be given either as *kilocalories* or *Calories* (with a capital C), because the nutritionist's unit of energy is one thousand times as large as the calorie (with a small c) used in chemistry and physics. One Calorie is the amount of energy equivalent to the heat needed to cause a specific temperature increase in a given amount of water. Specifically, one Calorie will cause one kilogram (somewhat over a quart) of water to increase in temperature one degree Centigrade.

However, the distinction between the Calorie and the calorie is so commonly overlooked that there is hardly a popularized article on the subject that uses the term correctly. Thus you may read of a "1000 calorie" diet when what is obviously meant is a *one million calorie,* a *1000 kilocalorie,* or a 1000 Calorie diet. A diet that actually furnishes only 1000 calories (small c) would consist of something like $\frac{1}{60}$ of a slice of bread, $\frac{1}{10}$ of an ounce of skim milk, or $\frac{1}{100}$ of a good-sized apple!

Another frequently made error is to refer to "calories and other nutrients." A calorie is *not* a nutrient, but an amount of energy obtained from the breakdown of a given quantity of certain nutrients. The term *energy nutrient* is perfectly acceptable, but to refer to "calories and other nutrients" makes no more sense than to speak of "heat and other sources of fuel."

One disadvantage of using the calorie as the basic unit of energy in nutrition is that it is defined in terms of heat. This may give the erroneous impression that heat is the form of energy useful for the performance of work in cells. Actually, the energy that cells can use to perform work is the chemical energy that is trapped in certain molecules such as ATP. When a cell oxidizes energy nutrients and simultaneously synthesizes ATP, or breaks down ATP to perform work, only part of the energy released is actually harnessed in ATP or used to do work; the rest is released as heat. Because energy in the form of heat is useless to the body except for maintaining the temperature of the body, it must continuously be excreted into the surrounding environment.

Because of this, as well as other objections that have been made, nutrition is at present abandoning the Calorie as a unit of measurement. In its place the *kilojoule* will be used. The kilojoule (or Joule with a capital J) is defined in terms of the amount of *work* that can be accomplished by a given amount of energy. Hence it is more accurate than is the Calorie with respect to the body's use of food energy. In addition, the kilojoule, unlike the kilocalorie, is defined in terms of the metric system, which is the system already used in most of the world today.

To convert from one system to another, numbers of kilocalories merely need to be multiplied by the factor 4.184, because one kilocalorie (one Calorie) is equal to 4.184 kilojoules. Thus a diet furnishing approximately 1800 Calories will instead be said to furnish some 7500 kilojoules. The numbers are rounded off in order to emphasize that measurements in nutrition are generally not accurate enough to justify the use of more exact values.

The flow of energy: a one-way street

Both materials and energy must continuously flow through living systems. However, there is one extremely important difference between the utilization of materials and the utilization of energy by organisms. Materials can be recycled indefinitely; an atom of some element in the soil today may be part of a complex molecule in a living cell tomorrow, appear in a still different form in some other place at a later time, and eventually return to the soil. The flow of any form of matter, in other words, is a cycle.

Energy, on the other hand, flows in one direction only. Once used to perform work in a cell, it becomes useless for any further purpose. The *first* law of thermodynamics states that energy is neither created nor destroyed, but merely changed from one form to another. When fuel such as coal is burned, for example, the chemical energy in the fuel molecules is released, largely as heat. The total amount of energy released is exactly equal to the total amount of potential energy present in the fuel before it was burned. Some of the heat released may be harnessed, as in a steam engine, and used to perform useful work. However, heat energy which is *not* trapped in such a manner escapes, and becomes useless for performing work. To put it another way, heat that is not trapped and put to work cannot be transformed to any other form of energy. This phenomenon is stated in the *second* law of thermodynamics: any time energy is changed from one form to another, at least part of the energy is changed to a form which cannot be further converted to other forms. Energy from food, just like energy from other types of fuel, obeys this law. As energy flows through a living system, a considerable portion of it is degraded to heat, which is of no further use to the organism.

Because energy is continuously being converted to a form that cannot be used for work by cells, it follows that there must be some energy source which continuously provides the earth with energy in a useful form. This ultimate source of useful energy is the sun. Of the enormous amounts of radiant energy released by the sun, a minute proportion reaches the earth, strikes the leaves of green plants, and is converted to the chemical energy of the bonds which hold atoms together in the molecules of energy nutrients. This process, whereby green plants harness solar energy, is known as *photosynthesis.*

Of all of the living things on earth, only green plants have the ability to use the energy of the sun to produce energy nutrients from simple materials such as water and carbon dioxide. Because of this ability, green plants are called *autotrophic* organisms; autotrophic means *self-nourishing,* and refers to the fact that the cells of green plants produce their own energy nutrients rather than requiring a supply from the environment.

Virtually all organisms other than green plants are *heterotrophic,* which means *nourished by others.* Directly or indirectly, heterotrophs must depend upon green plants for their energy, because they themselves are incapable of capturing the energy of the sun.

Food chains—or are they food pyramids?

The passage of energy through a series of living things occurs in a series of steps commonly known as a *food chain.* For example, plants may be eaten by insects, which in turn are eaten by birds, which in turn may be eaten by larger birds, or by humans. At each step of the food chain, only part of the energy obtained by the eater is retained in the form of energy nutrients which will be available to the next member of the chain. The rest is used to perform work by the cells of the eater, and is finally returned to the environment as heat. For this reason, the final members of a food chain obtain only a very small proportion of the useful energy originally trapped by the green plants at the beginning of the chain (Figure 12–1).

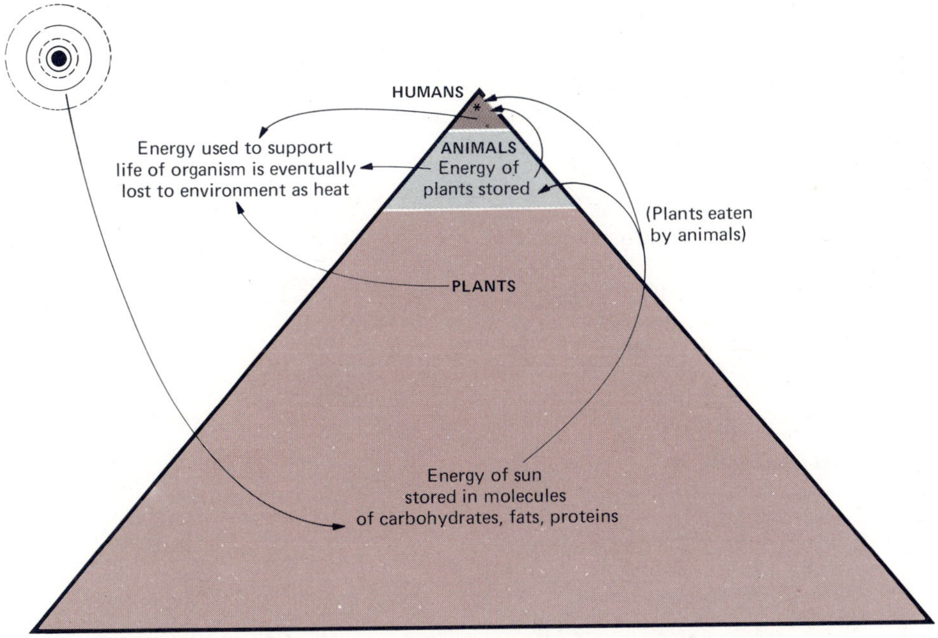

*Like other organisms, people use most of their energy intake to support their own lives.

FIGURE 12–1. The food pyramid. Organisms low in the pyramid use most of their available energy to keep themselves alive. Those higher up therefore obtain only the relatively small amount of energy stored in the bodies of their prey.

The energy values of foods

People can estimate the energy values of foods by consulting a handbook or a calorie chart, such as Table 12–1. How were these figures first obtained? The original measurement of the amount of energy furnished by a food is based upon the fact that when given amounts of

TABLE 12–1

Energy values of some common foods

Food and approximate amount*	Energy value (kilocalories)
Bread and cereal group	
1 slice enriched white bread	70
1 slice whole wheat bread	65
1 average corn muffin (1½ ounces)	125
½ cup cooked enriched white rice	110
½ cup cooked enriched macaroni, noodles, spaghetti	80–100
Meat group	
2 ounces cooked lean ground beef	120
2 ounces cooked regular ground beef	160
2 ounces broiled sirloin steak (lean only)	115
2 ounces broiled chicken (meat only)	80
2 ounces fried chicken (meat only)	120
2 eggs (raw or cooked without fat)	160
1 cup cooked navy beans	225
4 tablespoons peanut butter	380
Milk group	
1 cup whole milk (3.5% fat)	160
1½ ounces hard cheese (American, Swiss, cheddar, etc.)	160–175
1⅓ cup cottage cheese, creamed	380
1⅓ cup cottage cheese, low-fat	225
2 cups regular ice cream (10% fat)	510
Vegetable and fruit group	
1 medium apple	70
1 medium banana	100
½ cup cooked chopped broccoli	20
½ cup cooked diced carrots	25
½ cup cooked green beans	15
½ cup cooked green peas	60
½ cup cooked yellow corn	65
½ cup orange juice	55
½ cup tomato juice	25
1 cup chopped lettuce	10
Miscellaneous	
1 tablespoon white sugar	40
1 tablespoon jelly, jam, or syrup	50–60
1 tablespoon butter or margarine	100
1 tablespoon cooking or salad oil	125
10 medium potato chips	115
12 ounces cola-type soft drinks	145
12 ounces beer	150

* Within each of the four food groups, amounts of foods listed are equivalent to each other in the Basic Four Food Plan. For miscellaneous foods, amounts are not specified in the Basic Four Plan.

Adapted from "Home and Garden Bulletin No. 72," *USDA*, Washington, D.C., 1970.

energy nutrients are oxidized, a given amount of energy is released. Whether the oxidation occurs by actual burning, as in a fire, or by the controlled series of steps known as metabolism, the eventual outcome is the same:

$$\text{Energy nutrients} + \text{Oxygen} \longrightarrow CO_2 + H_2O + \text{Energy}$$

The energy released when foods are burned can be measured quite accurately by using an instrument known as a *bomb calorimeter,* which is essentially a box surrounded by water. A food sample is placed in the instrument, ignited, and allowed to burn completely. The water surrounding the combustion chamber absorbs the heat released from the burning food. By measuring the increase in temperature of the water, the amount of energy originally present in the food can be calculated.

Alternatively, the energy value of a food can be calculated by chemical analysis. In this method, the amounts of fat, carbohydrate, and protein in a food are determined. The energy value for each of the energy nutrients have been determined by repeated measurements of these in a bomb calorimeter. Knowing the amounts of energy nutrients in a given food sample therefore allows calculation of the energy value of the food.

The physiological fuel values of foods and nutrients

The amount of energy released when a food or an energy nutrient is burned in a calorimeter is somewhat greater than the amount of energy available to an organism which eats that food or nutrient. There are three reasons for this difference:

1. Some materials—notably cellulose—are combustible in a calorimeter but cannot be used as energy sources by people or by many other organisms. Thus the energy produced by burning a cellulose-containing food is greater than that available to an animal which cannot utilize cellulose.

2. Useful energy sources—fats, proteins, and carbohydrates other than cellulose—are digested and absorbed very efficiently, but not completely. Thus of the proteins present in the average American diet, approximately 92 percent are digested; of the fats, some 95 percent; and of the digestible carbohydrates, some 97 percent. Therefore, small proportions of energy nutrients remain in the digestive tract to be excreted in the feces, never reaching the cells where their energy could have been released.

3. The third reason for the difference between energy released in a calorimeter and energy available to the body is that the oxidation of amino acids in cells is incomplete. When carbohydrates and fats are metabolized within cells, they are completely oxidized; that is, all of their hydrogen is eventually removed. In contrast, the nitrogen-containing part (amino group) of an amino acid is converted to urea which is

TABLE 12–2
Calculation of physiological fuel values of energy nutrients

	Kilocalories per gram		
	Carbohydrates	Fats	Proteins
Heat of combustion	4.1	9.45	5.65
Energy unavailable to body because of incomplete digestion	0.1	0.45	0.45
Energy unavailable to body because of excretion of nitrogen-containing portion	—	—	1.3
Physiological fuel value (energy available to body) rounded off to nearest whole number	4.0	9.0	4.0

TABLE 12–3
Energy value of food calculated from energy nutrient content

Food	Grams energy nutrients	Kilocalories per gram	Approximate energy values (kilocalories)
Ice cream, regular, 1 cup			
Carbohydrates	28	4	110 (28 x 4)
Fats	14	9	125 (14 x 9)
Proteins	6	4	25 (6 x 4)
Total kilocalories			260
Ice cream, rich, 1 cup			
Carbohydrates	27	4	110 (27 x 4)
Fats	24	9	215 (24 x 9)
Proteins	4	4	15 (4 x 4)
Total kilocalories			340

then excreted in the urine. The energy of the urea molecule is thus lost to the body.

Physiological energy values are obtained by determining the heat of combustion in a calorimeter and then correcting for the factors just discussed, as shown in Table 12–2. The figures 4, 4, and 9 represent the number of Calories released in the body from one gram of carbohydrate, protein, and fat respectively. They are not absolutely precise, for not all of the members of a given nutrient class are digested or utilized to exactly the same degree. For example, less than 80 percent of the proteins in legumes, but fully 97 percent of the proteins in most meats, are digested. However, the figures 4, 4, and 9 are accurate enough to be useful in most situations which involve calculating the energy value of foods. An example of this is shown in Table 12–3.

Energy expenditure or output

Inside cells, energy in the chemical bonds of molecules obtained from food is transformed into other forms of energy, which can then do the work of the cells. Some of this work is vital to the continued life of the organism and must be performed more or less continuously; other types of work need to be performed only intermittently; still others may not be necessary to survival at all.

Broadly speaking, there are three general areas of energy expenditure in organisms such as humans: basal metabolism, physical activity, and specific dynamic effect (Figure 12–2).

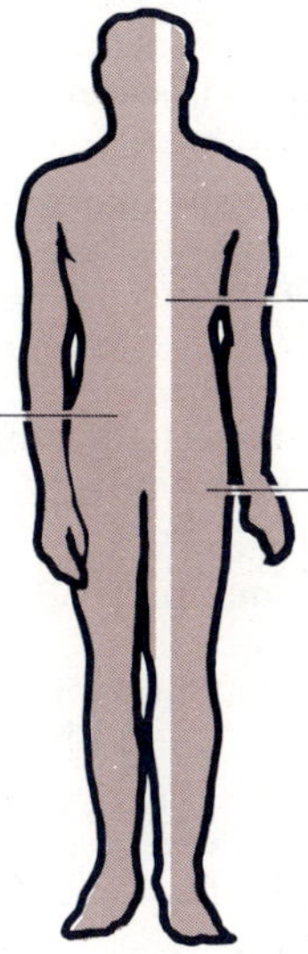

FIGURE 12–2. The three uses of energy in humans.

Basal metabolism

The basal metabolic rate, or BMR, represents the energy expended daily for so-called "vital life activities." Examples of such activities are the beating of the heart, the filtering activity of the kidneys, the synthesis of large molecules from smaller ones in all cells, the movements of the chest in breathing, the transmission of electrical impulses by the brain, and the ferrying of materials into and out of cells. Jumping out of the path of an oncoming truck might appear to be a "vital life activity" because continued life certainly depends upon the ability to perform this activity when the occasion demands. However, basal metabolism is defined as including only those internal activities that must take place automatically and continuously, and not those which are performed only occasionally or as the result of conscious muscular effort.

Basal metabolism is measured on a subject who is *awake* and at *physical, emotional, and digestive rest* in a comfortable environment. In practice, this means that the individual must be lying down, free of tension, after having gone at least twelve hours without eating. It would of course be difficult, if not impossible, to measure basal metabolism in some subjects; an infant or young child, for example, would be most unlikely to remain awake but quiet after twelve hours without food.

Although the term *basal* may seem to suggest a lower limit of en-

TABLE 12–4

Factors that influence the basal metabolic rate (BMR)

Factor	Comments
Aging	After maturity, the BMR declines, gradually at first but more rapidly as aging proceeds.
Body size	Total BMR is directly related to body size in people of normal weight.
Composition of body	Lean tissue is metabolically more active than fat tissue. Therefore obese people have a *lower* BMR and underweight people have a *higher* BMR than would be estimated by the usual rule of one kilocalorie per kilogram of body weight per hour.
Damp hot climate	Heat loss from the body is difficult when sweat does not evaporate readily, as it does in a *dry* hot climate; the body adapts to produce less heat. People adapt to other types of climate by means other than BMR adjustment; shivering, for example, produces the extra heat needed in a cold environment.
Endocrine gland secretion	Thyroxine is by far the most important hormone in regulating the BMR. Sex hormones affect the BMR indirectly for the most part, by altering the ratio of lean to fat. Adrenaline increases the BMR, but its action is short-lived.
Fever	The biochemical reactions which constitute metabolism occur more rapidly at higher temperatures, just as do chemical reactions in general.
Growth (including fetal and maternal growth in pregnancy)	The BMR increases when additional energy is needed to support the anabolic work of producing additional body materials.
Undernutrition (lack of adequate energy intake)	Chronic energy lack results in a decreased BMR; this helps to conserve the body's already inadequate energy supply.

Note: The alphabetical order of these factors, except for the last one, makes them easy to remember. Unfortunately, there seems to be no synonym for "undernutrition" that begins with the letter H.

ergy expenditure below which life cannot exist, this is *not* what BMR is. During sleep, energy expenditure goes down to a level even lower than that measured under basal conditions, which specify that the subject remain awake during the test.

The actual measurement of energy expenditure can be done in either of two ways. One method is similar to that used for studying the energy value of foods. The subject is placed in a large insulated water-jacketed chamber and the amount of heat produced by the body is determined by measuring the temperature increase in the surrounding water. This is called *direct* calorimetry because heat itself is measured. The second method, called *indirect* calorimetry, is done by measuring the amount of oxygen consumed, or of carbon dioxide produced, by the subject. Because gas exchange—oxygen consumption and carbon dioxide production—is proportional to the rate at which energy is being expended in the body, the basal metabolic rate can be calculated from these data.

A very rough approximation of the energy used daily by adults for basal metabolism can be obtained by multiplying the body weight in kilograms by 24. This is because the average adult expends one kilocalorie per kilogram of body weight per hour. Thus in an individual who weighs 121 pounds (approximately 55 kilograms) somewhere around 55 times 24, or 1300, kilocalories will probably be used for basal metabolism; in one weighing 165 pounds (75 kilograms), basal metabolism will represent some 1800 kilocalories. A glance at the RDA for energy—2000 kilocalories for young adult females (who average 58 kilograms), and 2700 kilocalories for young adult males (who average 70 kilograms)—shows that of the total energy intake recommended, more than half is intended to cover the needs for basal metabolism.

A number of factors, summarized in Table 12–4, cause the BMR to vary from one person to another, as well as from time to time within a given individual. Two of these factors are so frequently misunderstood that they deserve some comment.

First is the matter of hormones. An astonishingly large number of people believe that *glands* can somehow cause overweight, in defiance of all scientific laws. This is of course erroneous; although undersecretion of thyroid hormone can decrease the BMR so that weight will be gained unless energy intake is correspondingly decreased, in no case can any mysterious "glandular disorder" cause people to gain weight despite an energy intake less than the output.

A second frequently misunderstood point relates to the effect of age. It is sometimes assumed that weight gain is an inevitable consequence of aging, and that it is therefore pointless to try to combat this "natural" tendency. However, just as in the case of hormonal abnormalities, decreasing the energy intake to compensate for the decreased BMR and decreased activity will allow you to avoid excess weight regardless of age.

The specific dynamic effect

Basal metabolism is measured under conditions of digestive rest, because ingestion of food is soon followed by heat production over and above that associated with vital life activities. This phenomenon, known as the *specific dynamic effect* (or *action*) of food, represents the energy expended for the work of digesting the food, absorbing nutrients and carrying them to the cells, metabolizing the nutrients, and finally disposing of the end products. On the average, approximately 10 percent of the total energy expended is used for these purposes. In a sense, then, the specific dynamic effect operates somewhat like an income tax. A portion of people's income is withheld in order to support the society which allows them to use the rest of their income. In a similar manner,

TABLE 12–5

The energy cost of various activities

Type of activity	Examples	Estimated kilocalories (per hour)
Sedentary	Sitting with little or no body movement: reading; writing; watching television; eating; taking notes.	80–100
Light	Sitting or standing with some movement of arms and perhaps of other body parts: cooking; light housework such as dusting; personal grooming; walking slowly; office work such as filing and fast typing; ordinary laboratory work.	100–160
Moderate	Sitting with vigorous arm movements or standing with considerable movement of arms and perhaps of other body parts: walking at average speed; making beds; sweeping and mopping floors; polishing and waxing at a moderate pace; unusually vigorous laboratory work.	160–250
Vigorous	Moving body rapidly: heavy housework such as scrubbing floors or other surfaces; walking rapidly; heavy gardening; sports such as bowling, golfing, and moderately fast dancing.	250–350
Heavy	Moving body at maximum or near maximum capacity: rapid swimming; playing tennis vigorously; running; dancing many currently popular dances; skiing; cleaning house when guests or relatives are to arrive any minute.	350 and upwards

a portion of the energy intake is used for processes which enable the body to utilize the rest of the energy intake.

In experimental animals, the specific dynamic effect can sometimes be increased to as high as 30 percent of the total energy intake by feeding diets which consist entirely, or almost entirely, of pure proteins. This very high figure probably represents the energy which must be used to synthesize urea from ammonia, which is released in large amounts when the excess amino acids are deaminated.

The fact that diets of pure protein result in an increased specific dynamic action has led to the erroneous belief that all-meat or all-egg diets will have the same effect. According to this notion, people should be able to lose weight rapidly even if the energy intake is high because a large portion of the energy in meats and eggs will be used to digest and metabolize the nutrients in these foods. However, this idea is incorrect, because even lean meats contain far too much fat to constitute anything close to an all-protein diet. For example, a portion of lean steak (such as round steak) which contains 20 grams of protein also contains approximately 4 grams of fat, even if all the visible fat has been carefully cut away. As for eggs, the amount of fat is just about the same as the amount of protein present.

Resting metabolism, which is the sum of basal metabolism plus specific dynamic action, is often of great practical interest; it is the average metabolism during the night and for the periods of the day when no exercise is being performed, and thus represents a more normal situation than basal metabolism does. Resting metabolism, in short, is a measure of all energy expenditure except that used for exercise.

Physical activity, or exercise

Physical activity, the third area of energy expenditure, is the one that can vary the most from one person to another. The amount of energy required for a given amount of physical activity depends on body size to some degree, for more energy is required to move a large body than to move a small one, just as more fuel is required to operate a large automobile than a small one. Other factors that influence energy expenditure for exercise can introduce even more variation, because these factors—the kind, duration, and intensity of physical activity—are normally under the conscious control of the individual.

Estimating the energy expended for various types of physical activity is quite difficult to do accurately. Many of the values in Table 12–5 were based on studies of only a few subjects, and some of the activities themselves are described in terms that are not very helpful. "Moderately fast dancing," for example, could mean very different things to different people. Tables of energy expenditure associated with various types of activities should therefore be used as rough approximations, if they are used at all. Thus, although many people believe that they can determine their energy output down to the last fraction of a kilocalorie by using data such as these, such a degree of faith is not justified.

However, a real value of data on the energy cost of various activities is that they can help to dispose of some very common myths. One of these myths is that exercise is a negligible factor in energy output and hence in weight control. For example, it is often stated that "working off" 1 pound of body fat requires some thirty hours of walking, or five hours of running, or six hours of cycling at top speed. It is extremely unlikely that anybody would, or could, perform any of these activities *continuously* until a pound of body fat was lost. However, one hour of walking each day would result in the loss of 1 pound of fat per month; in a year's time, this would amount to a loss of 12 pounds.

While this rate of loss may be far too slow for those who hope for overnight results, it is nevertheless obvious that regular exercise can, over the long haul, be a valuable aid in weight control.

Another myth regarding exercise and weight control is that a single burst of vigorous or even violent exercise can cause a measurable amount of body fat to drop off like magic. A man may note that the scale registers a weight 5 pounds greater than that which he considers ideal. Grimly determined to remedy the situation, he spends several hours working away at the most energy-consuming activity he can think of, such as running, playing tennis, or digging furiously in a garden. Sweating profusely and feeling unusually virtuous for his perseverence, he steps back on the scale at the end of his ordeal and is delighted to see that he has lost a perceptible amount of weight, perhaps 2 or 3 pounds or even more.

However, he would be less pleased if he knew what had really happened. If this man is of average size, he may have expended perhaps 2400 kilocalories in three hours of running—assuming that the running was continuous rather than interrupted by frequent rest breaks, as it would have to be for almost anyone. This 2400 kilocalories represents only about ⅔ of a pound of fat tissue, and not several pounds, as he might think. Actually, most of the weight change was caused by the loss of fluid in sweating, and will return as soon as thirst drives him to drink enough water to replace it. Thus, although exercising can be very useful in a weight-loss program, it is important that people recognize that physical activity will not bring about results that can be seen immediately.

A third common misconception is that *mental* activity is as energy-consuming as is *physical* activity of the same duration. One reason for this belief may be that some people—by no means all—suffer a loss of appetite during times of anxiety, and erroneously attribute the resulting weight loss to the "increased activity" of the worrying brain. Actually, the nervous system is continuously active, and uses about the same amount of energy whether the person is sleeping, daydreaming, worrying, or studying furiously. Muscle tension, which commonly accompanies intense mental effort, can increase energy expenditure because muscles are partially contracted, but this has only a negligible effect on energy output. In fact, it has been calculated that the extra energy required to support one hour of the most extreme mental effort is furnished by approximately one-half of a peanut! The fatigue that commonly results from a long session of mental effort is primarily psychological, and should not be confused with the physical exhaustion which can be caused by prolonged physical activity.

Yet another myth is the belief that physical activity automatically causes increased appetite so that a greater energy intake, which offsets the energy cost of exercise, is inevitable. Actually, experiments with rats show that very sedentary animals eat *more* than their moderately exercised counterparts; and although increased levels of exercise do indeed cause rats to eat more, people can be assumed to possess a greater degree of self-control than rats.

ENERGY BALANCE AND WEIGHT CONTROL

Weight and *fat* are not necessarily the same thing. The "weight loss" brought about by sweating, for example, does not represent a loss of body fat. Nevertheless, the terms are so commonly used as if they were synonyms that "weight control" is generally understood to mean "control of body fat content."

Experts do not agree completely on the definitions of terms such as *underweight, overweight,* and *obesity.* Overweight individuals are generally defined as those whose body weight is greater than that which is considered ideal for the individual's height and sex. This does not *always* indicate excess body fat, because overweight can occasionally represent unusually heavy bones, unusually massive muscles, or abnormal accumulation of body fluid. However, differentiating these conditions from simple excess body fat is sometimes difficult, and for this reason the term *overweight* will be used here in the sense of *overly fat.*

The term *obesity* is somewhat more straightforward. Nutritionists agree that obesity means "excessively fat." Generally a person whose weight is more than 20 percent greater than the ideal weight can properly be considered obese, because an excess of this magnitude is rarely the result of heavy muscles, large bones, or other nonfat body components.

Underweight, like overweight, is somewhat difficult to define because a person whose weight may be less than that which is considered ideal may nevertheless be in very good health. The person with a delicate bone structure and smaller than average muscles may very well have an adequate amount of body fat and yet, on the basis of weight alone, appear to be too thin. As in the case for overweight, however, the term *underweight* will be used here in its usual meaning, namely, an abnormally small amount of body fat.

Energy balance—the difference between energy intake and energy output—is the key to controlling the fat content of the body (Figure 12–3). This point cannot be stressed too strongly, because attempts to control body weight in defiance of the concept of energy balance, although widely undertaken, are certain to fail. If energy intake is greater than energy output, the individual is said to be in *positive* energy balance, and the excess energy is stored as body fat. Conversely, if energy intake is less than output, energy balance is *negative* and body fat will be utilized to make up the necessary difference. There are no exceptions to these rules; the *first law of thermodynamics,* which states that energy is neither created nor destroyed, holds true in nutrition as it does in physics. There are no mysterious "metabolic conditions" or "miracle diets" which can circumvent this law, thereby causing excess energy to disappear into thin air.

One pound of body fat tissue, or adipose tissue, represents approximately 3500 kilocalories. This is less than the energy value of a pound of pure fat, because adipose tissue is only about 80 percent fat; the other 20 percent is protoplasm, which consists mostly of water and is therefore considerably lower in energy value than is fat.

An intake of 3500 kilocalories over and above the energy expended will result in the gain of 1 pound of fat tissue, and an intake which is 3500 kilocalories less than that expended will result in a loss of 1 pound. Whether the imbalance occurs over a period of days or of years is irrelevant; the time involved will affect the *rate* at which weight is gained or lost but not the total *amount* of weight lost or gained. Body fat can be compared to a bank balance; if the deposits put into a bank account are greater than the amounts removed, the account will increase. If the amount put in exceeds the amount removed by $10 each week, the account will obviously increase more rapidly than if the difference were only $1 per week. Ultimately, however, the final amount in the bank will depend entirely on the difference between deposits and withdrawals.

Energy balance depends on both intake and output, and not just one or the other of these. Let us consider the hypothetical "reference woman," upon whom the National Research Council bases the RDA for energy, as a concrete example. She is 23 years old, weighs 58 kilograms (approximately 128 pounds), and lives in an environment that does not require that she expend very much energy simply to keep herself warm. Her physical activity is described as "light," meaning that she is neither sedentary nor engaged in very heavy work much of the time. The recommended energy intake for this woman is 2000 kilocalories daily.

If this woman's average energy intake is 2000 kilocalories per day, that is precisely what she needs to keep her weight constant, and she

FIGURE 12–3. Energy balance.

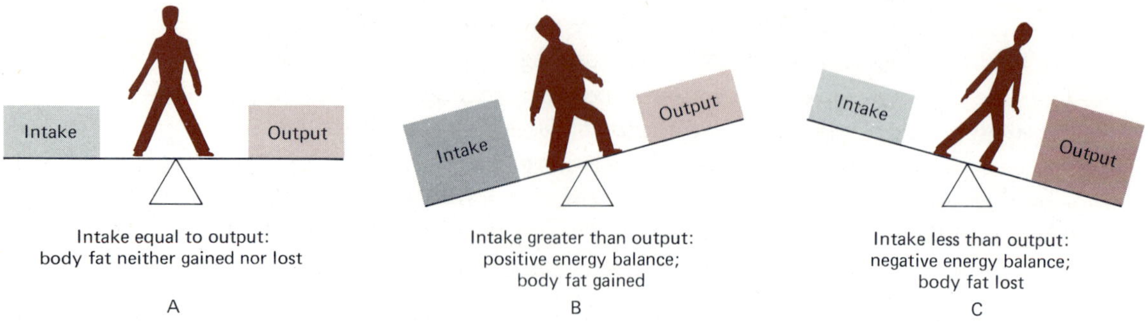

will neither gain nor lose body fat. However, perhaps she might acquire the habit of drinking a cup of hot chocolate every night, without making any other changes in her life. An average cup of hot chocolate made with whole milk would furnish approximately 250 kilocalories. Because this amount of energy represents an excess over and above the amount needed to maintain her weight, the extra energy will be stored as fat and she will begin to gain weight. This will, of course, occur very slowly; only about $\frac{1}{14}$ of a pound of body-fat tissue, or slightly more than 1 ounce, will be added each day. Consequently, it will take approximately two weeks for a pound of fat tissue (representing 3500 kilocalories) to be added, and many weeks may elapse before she notes that she has developed a "weight problem." If she does not do something about it at this point, she can expect to continue to gain slightly over 2 pounds per month, which would add up to the hefty figure of approximately 25 pounds in a single year!

If she *does* decide sooner or later to do something about her weight, more than one option is open. She could *decrease* her energy intake by omitting the hot chocolate, or by omitting something else of equal energy value from her diet, such as the gravy, butter, or margarine that she usually eats, or the leftovers she gleans from the table after dinner because she "can't stand seeing food go to waste."

Another possibilitiy is to *increase* her energy output by increasing her physical activity. Admittedly this would not be easy for many people; the reference woman would have to spend close to two extra hours daily in walking or some similar activity in order to expend the extra 250 kilocalories provided by her cherished bedtime snack. However, if she starts walking to work, to the shopping center, or to wherever else she formerly drove, she could expend enough energy to be in balance, despite the fact that her intake is as high as it was when she was gaining weight.

One problem remains: the fat gained previously is still there. In order to lose this weight, she must go into *negative* energy balance for a while. How she chooses to accomplish this will depend primarily upon how quickly she wishes to cast off her unwelcome burden. A look at her present energy balance shows the following:

> If she has omitted the hot chocolate or its energy equivalent, her intake is 2000 kilocalories daily, which is equal to the energy output for her as the reference woman.
>
> If she has not omitted the chocolate or its equivalent, her intake is 2250 kilocalories daily, which is equal to her energy expenditure, including the exercise of extra walking.

Suppose, moreover, that she had previously gained a total of 6 pounds and that she is determined to lose this amount of weight within a month. The total energy value of 6 pounds of fat tissue is 6 times 3500, or 21,000 kilocalories. If she is to lose this within 30 days, her daily energy deficit must be 21,000 divided by 30, or 700 kilocalories. A

TABLE 12–6
Various intake–output combinations for a given negative energy balance

Intake (kilocalories)	Output (kilocalories)	Balance (kilocalories)
1300	2000	−700
1500	2200	−700
2000	2700	−700
2250	2950	−700

deficit of this magnitude could result from a variety of intake-output combinations, such as any of those shown in Table 12–6.

In the first case, energy intake is greatly reduced and output is that of the reference woman without the additional walking.

In the second, the less drastic decrease in energy intake is offset by the output of extra exercise.

In the third situation, energy intake is that of the reference woman and energy output is increased to a level *much* higher than is likely for any woman except one accustomed to unusually heavy work.

The fourth case shows that the woman could, hypothetically, continue to have the energy intake of the reference woman *plus* the hot chocolate and still lose 6 pounds in a month if she could expend almost 3000 kilocalories daily. However, this would represent a level of physical activity *far* exceeding that which most women would, or indeed could, continue for long.

In summary, then, weight gain and loss are a matter of energy balance, and loss of fat can be accomplished only by achieving negative energy balance. This can be done by decreasing the intake, increasing the output, or both.

Despite the simplicity with which fat gain and loss can be explained, excess weight remains a problem for a very large number of people in developed countries. For this reason, although underweight may be no less serious than obesity as a health problem, nutritionists in developed countries concentrate mostly on the problem of excess weight.

Because energy balance involves intake and expenditure, it is helpful to look at some of the factors that regulate and influence these.

FACTORS AFFECTING ENERGY INTAKE

In the part of the brain known as the *hypothalamus* are feeding and satiety centers which are very important in regulating the total energy intake. When the feeding centers are active, the animal or person is motivated to eat; when the satiety centers are active the organism experiences a feeling of satiety, or satisfaction, and loses the desire for food until the feeding centers become active again. If these centers are damaged or destroyed, as occasionally happens in people as the result of certain types of brain injury, this physiological control can be lost. Injury to the satiety center can result in a permanent loss of the ability to be satiated by normal amounts of food; the resulting extreme overeating, or *hyperphagia,* can lead to obesity of an astonishing degree. If the feeding centers are damaged, the resulting *anorexia* (lack of appetite) may be so profound that the person or animal can literally starve to death in the presence of an abundance of food.

However, there is little evidence that a defect in this "appestat" mechanism is a common cause of abnormal appetite. Social and psychological factors, strong enough to offset the physiological controls, are more likely the usual causes. In our society, food is available in far greater quantities than needed for immediate use. Homes are normally stocked with a supply of food sufficient to last for several days or longer, and food can therefore be used for many purposes other than as a necessity to meet physical needs. It can provide a sense of security to the anxious; it may become the habitual accompaniment to social events, television viewing, and other activities; it can be used as a consolation in times of disappointment.

Deep-seated feelings regarding "proper" amounts of food are learned early, and are as resistant to change as are beliefs regarding specific kinds of foods. To some people, a meal without a rich dessert is hardly a meal at all; to others, liberal amounts of high-calorie additions such as butter, margarine, and salad dressings are absolutely necessary to make food edible; to still others, a plate must be heaped with food at each meal in order that life be sustained.

Because many people have little knowledge of the energy values of various foods, they may believe that their energy intake is much lower than it actually is. For example, it is not unusual to find people who believe that meat is virtually free of calories. However, their attempts to lose weight by restricting their evening meal to "only" a very large slab of meat and a salad are almost certain to fail because, contrary to popular opinion, most meats are not really low in energy value (Table 12–1). Information on the energy furnished by various foods can be very useful to those who would otherwise greatly underestimate their energy intake.

INDIVIDUAL VARIATIONS IN ENERGY OUTPUT

Of the three components of energy expenditure, specific dynamic action varies so little under ordinary conditions that it need not be considered further. Variations in the other two, however, can significantly affect energy output.

The basal metabolic rate is regulated in large part by the hormone, thyroxine. Hypothyroidism, a condition in which thyroxine secretion is abnormally low, can result in a decrease as great as 30 percent in the BMR. For the reference woman, with a BMR of approximately 1350 kilocalories, this could amount to a decrease as great as 400 kilocalories per day in energy output. The possibilities for weight gain are readily seen. However, hypothyroidism of this degree is seen in only a small proportion of people.

The greatest variations in energy output are seen as the result of *differences in physical activity.* Except for those with unusual conditions which make exercise difficult or inadvisable, the reasons for the low levels of physical activity commonly seen in countries such as the United States are social and psychological rather than physical. In the minds of many, success is equated with freedom from the necessity to use muscle power. One who drives has more prestige than one who walks; people who use their brains are socially above those who must work at a physically demanding job; the successful woman is one who can hire somebody to do the heavy housecleaning for her. For the most part, the need to move about to relieve monotony and to seek something new has been filled for modern humans by the ready availability of television and reading materials, which are capable of keeping people immobilized for hours. Students, from kindergarten through college, are systematically trained to be physically inactive for long periods of time, and the activity performed outside of classes is often far too little to make up for the hours spent doing nothing more active than writing notes and turning the pages of the notebook. Women, from adolescence on, have been subjected to one further influence: Traditionally, strenuous or vigorous exercise has been considered "unfeminine." Croquet and lawn tennis were at one time believed to be the most heavy exercise suitable for "the ladies." Fortunately, in more recent generations, common sense has prevailed in this respect.

DETECTING OVERWEIGHT AND OBESITY

People are sometimes surprised to learn that a problem exists regarding the detection of overweight or obesity. It is commonplace to believe that one's ideal weight is easily determined, and that weight significantly higher or lower than the ideal is automatically undesirable. Actually, the amount of body fat that is considered desirable varies greatly. In some cultures, fatness is considered a sign of success and is therefore attractive; "How fat you are!" may be the highest compliment that can be paid. In some Western societies, the opposite situation is prevalent; fat is considered so unattractive that many people consider themselves overly fat even though, medically, their weight is normal. Younger women in particular are under a good deal of cultural pressure to conform to the "right" feminine weight, even if current fashion demands a degree of slenderness that actually constitutes undernutrition.

Methods for determining whether an individual is overweight range from those which are very simple, even crude, to techniques so complex that they can be performed only in research centers that possess specialized equipment. The simpler methods available are the following:

1 **Visual inspection.** In many cases, it is possible to detect excess fat simply by looking at a person. However, not all large people are necessarily fat, and visual inspection cannot detect slight degrees of excess fatness.

2 **Use of body weight standards.** Table 12–7 shows desirable weights based on statistics obtained from an insurance company. "Desirable" in this case means "associated with the lowest mortality rates." The weights were obtained by weighing people dressed in "normal" clothing, and the heights are those obtained with shoes on; heels were two inches high for women and one inch high for men. The greatest problem in using these tables is that the individual decides which body frame category he or she fits into—and it is very tempting for overweight people to decide that they have a large frame and therefore are not truly overweight! Excesses as great at 30 pounds or more can easily be rationalized away in this manner.

3 **Skinfold measurements.** People sometimes attempt to measure the thickness of subcutaneous fat by an informal method described in magazines as the "pinch test." Essentially this consists of measuring the thickness of the tissue which can be pinched between the thumb and fingers at certain sites on the body. Measurements made with special constant-pressure calipers are much more accurate, although still not capable of identifying obesity in all cases.

These methods are simple compared to some of the techniques used in research on obesity. In body-density studies, for example, the individual is weighed in air; then, using special equipment, he or she is weighed under water. The difference between the two weights is the weight of water the body displaced, which is related to the body's volume. It is then possible to calculate the body's density by dividing the weight (obtained in air) by the volume of the body. Fat is less dense than water, which is the most abundant component of lean tissue; this is why cream rises to the top of milk, and why the oil layer rather than the water layer is on top when salad dressing separates. Knowing the density of the body therefore allows one to calculate the relative amounts of fat and lean present.

Other techniques are also available for estimating the amount of fat in the body, but the example of body-density determination should suffice to explain why simpler techniques must be used routinely, even though they are not always highly reliable indicators of obesity.

People with abnormally *small* amounts of body fat can, of course, also be studied by any of the methods used to study obese people. The emphasis has been placed upon overweight rather than underweight because of the greater concern about overweight in our society.

TABLE 12–7
Table of desirable weights, with three frame categories

Desirable weights for women 25 years of age and over*†

Height with shoes on (2-inch heels) (Feet)	(Inches)	Small frame	Medium frame	Large frame
4	10	92–98	96–107	104–119
4	11	94–101	98–110	106–122
5	0	96–104	101–113	109–125
5	1	99–107	104–116	112–128
5	2	102–110	107–119	115–131
5	3	105–113	110–122	118–134
5	4	108–116	113–126	121–138
5	5	111–119	116–130	125–142
5	6	114–123	120–135	129–146
5	7	118–127	124–139	133–150
5	8	122–131	128–143	137–154
5	9	126–135	132–147	141–158
5	10	130–140	136–151	145–163
5	11	134–144	140–155	149–168
6	0	138–148	144–159	153–173

Desirable weights for men 25 years of age and over*†

Height with shoes on (1-inch heels) (Feet)	(Inches)	Small frame	Medium frame	Large frame
5	2	112–120	118–129	126–141
5	3	115–123	121–133	129–144
5	4	118–126	124–136	132–148
5	5	121–129	127–139	135–152
5	6	124–133	130–143	138–156
5	7	128–137	134–147	142–161
5	8	132–141	138–152	147–166
5	9	136–145	142–156	151–170
5	10	140–150	146–160	155–174
5	11	144–154	150–165	159–179
6	0	148–158	154–170	164–184
6	1	152–162	158–175	168–189
6	2	156–167	162–180	173–194
6	3	160–171	167–185	178–199
6	4	164–175	172–190	182–204

* Courtesy Metropolitan Life Insurance Co., Four Steps to Weight Control, 1969. Based on 1959 Build and blood pressure study.
† Weight in pounds, according to frame (in indoor clothing).

CHOOSING AND FOLLOWING A WEIGHT CONTROL PROGRAM

Is there any "secret" to weight control? Yes, and it is energy balance. Weight cannot be controlled through the use of steam baths, massages, gadgets which jiggle the body fat around, special belts or suits which purportedly "break down" body fat, or any other such gimmicks.

The basic facts regarding energy balance are among the most firmly established verities in the field of nutrition. However, the prevalence of overweight even among health professionals (including nutritionists) shows that an *understanding* of the relationship of energy balance to obesity is not in itself sufficient to prevent or treat obesity. Weight control involves three basic steps, all of which are related to human behavior:

1 Deciding to lose weight (or gain it, if this is the problem).
2 Deciding on a particular program or method.
3 Following through with appropriate alterations of behavior.

The decision to lose or gain weight is best made with the help of a physician. In addition to providing nutritional information, the physician can offer emotional support and can guide the individual toward a type of diet suited to his or her particular physical and psychological needs. Past dietary habits, snacking habits, previous unsuccessful attempts at weight control, age of onset of the weight problem, activity patterns, the present state of physical and emotional health, and many other factors can determine the success or failure of a weight-control program.

The particular method should then be selected on the basis of the individual's characteristics. All weight-control programs, however, should supply adequate amounts of essential nutrients but should provide a deficit of energy. This means decreased amounts of additional foods (including alcoholic drinks), and moderate portions of foundation foods. No single food need be omitted completely; the secret is moderation, not ruthless austerity. Nor are any special diet foods or nutrient supplements necessary.

An individual weight-loss program can be devised by anyone who is familiar with the Basic Four Food Group Plan. Information on the calorie values of specific foods within each group can be obtained from food labels, from the U. S. Department of Agriculture, or from books and pamphlets which list the energy values of common portions of foods. Actually, however, it is highly probable that the kinds and amounts of foods recommended in the Basic Four guide will automatically constitute an effective weight-loss diet, regardless of the individual choices made within each group. As shown in Table 12–8, a high-energy diet based on the Basic Four is likely only if (a) very unusual choices are made, or (b) foundation foods are prepared with added ingredients such as sugar or fat, which increase the foods' original energy value.

For some people, group methods such as Weight Watchers or TOPS (Take Off Pounds Sensibly) are highly successful. Admittedly, there are a few disadvantages to such programs. They are expensive, both because they charge a fee for membership and because they may specify unnecessarily large amounts of certain high-cost foods, especially meat. In addition, the super-strict regimen can be questioned; dedicated members of Weight Watchers, for example, must eat fish five

TABLE 12–8
Variation of energy values from the Basic Four Plan

Lower energy choices: Food	Kilocalories	Higher energy choices: Food	Kilocalories
Bread and cereal group			
Bread, enriched white, 4 slices	280	Corn muffin, enriched, 1	125
		Rice, enriched, cooked, ½ cup	110
		Doughnut, enriched, 1	125
		Biscuit, enriched, 1 (2 in. diameter)	105
Meat group			
Chicken, broiled, 3 ounces	115	Steak, sirloin, 3 ounces	330
Egg, 1 medium, boiled	80	Sausage, cooked, 1 ounce	125
Milk group			
Skim milk, 2 cups	180	Whole milk, 1 cup	160
		Cheddar cheese, ¾ ounce	90
		Ice cream, 1 cup	200
Vegetable and fruit group			
Potato, baked, 1 medium	100	Potato, french fried, 1 medium	250
Cucumber, ½ medium	15	Avocado, 1 medium	190
Spinach, ½ cup	20	Orange juice, ½ cup	55
Lettuce, 2 large leaves (1 cup chopped)	10	Sweet potato, 1 boiled	170
Total	800	Total	2035

Note: *Ordinary* choices, neither unusually low nor unusually high in energy value, furnish approximately 1200 kilocalories daily.

times a week and liver once a week, regardless of whether they like these foods. Because a weight-control program should create good eating habits that people can enjoy for the rest of their lives, a more flexible program is needed by many. However, others find group methods extraordinarily successful by *learning* to like previously disliked foods; they actually change their tastes in the direction of good eating habits and enjoyment of nutritious low-calorie foods.

Liquid-formula diets, although they provide adequate amounts of essential nutrients and only some 900 to 1000 kilocalories, are not recommended because they do not bring about the permanent changes in eating habits that are needed to maintain normal weight once this is achieved.

Although *anorexic* (appetite-depressing) drugs are available, they act at best as a temporary aid. The same is true of nonprescription items, such as candy-type supplements and methylcellulose-containing products that "swell up in the stomach." At any rate, these are of questionable effectiveness, despite the prominent role of testimonials in their advertising.

The most valuable aids in successful weight control are based, not on chemical crutches, but on behavioral modifications such as the following:

1 Eating in one place only, specifically the table, forces the person to give conscious thought to eating and to give up certain practices such as nibbling during television programs.
2 Keeping "problem foods," such as potato chips, soft drinks, and candy, out of sight (or even out of the house) minimizes the chance of giving in to a sudden moment of temptation.
3 Eating only those foods that require preparation automatically discourages impulse eating. If a food must be peeled, cut up, or cooked before eating, it is less likely to be eaten than something that offers instant gratification.
4 Prolonging the eating time, by pausing frequently during each meal or by putting the fork down after each bite, commonly allows a person to avoid overeating. People who eat very rapidly may overeat before they realize that they are no longer hungry.
5 Leaving the last bite of each food on the plate represents, for many people, a psychological victory over the common feeling that one *must* eat everything available (or even everything in sight).

The successful dieter should never be discouraged if the expected rewards of dieting are not immediately forthcoming. People often have unrealistic expectations ("If I could only lose 25 pounds, I'd be happy"; "Surely everybody will notice how much weight I've lost by next week"). No single factor, including normal weight, can guarantee happiness; and since the *individual* benefits from weight control, why should rewards come from others, in the form of compliments? Many behavioral scientists believe that self-awarded prizes are a legitimate means of rewarding desirable behavior. The prospect of a new suit or dress for losing 10 pounds, or a weekend trip for staying on the diet during the week, may provide the continued motivation which is the really important factor in success or failure of weight control.

SUGGESTED READINGS

Calloway, D. H. "Dietary Components that Yield Energy." *Environmental Biology and Medicine* 1 (1971):175.

Christakis, G. and R. K. Plumb. *Obesity.* New York: The Nutrition Foundation, Inc., 1966.

"Food and Your Weight." USDA: Home and Garden Bull. No. 74, Washington, D.C., 1969.

Harger, B. S., J. B. Miller, and J. C. Thomas. "The Caloric Cost of Running: Its Impact on Weight Reduction." *Journal of the American Medical Association* 228 (1974):482.

Hoch, F. L. *Energy Transformations in Mammals: Regulatory Mechanisms.* Philadelphia: Saunders, 1971.

Konishi, F. *Exercise Equivalents of Foods.* Carbondale, Ill., Southern Illinois University Press, 1974.

Mann, G. V. "Relationships of Age to Nutrient Requirements." *American Journal of Clinical Nutrition* 26 (1973):1097.

Meyer, J. *Overweight: Causes, Cost and Control.* Englewood Cliffs, N. J., Prentice-Hall, 1968.

Moore, T. "The Calorie Versus the Joule." *Journal of the American Dietetic Association* 59 (1971):327.

Stunkard, A. "New Therapies for the Eating Disorders: Behavior Modification of Obesity and Anorexia Nervosa. *Archives of General Psychiatry* 26 (1972):391.

Tullis, I. F. "Rational Diet Construction for Mild and Grand Obesity." *Journal of the American Medical Association* 226 (1973):70.

13

proteins: problems and proposals

In the past twenty-five years, interest in proteins has increased tremendously. Much of this interest has been generated by the discovery that, next to sheer lack of food energy, protein deficiency is the most serious nutritional problem in the world today. Particularly among children in the developing countries, malnutrition caused by a lack of both adequate amounts and adequate kinds of protein is a major cause of disease and death. Because protein malnutrition is often accompanied by energy undernutrition, the term *protein-calorie malnutrition* (PCM) is often used to describe the pathetically malnourished victims.

By contrast, most people in the developed countries consume far more protein than they actually need. They do this partly because of

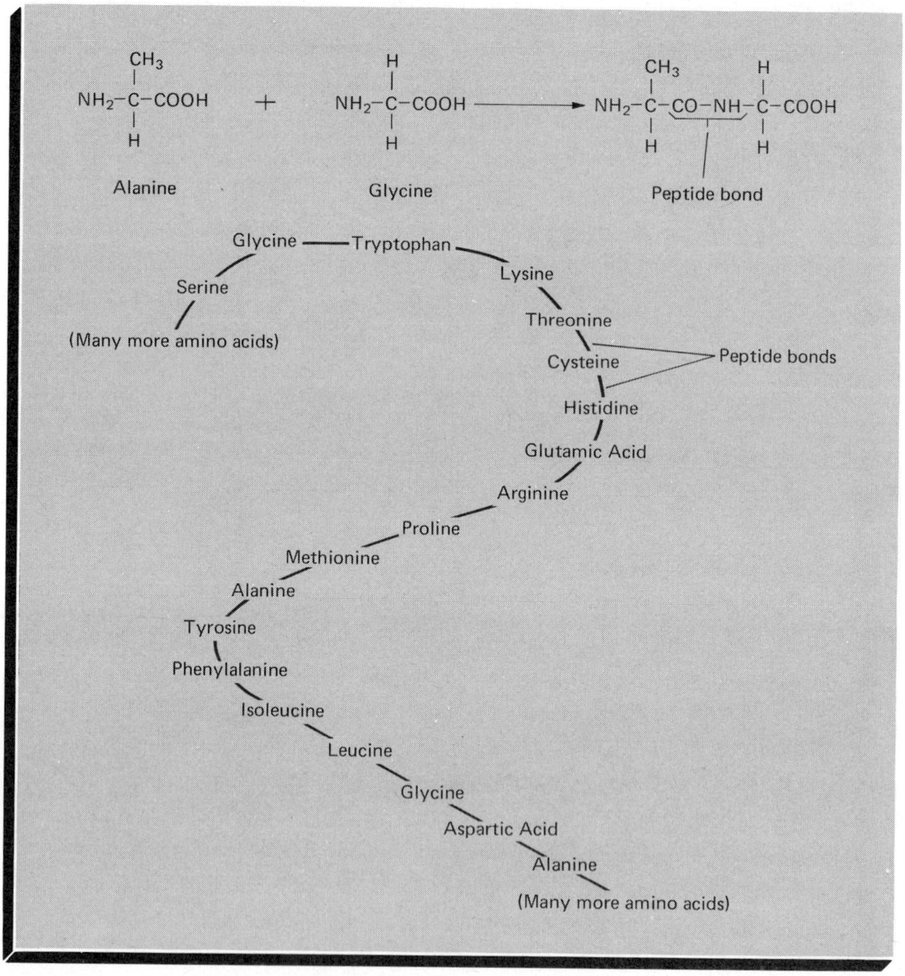

FIGURE 13–1. A protein is a giant molecule formed from amino acids linked together.

habit, having generally had an abundant supply of high-protein foods available in the past; partly for prestige, because certain high-protein foods are among the most expensive foods available; and partly on the basis of health beliefs, many of which are not founded on fact.

Proteins are giant molecules constructed of many amino acids fastened together by linkages called *peptide bonds* (Figure 13–1). Although there are only about 20 amino acids, a fantastic variety of protein molecules can be built from these, just as all of the words in the dictionary can be constructed from the 26 letters of the English alphabet. One protein can differ from another with respect to the total *number* of amino acids, the *kinds* of amino acids, the relative *proportions* of the various amino acids, or their *order or sequence* along the chain. It is because of this tremendous possibility for diversity that a single human cell can contain thousands of different kinds of proteins which, in turn, are different from the thousands of different proteins found in each of the millions of other forms of life with which we share the earth.

Of the 20 amino acids found in proteins, 8 are essential for adult humans; a ninth one, *histidine,* is also essential for infants (Table 13–1). An essential amino acid is one which the organism cannot produce in amounts sufficient to meet its needs; it does not necessarily play more important roles than the nonessential ones do. Indeed, many nonessential amino acids participate in roles so vital to life that lack of them would be disastrous to the organism (Figure 13–2).

Two aspects of the need for protein can be identified. First, there is a minimum *total amount* of protein required for growth and renewal of body structures. Although the body of an adult may contain only

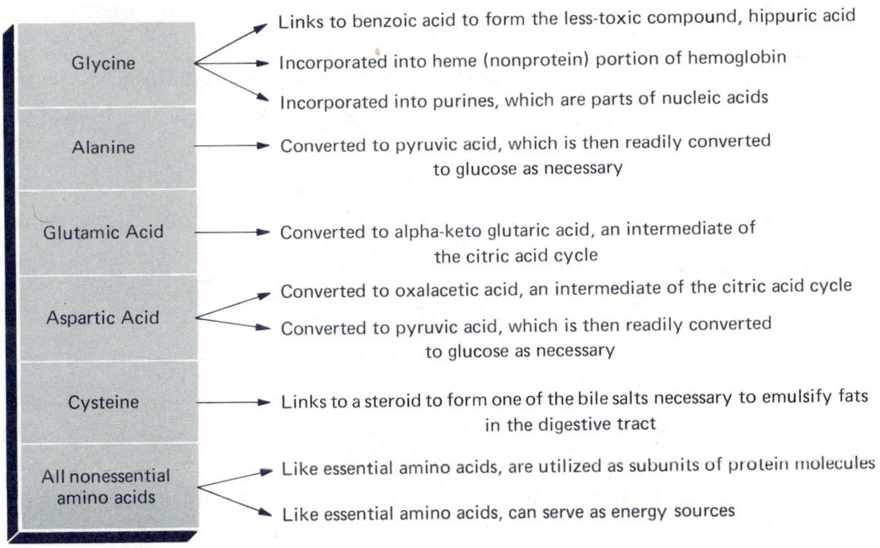

FIGURE 13–2. Examples of the importance of some nonessential amino acids.

TABLE 13–1

Essential and nonessential amino acids for humans

Essential	Nonessential
Isoleucine	Alanine
Leucine	Arginine
Lysine	Aspartic acid
Methionine	Cysteine
Phenylalanine	Cystine
Threonine	Glutamic acid
Tryptophan	Glycine
Valine	Histidine
	Hydroxyproline
	Proline
	Serine
	Tyrosine

Note: Other classifications may be found in other books. For example, histidine is often listed as essential because it is required by infants although not by people beyond infancy. Other compounds, such as hydroxylysine and norleucine, are considered amino acids by some but dismissed as mere variants of amino acid structures by others. Therefore, let us relax and say that there are *approximately* 20 amino acids, 8 of which are essential for all people.

some 25 pounds of protein, a total of *500 pounds or more* may have been synthesized during the years of growth. However, practically all of this was used to replace other protein molecules which were simultaneously being broken down. Second, *minimum amounts of the essential amino acids* are needed, and deficiency can result from the lack of any one of these, as well as from the lack of a sufficient total amount of protein.

No single specific protein is essential in the diet, for reasons which can be seen in Figure 13–3. The two proteins shown at the top are different in the sequence of amino acids along the chain, as well as in the relative proportions of some of the amino acids. When they are digested, however, only the liberated amino acids are absorbed, and the result in each case is similar: approximately the same amounts of each essential amino acid, and approximately the same number of total amino acids. The differences in the original proteins may have been vitally important to the organisms from which these two proteins came. For example, one protein may have been an enzyme that catalyzed one of the reactions of the citric acid cycle, and the other may have been a structural muscle protein, a hormone, or some other type of important biochemical. To the cells of the organism which eats these proteins, however, it makes no difference what the original structures of the two proteins were.

For this reason, although it is common to speak of *protein* as an essential nutrient, it is, actually, only certain of the amino acid *subunits*, not one of the intact proteins themselves, which must be obtained in the diet.

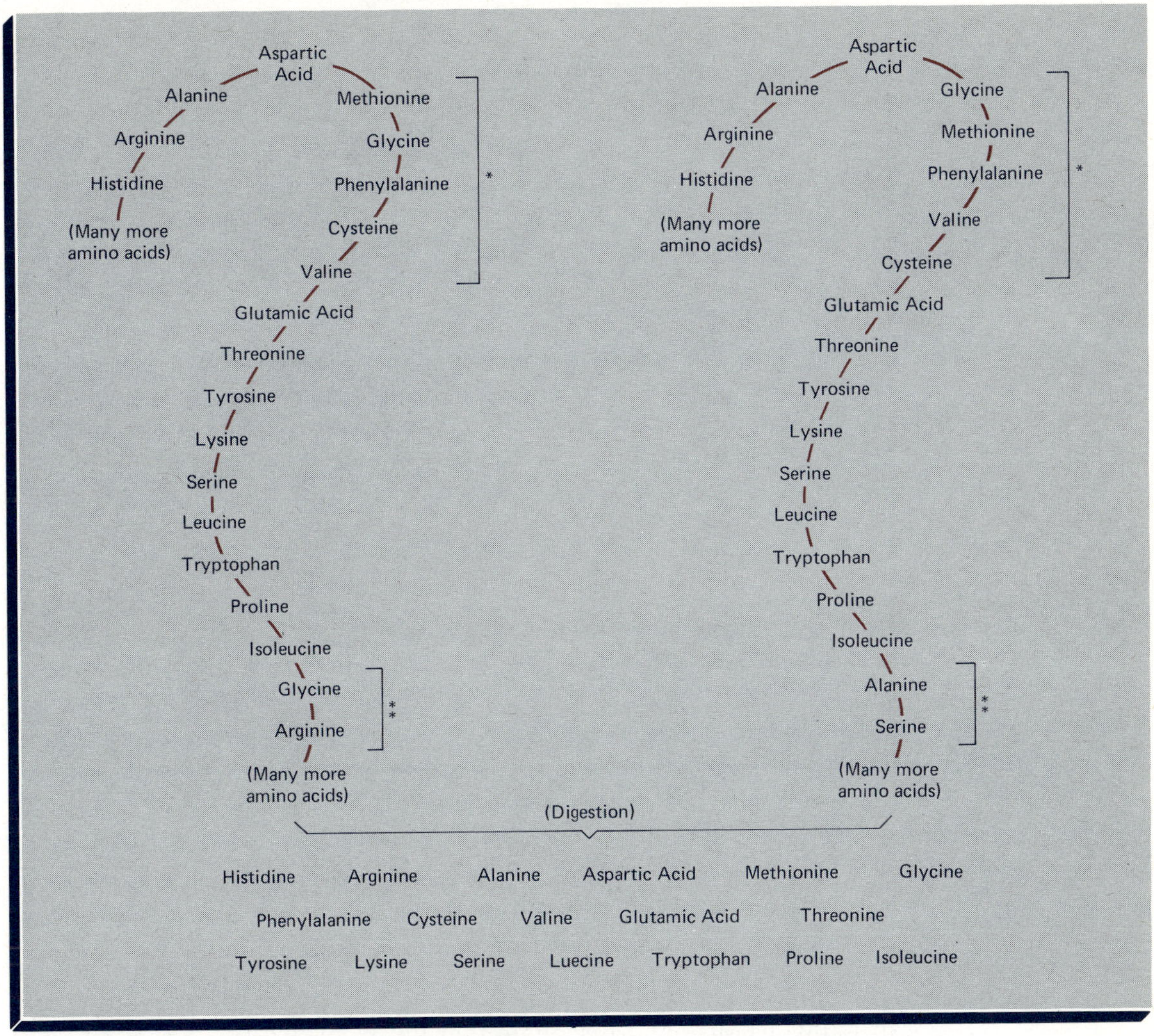

*Difference in sequence or order of amino acids along the chain.

**Difference in proportions of certain amino acids; the protein on the left has twice as much glycine and arginine, and half as much alanine and serine, as the protein on the right.

FIGURE 13–3. No specific protein can be essential in the diet.

PROTEIN QUALITY

Except for the presence of the essential amino acid, *lysine,* the two proteins represented in Figure 13–4 are identical in composition. One, however, is a *complete* protein, of high quality nutritionally, because it contains adequate amounts of all of the essential amino acids. The other is an *incomplete* protein in that it is lacking in the essential amino acid, lysine. In fact, the second protein is, by itself, no better than a protein that lacks several or even all of the essential amino acids. If amino acids are to be used for protein synthesis in the cells of the animal which consumed the protein, all of the amino acids from which the protein is to be constructed must be present at the same time.

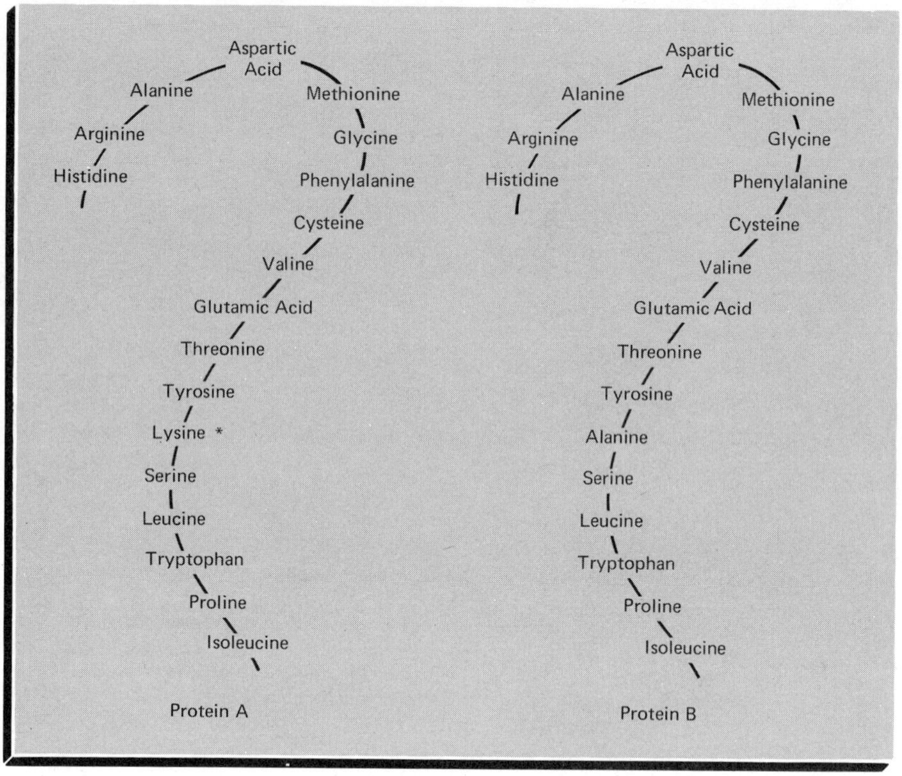

*Note presence of lysine in protein A but not in protein B.

FIGURE 13–4. Hypothetical examples of a complete protein and an incomplete protein. In reality, proteins are much longer amino acid chains than the ones shown here.

Otherwise, the problem is the same as that of a builder who is constructing a house and discovers that he is out of nails. Even if he has enough of all the other necessary materials, construction must halt until the nails become available. Similarly, cells cannot proceed to construct protein molecules unless all of the necessary amino acids are available.

As a general rule, proteins in foods of animal origin are complete, and proteins from foods of plant origin are incomplete. This is to be expected in view of the fact that humans are genetically much more similar to animals than to plants; because genes control protein structure, the proteins of animals are more likely than plant proteins are to contain amino acids in the proportions needed by humans. There are, however, a few notable exceptions to this general rule on protein quality. The amounts and kinds of proteins in nuts and in mature legumes are such that these foods are considered alternates to meats. But gelatin, which is derived from the connective tissues of animals, is so lacking in several essential amino acids that animals die if gelatin is the sole protein in their diets.

Different species of animals have qualitatively different requirements with respect to amino acids. The rat, for example, requires *arginine* and *histidine* in addition to the eight amino acids required by adult humans, and the chick requires *glycine* as well. By and large, however, nonhuman animals are quite similar to humans in being unable to synthesize sufficient amounts of a number of amino acids. Obviously, then, animals must ultimately obtain these essential amino acids from plants. Here we see an apparent paradox: plant proteins are the ultimate sources of essential amino acids, yet plant proteins are lacking in essential amino acids. In order to explain this seeming paradox, it is necessary to go back to the real beginning of protein synthesis: the nitrogen in the air and the simple nitrogen-containing compounds in the soil.

The nitrogen cycle and the carbon cycle

Unlike energy, which becomes useless for further work as it flows through a living system, various forms of matter are used in a cyclic manner. Each form of matter can be discussed in terms of a cycle whereby atoms repeatedly enter a living system and are returned to the environment. In the production of amino acids and proteins, two great cycles, that of carbon and that of nitrogen, are important (Figure 13–5).

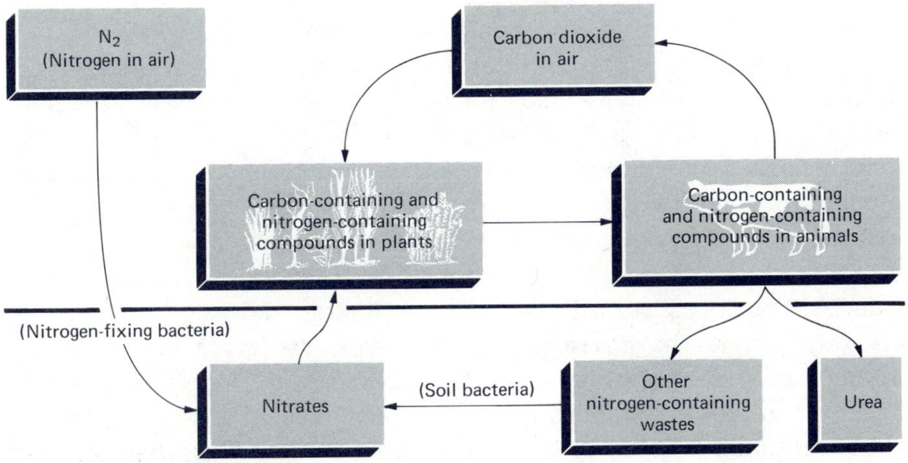

FIGURE 13–5. The nitrogen cycle and the carbon cycle.

Four-fifths of the air we breathe is nitrogen gas, but of all the organisms on earth only a few kinds of microorganisms can utilize nitrogen in this form. These organisms, soil bacteria in the earth and certain blue-green algae in aquatic environments, can convert atmospheric nitrogen to nitrogen-containing compounds which can then be utilized by green plants. Of the soil bacteria capable of this process, called *nitrogen-fixation,* some are capable of fixing nitrogen while living free in the soil. Others cannot fix nitrogen alone, but become able to do so in combination with cells in the roots of leguminous plants. Root nodules form where the nitrogen-fixing bacteria enter the roots, and the resulting legume cell–bacterial cell combination can fix up to 5 pounds of nitrogen per acre per year. It is for this reason that legumes such as peas and beans are sometimes planted on fields to increase their fertility. Indeed, before the development of modern chemical fertilizers, nitrogen fixed in this manner was very important in replenishing land that had been depleted of its nitrogen supply.

A great deal has been said and written of the supposed superiority of "organic fertilizers," such as compost or manure, to the inorganic forms of nitrogen supplied in commercial chemical fertilizers. Actually, organic nitrogen compounds must be broken down to inorganic forms before they can be used by plants. This breaking-down process is carried out by soil bacteria other than the nitrogen-fixers. All organic nitrogen-containing materials—those in the nitrogen-fixing bacteria, the urea excreted in the urine of animals, and the nitrogen-containing compounds in the bodies of dead plants and animals as well as in manure—are converted to ammonia. Ammonia is then converted to nitrates by still other bacteria, and it is in this inorganic form that nitrogen is finally absorbed by the roots of plants (Figure 13–5).

The plants then incorporate the nitrogen into amino acids, which are used for plant protein synthesis. Animals that eat the plants digest the proteins and use many of the liberated amino acids for synthesis of their own proteins. Sooner or later, the nitrogen returns to the earth in the form of organic compounds present in excretions or the bodies of dead organisms, and so the cycle goes on.

Through photosynthesis, green plants produce the carbon-containing parts of amino acids from carbon dioxide, absorbed directly from the air, and from water, absorbed from the soil, just as they manufacture all of their other organic compounds from these simple starting materials. As is true for nitrogen, carbon dioxide and water are eventually returned to the environment. However, the route back may be roundabout and lengthy because of the passage of organic compounds through complex metabolic cycles in the bodies of many organisms, which eat and are eaten in turn. As long as animals live, they convert energy nutrients to carbon dioxide and water; and after they die, the energy nutrients present in their bodies at the moment of death are broken down to the same end products by bacteria.

To a green plant, there is no such thing as an essential amino acid. This is reasonable in view of the fact that these organisms are rooted in the soil, on which they are dependent for their nutrients. A green plant which lost the ability to synthesize one or more amino acids could not move to a new environment in which the amino acid might be present; it would simply perish. Therefore, green plants must synthesize *all* of the amino acids, including those which are essential to animals. The reason that plant proteins are incomplete is not that they are totally devoid of essential amino acids, but rather that plant proteins generally contain small amounts of essential amino acids compared to the quantities needed by animals. This is of course of no concern to the plant, which synthesizes proteins in accordance with its own needs for survival and not for the purpose of providing food needed by animals.

When plant proteins are eaten by an animal, the amino acids are made available for synthesis of proteins in the animal's cells. However, the proteins the animal produces generally contain a much higher proportion of essential amino acids than did the ingested plant proteins. This difference is possible because animal cells use most of the plant's sparsely distributed essential amino acids for protein synthesis, and oxidize most of the excess nonessential amino acids as energy sources (Figure 13–6). In effect, then, a plant-eating animal acts as a concentrating mechanism, retaining a larger proportion of the essential amino acids than of the nonessential ones. The proteins in foods of animal origin, including eggs and milk as well as flesh, are therefore complete, and are said to be of high biological value, because they supply adequate amounts of essential amino acids.

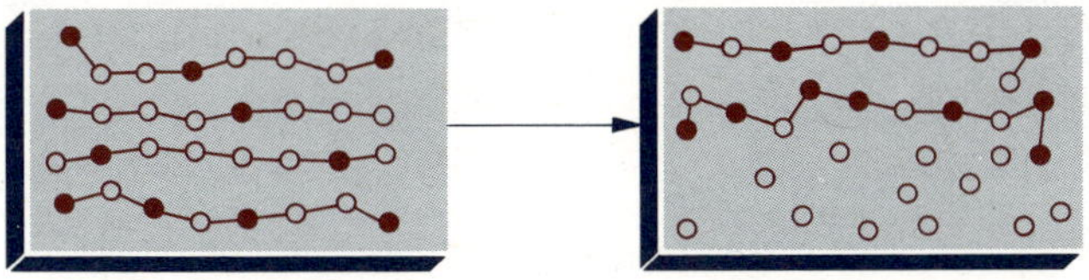

FIGURE 13–6. An animal concentrates the essential amino acids obtained from plants.

USES OF AMINO ACIDS IN THE BODY

The general features of amino acid metabolism are shown in Figure 13–7. The use of amino acids as energy sources is generally the least important aspect of their metabolism, for fats and carbohydrates can be used for this purpose as well. Under certain circumstances, however, amino acids are very important as energy sources. This is the case whenever the intake of carbohydrate is severely curtailed, as during starvation or when diets consist almost entirely of low-carbohydrate foods. At these times, the stores of glycogen in the body are soon exhausted, and the level of glucose in the blood would decrease to a

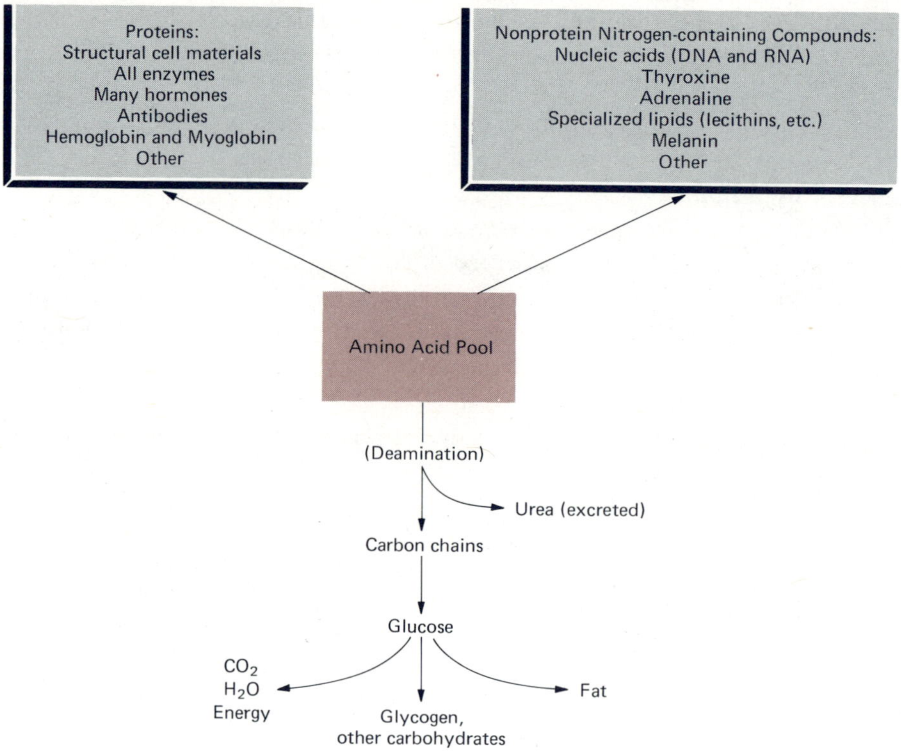

FIGURE 13–7. The overall picture of amino acid metabolism.

dangerously low value if some other materials could not be converted to glucose. Fats cannot be used for glucose synthesis because one very important step in metabolism—the conversion of pyruvic acid to acetic acid—is essentially irreversible. Therefore, amino acids are the only materials that can provide a continuing glucose supply in the absence of dietary carbohydrate.

Amino acids are also utilized for the production of a number of important biochemicals which, although they contain nitrogen, are not proteins. Examples are the nucleic acids, DNA and RNA; the skin and hair pigment, melanin; the hormones, adrenaline and thyroxine; and the specialized nitrogen-containing lipids in the membranes of cells. However, the principal function of amino acids in cells is protein synthesis. Under the control of the genes, cells put amino acids together in certain preordained sequences to form the particular protein structures needed. Temporary lack of a nonessential amino acid is generally no problem to the cell. It simply produces the necessary amino acid; the carbon chain can be made from glucose, and the nitrogen-containing amino group can be donated by any of a number of amino acids present in excess of what is needed for immediate use. This assumes, of course, that the *total* supply of amino acids—nonessential as well as essential—is adequate to donate amino groups as needed.

However, if one of the *essential* amino acids is missing, the situation is very different. Because an essential amino acid is one that the organism *cannot* synthesize in amounts sufficient to meet its needs, protein synthesis is curtailed if an essential amino acid is lacking. The cell cannot decide simply to omit the missing amino acids from the structure of the finished protein molecule, for protein structure is dictated by the genes. Protein structures are synthesized according to genetic directions, or they are not synthesized at all.

Figure 13–8 shows an example of the synthesis of a nonessential amino acid. Pyruvic acid serves as the carbon chain of the amino acid,

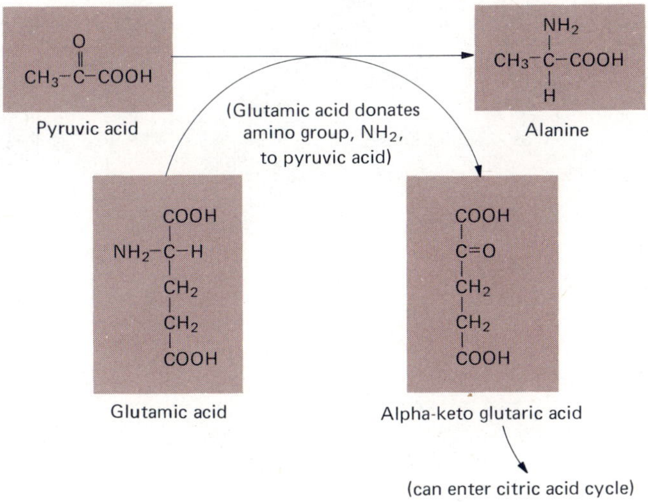

FIGURE 13–8. The synthesis of a nonessential amino acid.

alanine; by means of similar reactions, many other compounds produced during metabolism can accept amino groups from any of a number of amino acids, forming other amino acids. The reason that some amino acids are essential, then, is that cells are incapable of producing some of the organic compounds (carbon chains) which, if present, could accept an amino group and thereby become an amino acid. Green plants have the ability to produce *all* of the carbon chains needed for amino acid synthesis, whereas animals, through gene mutations, have lost the ability to produce a number of them.

When the necessary complement of amino acids is present, as it is in the normal well-nourished organism, synthesis of protein molecules proceeds at a rate that is almost beyond belief. The swiftness of protein synthesis during periods of rapid growth is fairly obvious; less generally appreciated is the rate at which proteins are built up to keep pace with their continuous breakdown in the body. For example, in order to replace the hemoglobin molecules degraded as the result of

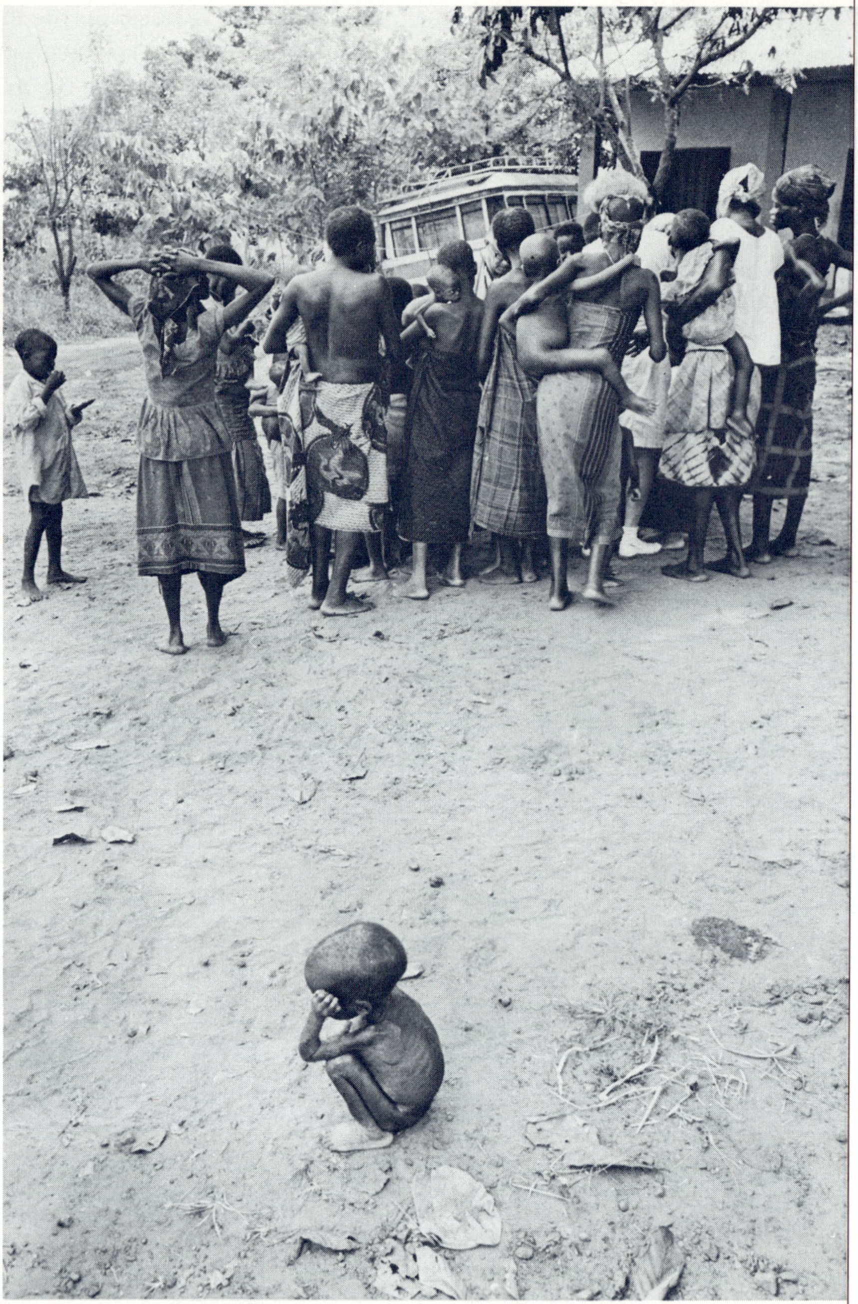

FIGURE 13–9
An all-too-typical victim of Kwashiorkor. (UNICEF photo by R. Farquharson.)

normal red blood cell destruction, the average adult human must synthesize approximately *50 billion billion* molecules of hemoglobin daily.

FUNCTIONS OF PROTEINS IN THE BODY

Practically everything outwardly visible in an animal—skin, hair or fur, nails or claws, scales, feathers—is largely protein. Inside the body as well, protein makes up a major part of all structures; the matrix or framework of bones consists largely of the connective-tissue protein, *collagen,* and proteins are found dissolved in cells and body fluids, as well as in the *mitochondra, endoplasmic reticulum,* and other organized structures within cells. In fact, proteins collectively constitute the principal structural solids of animals, accounting for approximately one-sixth of the total weight of the average person.

Enzymes, which are all proteins, catalyze the biochemical reactions in cells; hormones, many of which are proteins, act to regulate and integrate biological processes; antibodies, special protein molecules generated in response to foreign proteins, combat infectious microorganisms or neutralize the toxins they produce. Proteins in the bloodstream assist in regulating fluid balance by controlling the passage of water across the walls of blood vessels; if these plasma proteins are greatly reduced in concentration, fluid leaves the blood vessels and accumulates in tissue spaces, resulting in a condition known as *edema.*

Certain uses of proteins and amino acids in the body have higher priority than others. Thus, one of the first signs of protein deprivation is lack of growth in the young, because synthesis of new protoplasm is less important to survival than maintenance of tissues already present. If protein deficiency is severe and prolonged enough, cells of various organs are broken down and their proteins degraded in order to make amino acids available for the synthesis of those proteins with highest priority. Although the loss of muscle tissue is outwardly most obvious, internal organs such as the liver, kidneys, and heart are also decreased in size during prolonged protein deprivation. The brain is the organ most resistant to change in size. This phenomenon, known as "brain sparing," protects that organ—which is most vital to life—at the expense of other organs.

Kwashiorkor is the disease resulting from extreme protein deficiency (Figure 13–9). The term was derived from an African word meaning "first-second" or "displaced," because the disease most commonly develops soon after a young child is displaced from the breast, often because of the mother's next pregnancy. Displacement from the breast does not create a serious problem in developed countries, because many excellent protein sources other than human milk are available. In many developing countries, however, alternative high-quality protein sources are either unavailable or are by custom not given to the young. The foods considered suitable for a young child, although commonly adequate as energy sources, may be lacking as to both quality and quantity of protein. The observed effects of such a diet are clearly related to the functions of proteins, as follows:

1 Growth failure, in both weight and height, is one of the earliest signs, and tissues already present become wasted or atrophied.
2 Edema, resulting from abnormal fluid balance, is sometimes so extensive that the child's weight may be normal despite the great reduction in the size of muscles and other tissues.
3 The skin becomes very flaky and dry and loses its normal pigmentation, presumably because of impaired production of melanin. The hair may also become scanty and lighter in color.
4 Behavioral changes develop, and the child may become too profoundly apathetic to show any of the curiosity characteristic of normal children.
5 Appetite is decreased and digestion is impaired; the diarrhea and vomiting which frequently result may precipitate an even more severe degree of malnutrition.
6 The ability to combat infection is drastically lowered, probably as the result of impaired antibody synthesis. This can tip the balance between survival and death, because diseases which healthy children can withstand may prove fatal to a victim of kwashiorkor.

The treatment of advanced cases of kwashiorkor can be a difficult medical problem because of the resulting severe damage to many organs. However, the *prevention* of protein deficiency is almost entirely a matter of applying the nutritional knowledge which already exists.

MEETING THE NEED FOR PROTEIN

One way to insure that the protein intake is adequate in both quantity and quality is through diets similar to those consumed in countries such as the United States. Even the minimum number of servings of foods recommended by the Basic Four Plan provides much more protein than the average person actually needs, as shown in Figure 13–10. The quality of the protein is also excellent because a large proportion comes from foods of animal origin.

However, the fact that the American diet provides such an abundance of protein does not necessarily make it a practical means of meeting protein needs throughout the world. In cultures that forbid the eating of flesh, as well as perhaps eggs and milk, the American diet would not be acceptable. In many other cultures, these foods may be acceptable and to some degree available, but may be economically beyond the reach of most of the population. Although it is hoped that the economic development of these nations will eventually allow their people to obtain more protein from foods of animal origin, this is not likely for some time in the future.

However, a number of ways have been devised to improve diets

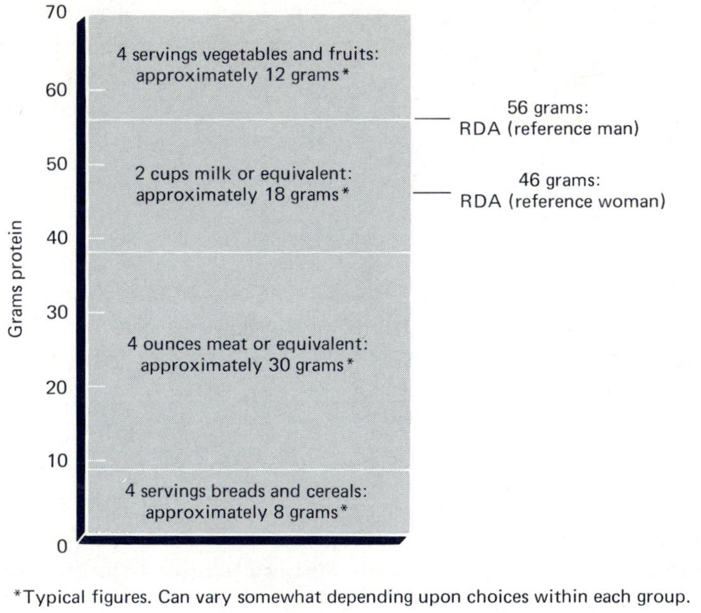

FIGURE 13–10. Protein furnished by the Basic Four Plan.

both as to quality and quantity of protein without increased use of foods of animal origin. Some of these methods increase the total amount of food available and are therefore valuable in solving the problem of energy deprivation as well as the problem of protein deficiency, whereas others are useful in improving protein intake specifically, but have little impact on the remaining problem of calorie undernutrition.

Simulated foods

Simulated meats are already being used to a limited extent in the United States. These are made by spinning plant proteins, such as those from soybeans, into fibers which can be shaped, colored, and flavored so as to resemble beef, chicken, or other meats. Because the proteins of soybeans compare favorably in biological value to the proteins of animal tissues, it is possible to produce a suitable meat substitute without the use of livestock. Converting plant products directly to artificial "meat" is much more efficient than feeding plants to animals, which use much of their feed for maintenance and convert only a small proportion to edible products.

Simulated dairy products can also be used in place of products traditionally derived from livestock. The most familiar example in the developed countries is oleomargarine, which competes very successfully with butter; other imitation dairy products include whipped toppings and coffee whiteners used as substitutes for cream. However, none of these is a significant protein source. It is therefore in the development of milk substitutes that food technology has made its most valuable contribution to nutrition. A variety of beverages based on plant proteins but having the nutritional value of milk are currently being produced in developing countries. Some are intended to be used as milk is, primarily in the diets of infants and children; others are sweetened and flavored so as to be used as soft drinks by people of all ages.

Genetically improved crops

Although many foods of plant origin contain reasonably good *quantities* of protein, the *quality* is commonly poor because one or more of the essential amino acids is lacking. The proteins of grains, for example, contain very little lysine; corn is, to a lesser extent, also deficient in tryptophan. People who depend heavily upon corn as a staple food are therefore likely to lack these two amino acids. In the 1960s, high-lysine corn was developed by selective breeding of mutants which contained unusually high lysine levels. Research with other grains has shown that the quality of protein in wheat and rice can also be improved by selectively breeding those genetic varieties which produce the highest levels of the most limited amino acids.

The total *quantity* of protein in plants can also be improved by selective breeding. Generally this is a matter of increasing the yield of edible food per plant, as for example the number of grains of rice on a single stalk. However, in other cases, selective breeding results in faster-maturing plants, allowing two crops to be grown in the time formerly required for one. If all of the desirable qualities that have already been developed in different varieties of the same plant—high yield, increased protein content, and better protein quality—could be incorporated into a single variety, the resulting plant could be of tremendous value in improving nutritional status with respect to protein.

Fortification of foods with amino acids

Amino acids, like other organic compounds, can be synthesized in the laboratory at very little expense. Thus it is feasible to improve the nutritional value of foods such as grains by adding the amino acids which are not naturally present in adequate amounts. One advantage of this method over the genetic improvement of crops is that it can be done with the technology available now, whereas genetic improvement requires years of painstaking crossbreeding experiments. Adding the necessary small amount of synthetic lysine to a ton of wheat costs only a few dollars, and greatly improves the suitability of wheat as the principal source of dietary protein. It does not, however, significantly increase the total quantity of protein in the diet.

Combination of foods containing incomplete proteins

Still another approach is to combine foods that contain incomplete proteins so that the shortcomings of one are offset by the strengths of another. This method takes advantage of the *supplementary value* of various incomplete proteins. One of the best-known examples of a product resulting from this approach is *Incaparina,* developed at the Institute of Nutrition of Central America and Panama, or INCAP. At a cost of only a few cents per day, Incaparina can prevent and treat protein deficiency in infants and children as effectively as milk or meat can. The low cost is possible because Incaparina is made from the indigenous plant products corn, sorghum, and cottonseed meal, with yeast, vitamin A, and calcium added in order to make the mineral and vitamin content the same as that of milk.

A similar approach is the use of *small* amounts of foods of animal origin in combination with *large* amounts of foods of plant origin. For example, the proteins of grains are particularly low in lysine, which the proteins of foods of animal origin contain in abundance. Therefore, eating a cereal food with even a small amount of milk, meat, or eggs in the same meal can result in a vastly improved pattern of amino acids and, consequently, in much better utilization of the amino acids of grains, without any loss in quality of the animal proteins.

DETERMINING PROTEIN REQUIREMENTS

The most common approach to determining the amount of protein needed is the method known as the *nitrogen balance* determination. The principles are similar to those of an energy balance determination in that the difference between intake and output is studied. Of course, in the nitrogen balance method actual chemicals are studied, whereas in an energy balance study the intake and output of units of energy are determined. In order to determine nitrogen balance, two things must be found: the amount of nitrogen in the diet, and the amounts of nitrogen-containing compounds subsequently excreted in the urine and feces. The output is then subtracted from the intake. Small amounts of nitrogen-containing materials are lost via routes other than urine and feces, for instance, through the growth of hair and the sloughing off of cells from the surface of the skin. However, these amounts are generally small enough to be ignored in a nitrogen balance study.

If intake is just enough to replace losses from the body, the subject is said to be in *nitrogen balance,* or equilibrium. If intake is greater than output, balance is positive, indicating a net gain of body protein. If intake is less than output, balance is negative, indicating that intake is too low to meet the individual's needs and that a net loss of body protein is occurring.

FACTORS THAT ALTER THE NEED FOR PROTEIN

The amount of protein required by a given individual depends upon a number of factors, as follows:

1 **Adaptation.** People have some ability to adapt to a low protein intake over a long period of time, via metabolic adjustments which allow limited supplies of amino acids to be used more efficiently than when the supply is generous.

2 **Quality of dietary protein.** A protein of low nutritional quality, lacking relatively, or absolutely, in one or more essential amino acids, cannot be used efficiently for protein synthesis in cells. A large proportion of the amino acids are therefore useful only as energy sources unless the protein is supplemented with another which contains the lacking amino acids.

3 **Total energy value of the diet.** If energy intake is *very* low, as during "crash" dieting, a disproportionate number of amino acids will be used as energy sources, and the amounts available for protein synthesis will be correspondingly decreased.

4 **Carbohydrate content of the diet.** Even if the *total* energy value of the diet is sufficient, increased amounts of amino acids will be converted to glucose if the carbohydrate intake is not sufficient to maintain normal blood glucose levels.

5 **Previous protein undernutrition.** If tissues have become wasted or atrophied as the result of previous protein deficiency, protein is required to replace these tissues, in addition to that needed to maintain those present.

6 **Growth.** During infancy, childhood, and adolescence, gain in body weight represents an increase in protoplasm as well as an increase in fat; of the protoplasm gained during growth, approximately one-sixth consists of proteins.

7 **Pregnancy.** Extra protein is required during pregnancy for the growth of the fetus and placenta, as well as for maternal tissues such as increased breast tissue.

8 **Lactation.** Extra dietary protein is required to replace that lost in the milk. The amount of protein is approximately 10 to 15 grams daily in the average lactating woman.

9 **Stress.** During prolonged stress, people commonly secrete increased amounts of *corticoids,* hormones that stimulate the enzymatic breakdown of amino acids to glucose and urea. Increased protein intake is necessary to compensate for this increased enzyme activity.

10 **Certain drugs.** Compounds such as *cortisol,* a *glucocorticoid* used medically in the treatment of diseases such as arthritis, increase the breakdown of amino acids exactly as do endogenously produced glucocorticoids.

11 **Kidney disease.** Amino acids in excess of actual needs are used as energy sources, and urea is produced from the amino groups. Because the kidneys must excrete urea, a high protein intake must be *avoided* by people whose kidney function has been impaired, as through disease.

12 **Major surgery and extensive burns.** Surgery and burns increase the need for protein to support the necessary synthesis of new tissue formed in healing.

The RDA for protein is set high enough to cover the increased needs associated with many of these factors. However, the needs of some individuals, such as those receiving glucocorticoid therapy or recovering from surgery, burns, or previous malnutrition, may not be met by the protein intake recommended for the majority of normal people. Special dietary treatment under medical supervision is required in these special cases.

PROTEIN FALLACIES

Some common misconceptions people have about dietary protein are these.

The flavor of protein. Pure proteins are completely tasteless. Thus, although many people assume that the flavor of meat is because of its high protein content, meat flavor is largely the result of the fat, in which are found various organic flavor components, none of which are proteins.

The high protein content of foods that taste "meaty." This idea may have originated from the common hospital practice of serving meat-flavored hot beverages, such as broth and boullion, to convalescing patients. Although these drinks provide fluid and salts, as well as comfort, as a source of protein they are of little value; 1 cup provides only about 1 gram of protein.

The superiority of meat proteins over those of eggs and milk. Many people believe that the proteins of meats have greater nutritional value than those of any other foods of animal origin. Actually, the nutritional quality of egg proteins is somewhat greater than that of meat proteins, and the value of milk proteins is approximately the same as that of meats. An all-meat weiner may be more expensive than one "adulterated" with dry milk solids, but it is no better as a protein source.

The superiority of "red meat" proteins. Although the color of red meat may suggest life, vigor, and masculinity more than white does, proteins from white meats such as fish and poultry have the same nutritional value as the proteins in the most masculine looking slab of beef.

The necessity of white meats for invalids. White meats and red meats are digested with equal ease and efficiency, and there is therefore no advantage in one or the other for invalids or others who are assumed to have a "delicate" digestive system.

Meat proteins and aggressiveness. A good many vegetarians believe that people become more spiritual and gentle by avoiding proteins from animal sources, especially from meats. In some Eastern religions, reverence for life is associated with both control of aggressive behavior and a ban on the use of animals for food. However, the writings of such famous vegetarians as George Bernard Shaw testify to the lack of any relationship between vegetarianism and gentleness.

"Necrones" from meat proteins. Although few people take this seriously today, the idea keeps cropping up in food faddists' writings. Necrones were once believed to be poisonous materials resulting from the breakdown of meat proteins by bacteria in the colon, and absorp-

TABLE 13–2

Protein content of a typical lacto-ovo-vegetarian diet

	Approximate protein content (grams)
Bread and cereal group	
Enriched white bread, 3 slices	6
Enriched white rice, cooked, ½ cup	2
Meat group	
Egg, 1 medium	6
Cheese, cheddar, 1 ounce	7
Peanut butter, 2 tablespoons	8
Cooked dried navy beans, ½ cup	8
Milk group	
Whole milk, 2 cups	18
Vegetable and fruit group	
Apple, 1 medium	trace
Carrot, 1 medium	1
Orange, 1 medium	1
Potato, boiled, 1 medium	2
Total	59

From "Home and Garden Bulletin No. 72," USDA, Washington, D.C., 1970.

tion of these toxins was believed to be the cause of headaches and other discomforts.

Protein intake and athletic performance. There is no question that athletic ability is impaired by actual protein deficiency, and that a *small* amount of extra dietary protein is required in order for muscles to enlarge during prolonged physical training. However, exercise does not "break down the muscles," because glycogen and fat are the main sources of energy used for muscle contraction. The enormous protein intakes commonly advocated for athletes may be of *psychological* value, in that they make the athlete feel important and deserving of special treatment. However, rituals such as the pregame steak for breakfast could not possibly have any *physiological* effect on an athlete's performance, although the sight of a big chunk of almost-raw meat might well suggest inflicting injury on one's opponents.

Protein intake and physically demanding work. Heavy labor of any kind, such as that performed by lumberjacks or construction workers, has no more effect on protein requirements than athletic activity has. Nevertheless, people in such occupations often have strong ideas regarding the amounts of meat proteins needed to support the heavy work of a "real man." Woe be to the wife who offers such a man a diet providing just enough protein to meet his physiologic needs alone.

The "slenderizing" effect of high-protein diets. A large number of people believe that high-protein foods, especially meats, are very low in energy value compared to those "fattening" less expensive carbohydrates. Even if lean meats were low in fat—and they are not—

protein itself furnishes 4 kilocalories per gram, just as carbohydrates do. Although it is true that obesity is commonly associated with high carbohydrate intakes and low income, this appears to be related to educational and motivational factors, not to the need of low-income people to depend on supposedly "fattening" foods of high carbohydrate content and low price.

The "slenderizing" effect of *low*-protein diets. Low-protein diets for "taking inches off" have actually been advocated by a writer who also advocated high-protein diets for losing weight. The writer contended that high protein intakes cause one to lose *fat,* whereas low protein diets reduce "protein bulges" by forcing one to "pull fat out" of muscles. This diet is alleged to supply plenty of protein to maintain vigor and health, and merely avoid *excess* protein intake. However, if you were to examine the diet, you would find that dried legumes, cheeses, milk, poultry, fish, shellfish, meats, and eggs are *all* on the list of forbidden foods. The sample menus that are given provide only a small fraction of the RDA for protein and, in addition, the proteins are of low quality nutritionally. Although a healthy adult would probably not be harmed by following such a diet for a period of days or perhaps even weeks, long-term use of such a plan could not possibly be recommended. In addition, the plan causes weight loss only because it is a low-energy, as well as a low-protein, diet. Sample "inches-off" menus typically provide only some 500 to 600 kilocalories daily, forcing the body to use most of the limited protein intake as fuel.

Gelatin to strengthen fingernails. The belief that eating or drinking unflavored gelatin strengthens the nails is based on the following line of reasoning: gelatin is 100 percent protein; nails consist largely of protein; therefore gelatin will be used to build nails. Actually, the amino acids in gelatin are very unsuitable for building fingernails. Gelatin is derived from collagen, a connective tissue protein with a very low content of sulfur-containing amino acids, whereas the main protein found in nails is *keratin,* which has an unusually high content of sulfur-containing amino acids. Gelatin is therefore of very little value for synthesis of body proteins of any kind, and of even less value for producing the proteins in fingernails specifically.

PROTEIN INTAKE AND VEGETARIANISM

Americans are so accustomed to eating meat every day that people who choose vegetarianism are considered decidedly strange, and probably in danger of poor health. However, it is important to distinguish the several distinct types of diets consumed by those who may consider themselves vegetarians:

Nonmeat eaters. Many of these people do not really avoid all forms of flesh, just those derived from mammals, such as beef and pork.

If they accept fish, shellfish, and perhaps poultry as well, they are under no nutritional disadvantage, because in fact they are not really vegetarians.

Lacto-ovo vegetarians. These people accept milk and eggs, but reject all forms of flesh.

Lacto-vegetarians. To these people, milk is the only permissible animal-derived food; eggs, because they are considered a potential form of flesh, are shunned, as are all forms of actual flesh.

Vegans. The strictest of the vegetarians, vegans eschew milk as well as eggs and flesh, on the basis that milk is obtained by robbing the calf of its rightful food and therefore represents potential flesh, just as eggs do.

The diets of lacto-ovo-vegetarians can rather easily provide protein which is adequate in both quality and quantity (Table 13–2). The same is true of lacto-vegetarian diets, especially if larger amounts of milk are used to compensate for the absence of any other foods of animal origin. Vegans, however, may have a problem in getting protein of sufficient quantity, to say nothing of the problem of protein quality. A vegan who is willing to learn about the amino acid composition of foods may be able to avoid these problems by combining plant proteins of supplementary value. However, because several vitamins and minerals, as well as protein, are often lacking in the diets of vegans, low protein intake is far from the only nutritional problem seen in these individuals. In any event, many vegans seem to be primarily concerned with the "spirituality" of the diet, dismissing the scientific aspects of nutrition as irrelevant. For these reasons, even nutritionists who approve of other well-planned types of vegetarian diets generally draw the line at vegan diets, which reject all foods of animal origin.

SUGGESTED READINGS

"Amino Acid Content of Foods and Biological Data on Proteins." United Nations: FAO Nutritional Studies No. 24, Rome, 1970.

Dwyer, J. T., L. D. V. H. Mayer, R. F. Kandel, and J. Mayer. "The New Vegetarians: Who Are They?" *Journal of the American Dietetic Association* 62 (1973):503.

Handbook on Human Nutritional Requirements. FAO/WHO, Rome, 1974.

Hardy, R. W. F. and U. D. Havelka. "Nitrogen Fixation Research: A Key to World Food?" *Science* 188 (1975):633.

Harper, A. E., P. R. Payne, and J. C. Waterlow. "Assessment of Human Protein Needs." *American Journal of Clinical Nutrition* 26 (1973):1168.

"Nutrition for Athletes." American Association for Health, Physical Education, and Recreation. Washington, D.C., 1971.

14

carbohydrates and fats

Because the worst aspects of carbohydrates and fats are usually the most newsworthy, what is written and believed about them is largely negative. Fats and carbohydrates are therefore credited with more than their fair share of detrimental effects on health. These greatly underrated nutrients deserve a much better reputation than they have, for they actually serve a number of useful functions.

The characteristics carbohydrates and fats have in common are as follows:

They are energy nutrients; 1 gram of fat supplies 9 kilocalories, and 1 gram of carbohydrate supplies 4 kilocalories. In this regard, they are similar to proteins, which also furnish energy.

They are composed of carbon, hydrogen, and oxygen and, in metabolism, are completely oxidized to carbon dioxide and water. This distinguishes them from proteins, because amino acid metabolism results in the production of urea as well as carbon dioxide and water.

The National Research Council has never set a Recommended Die-

FIGURE 14–1. Nutritionally significant carbohydrates.

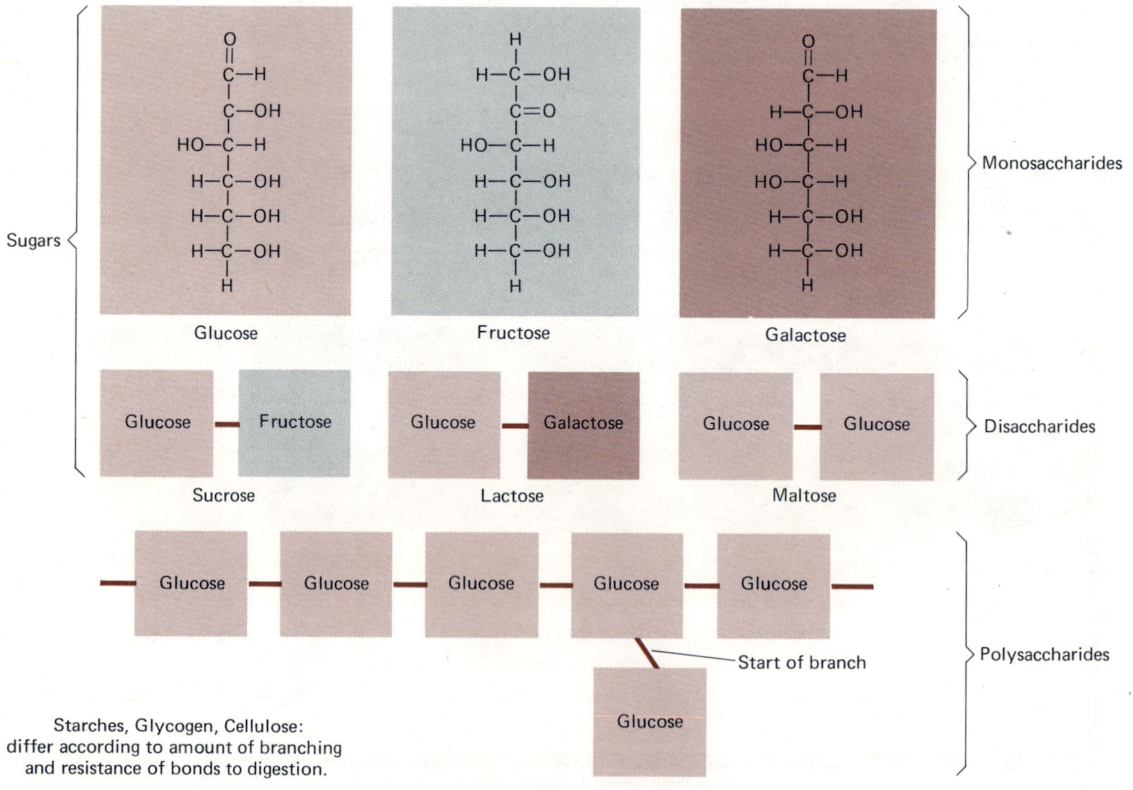

tary Allowance for either fat or carbohydrate, in contrast to dietary protein. The reason is that, given an adequate supply of protein, you can vary carbohydrate and fat intake within wide limits to obtain the rest of your total energy intake in accordance with your preferences. Typically, an American diet furnishes about half of its total energy from carbohydrates, somewhat over one-third from fats, and approximately one-sixth from proteins.

Besides having certain characteristics in common, fats and carbohydrates differ sharply from each other in several respects. These unique features will be emphasized in the following discussion.

CARBOHYDRATES IN FOODS

Carbohydrates, it will be recalled, exist in foods as sugars and polysaccharides (Figure 14–1). The polysaccharides, starch and cellulose, are present in practically all foods of plant origin: grains, legumes, vegetables, and fruits. Although sugars are generally found in smaller amounts than polysaccharides are, the sugar content of milk and of many fruits is great enough to impart a decidedly sweet taste to these. In fact, meats and eggs are the only common foods that are virtually free of carbohydrates, and the small amount of carbohydrate present is mostly glycogen.

It is, of course, easy to increase the amount of carbohydrate to far above that which is present in a food as it is harvested, as when sugar is added for flavor. Presweetened breakfast cereals, for example, may actually contain more sugar than cereal; and even if the processor has not presweetened the cereal, the consumer may sprinkle sugar with such a heavy hand that the end result is the same.

Although much has been written about the supposed nutritional advantages of "natural" sugars over refined table sugar, in reality the only advantage of sugars found naturally in foods is the limited amounts in which they occur. This makes it much more difficult to eat excess amounts of natural sugars than to eat excess table sugar, which is relatively inexpensive and readily available. Of course, natural sugars in fruits and milk are *accompanied* by the minerals, vitamins, proteins, and other nutrients in these foods. However, this is a nutritional advantage of the whole foods, not of the sugars they contain. A given amount of a natural sugar has the same effects as an equal amount of refined sugar in furnishing energy and in contributing to any associated health problems.

People often assume that brown sugar, which is less highly refined than white sugar, must contain large amounts of certain vitamins and minerals (as brown rice contains more nutrients than *unenriched* white rice does). However, the substances that give brown sugar its color are largely impurities of no nutritional significance, and the nutrient content of both brown and white sugar is trivial (Table 14–1).

TABLE 14–1
Nutrient content of white sugar and brown sugar

	White sugar, one tablespoon	Brown sugar, one tablespoon
Kilocalories	45	50
Protein (grams)	0	0
Vitamin A value (IU)	0	0
Calcium (milligrams)	0	12
Iron (milligrams)	Trace	0.5
Thiamin (milligrams)	0	Trace
Riboflavin (milligrams)	0	Trace
Niacin (milligrams)	–	Trace
Vitamin C (milligrams)	0	0

Note: The supposed nutritional value of brown sugar and of "natural" sweets such as honey is unimpressive when nutrient contents are examined. For example, an adult could meet the RDA for calcium by eating a mere 66 tablespoons (over 2 pounds) of brown sugar—but look what would happen to energy intake.
From "Home and Garden Bulletin No. 72," *USDA*, Washington, D.C., 1970.

TABLE 14–2
Energy values of different types of milk

Type of milk	Amount	Energy (kilocalories)
Whole, fluid, 3.5% fat	1 cup	160
Nonfat (skim)	1 cup	90
Partly skimmed, 2% nonfat milk solids added	1 cup	145

From "Home and Garden Bulletin No. 72," *USDA*, Washington, D.C., 1970.

FATS IN FOODS

In contrast to carbohydrates, found in large amounts in the less expensive foods of plant origin, fats are abundant in foods of animal origin. Practically all meats contain considerable fat, whether it can be seen or not; even very lean beef, broiled so as to allow much of the fat to drip out, may be one-tenth fat or more. Certainly you can *decrease* the intake of fat by cutting away all of the visible fat, but the resulting meat is still far from fat-free. The same holds true for eggs; although boiled or poached eggs have a lower fat content than eggs fried or scrambled in fat, the egg itself, prepared without any fat, is almost one-eighth fat.

The one common food of animal origin that can be made virtually fat-free is milk. Whole milk is approximately 3.5 percent fat (much lower than many consumers believe; people commonly guess 10, 20, or even 30 percent). Skim milk, from which as much fat as possible has been removed, is the lowest-calorie form of milk available, whether in fluid form or as powder reconstituted by adding water. Other "low fat" milks may contain varying amounts of fat, and the energy value of these can vary accordingly (Table 14–2). Two percent milk is produced by removing approximately half of the fat from whole milk. A very common assumption is that the energy value of 2 percent milk must be approximately half of that of whole milk. This is incorrect, because it is half of the *fat*—not half of the total energy nutrients—which has been removed. In addition, dry skim-milk solids are commonly added to improve the palatability of low-fat milks; the lactose and proteins of these added solids raise the energy value of 2 percent milk almost up to the original level of whole milk.

Unlike sugars, which are easily tasted even in small amounts, fats can be added to foods in surprisingly large amounts without being detected. Consequently, total fat—the sum of naturally present fat plus that added in food preparation—can easily provide over 40 percent of the total energy in a diet. This does not mean that over 40 percent of the total *weight* of energy nutrients consists of fat. Because 1 gram of fat furnishes more than twice the energy of a gram of carbohydrate or protein, fats can account for only about one-fourth of the total weight of energy nutrients although furnishing over 40 percent of the total energy intake. People sometimes find it difficult to believe that 35 to 40 percent or more of their energy comes from fat, but it is nevertheless true for most of the people of developed countries.

Most foods of plant origin—grains, vegetables, fruits, and legumes—are low in fat content at harvest. For example, only about one one-thousandth of the weight of a potato consists of fat. However, by the time it has been fried, mashed with milk and butter or margarine, or glorified with sour cream, butter, and/or margarine at the table, the fat content can easily be a hundred times as great as it was originally. Therefore, although plant products are generally low in fat as they are obtained from nature, they are commonly *made* rich in fat as a result of people's food habits.

ARE CARBOHYDRATES AND FATS ESSENTIAL?

No one specific carbohydrate is essential in the diet. In fact, it is possible to adapt to a diet which contains virtually no carbohydrates, as native Eskimos have done. However, if not obtained in the diet, glucose must be derived from amino acids, which are obtained by breaking proteins down. Economically, the use of protein as an energy source is analogous to using furniture as firewood.

Those adapted to the usual American diet require approximately 100 grams of carbohydrate per day to prevent undesirable metabolic effects such as excessive protein breakdown. However, any starch or sugar, and not any one particular carbohydrate, serves well for this purpose. Because one hundred grams is less than a third of the amount of carbohydrate most Americans eat daily, it appears that few people need worry about the possibility of getting too little carbohydrate.

Fats, like carbohydrates, exert a "protein-sparing effect"; that is, they spare protein from the fate of being burned as fuel. Any kind of fat can be used for this purpose: meat fats, milk fats, vegetable fats, and so on. However, as was explained in the discussions of metabolism and of energy, fat *cannot* be converted to glucose to any significant degree. It thus cannot spare protein from being, to some extent, sacrificed as necessary in the service of the brain, which specifically requires glucose as an energy source.

Also, unlike carbohydrates, fats contain one specific component which the body cannot synthesize in sufficient amounts. This essential substance is a fatty acid called *linoleic acid.* At this point, it is necessary to define certain terms that are familiar to the public because of advertising. Among these terms, the most familiar is probably "polyunsaturated."

FATS AND OILS, SATURATED AND OTHERWISE

Both fats and oils are *triglycerides;* that is, they are made up of three fatty acids linked to glycerol. Those triglycerides that are solid at ordinary room temperatures are called fats and those that are liquids at ordinary temperatures are called oils. In general, triglycerides from animal sources are solids, and those from plant sources are liquids.

One triglyceride can differ from another according to the identity of the fatty acids. Different fatty acids may contain different numbers of carbon atoms—as few as 4 or more than 20.

Another way in which fatty acids vary is with respect to the presence or absence of a certain type of chemical bond known as a *double bond.* Each carbon atom in a fatty acid may have either one or two hydrogen atoms linked to it. If there are two hydrogens on each carbon, the fatty acid is said to be saturated, because each carbon has the maximum possible number of hydrogens it can hold. In some fatty acids, however, some of the carbon atoms are joined to only one hydrogen atom rather than to two. These are called unsaturated fatty acids. If only one hydrogen atom is attached to each of two adjacent carbons, the carbons are free to form an additional bond between themselves, thereby becoming linked by a double bond rather than by the usual single bond (Figure 14–2). If a fatty acid contains even one double bond, it is said to be unsaturated; the presence of two or more double bonds make it a polyunsaturated fatty acid.

Fats are classified as saturated or unsaturated on the basis of the fatty acids they contain. However, very few fats contain *only* saturated fatty acids or *only* unsaturated ones. An unsaturated fat is therefore one that is *relatively* high in unsaturated fatty acids, and not one that is absolutely devoid of saturated fatty acids. Most liquid triglycerides (oils) contain larger amounts of polyunsaturated fatty acids than do

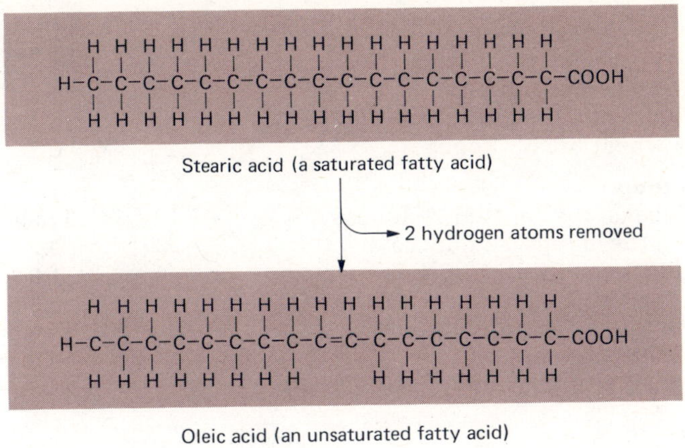

FIGURE 14–2. An unsaturated (double-bond containing) fatty acid.

most solid triglycerides. However, there are exceptions. Coconut oil, for example, is a liquid that contains very few polyunsaturated fatty acids. Advertisers sometimes take unfair advantage of consumers by emphasizing that their product contains no "animal fats," which are generally saturated and which the public associates (correctly or not) with certain health hazards. People need to be informed that there is no advantage whatsoever in using products in which coconut oil has replaced animal fats. However, plant oils other than coconut oil *are* rich in polyunsaturated fats.

The one essential fatty acid, linoleic acid, is a polyunsaturated fatty acid, and the richest food sources are therefore plant oils and foods made from these oils, such as those included in Table 14–3. The amount of linoleic acid generally needed is that amount which provides approximately 2 percent of the total energy value of the diet. For example, if a diet furnishes 2500 kilocalories, linoleic acid should provide 50 of these. This represents approximately 5 grams of linoleic acid, an amount easily obtained from common foods. Because ordinary diets readily provide the necessary amount, linoleic acid deficiency is rare in humans, although infants fed solely on skim milk have developed an essential fatty acid deficiency. This does not mean that skim milk is not suitable as a food; it means only that other sources of linoleic acid must be provided if linoleic acid is removed from milk, as is the case when the cream is skimmed off.

Unsaturated fatty acids can be converted to saturated fatty acids by a process known as *hydrogenation*. In the production of margarine from corn oil or other plant triglycerides, for example, hydrogen is added to the double bonds of many of the unsaturated fatty acids. This makes a more solid product, which of course contains fewer unsaturated fatty acids than did the original oil. *Partially* hydrogenated fats still contain valuable amounts of linoleic acid and other unsaturated

TABLE 14–3
Food sources of linoleic acid

Food	Linoleic acid (grams)
Bread and cereal group	
Enriched white bread, 1 slice	0.1
Whole wheat bread, 1 slice	0.2
Meat group	
Beef (steaks, roasts, etc.), 2 ounces	Trace to 0.7
Chicken (flesh only), 2 ounces	0.7
Ham, luncheon meat, 2 ounces	1.0
Pork, roasted, 2 ounces	0.8
Eggs, raw or prepared without fat, 2	Trace
Peanut butter, 4 tablespoons	8.0
Cooked mature (dry) navy beans, 1 cup	———*
Milk group	
Whole milk, 1 cup	Trace
Cheese, hard, 1½ ounces	Trace
Cottage cheese, 1⅓ cups	Trace
Ice cream, regular, 2 cups	Trace
Ice cream, rich (16% fat), 2 cups	2.0
Vegetable and fruit group	
Most common types	———
Avocado, 1 average	5.0
Miscellaneous	
Bacon, 2 slices	1.0
Butter, 1 tablespoon	Trace
Lard, 1 tablespoon	1.0
Margarine, 1 tablespoon	3.0
Oils (salad or cooking, 1 tablespoon)	
Corn, cottonseed, or soybean	7.0
Olive	1.0
Peanut	4.0
Safflower	10.0
Salad dressings (mayonnaise, French, thousand island)	3.0–4.0
Sugars, syrups, etc.	———

* Dashes in the column indicate that no suitable value could be found.
Note: Most rich linoleic acid sources are foods other than those in the Basic Four food groups.
From "Home and Garden Bulletin No. 72," *USDA*, Washington, D.C., 1970.

fatty acids; very extensive hydrogenation can, however, produce a very hard fat which is almost devoid of unsaturated fatty acids.

FUNCTIONS OF CARBOHYDRATES AND FATS IN THE DIGESTIVE TRACT

Even before they are digested and absorbed into the body proper, carbohydrates and fats exert certain favorable effects through their actions in the digestive tract.

One very important function of a carbohydrate in the digestive process is that of cellulose, also called *fiber, bulk* or *roughage.* Because it is indigestible, cellulose remains in the intestinal lumen, where it stimulates the walls of the digestive tract. This mildly irritating action causes muscles in the digestive system to contract, moving the partially digested mass along the intestine. Most ordinary diets provide a sufficient amount of cellulose for this purpose; only about 5 grams of cellulose daily will suffice. Under certain conditions, for instance, following some types of surgery, it is important to slow down intestinal action drastically. A low-residue diet, containing very little indigestible material, is effective for this purpose.

Various carbohydrates, small amounts of which remain in the digestive tract because they are not quite completely absorbed, serve as energy sources for useful intestinal bacteria. These bacteria produce vitamins, some of which can then be absorbed by the host (the person in whose intestine they are harbored).

A major role of fat in the digestive system is to aid in the absorption of the fat-soluble vitamins. Because the amount of fat required for this purpose is very small compared to the fat in the average American diet, impaired vitamin absorption is rarely caused by a lack of dietary fat. More often it is seen when fats themselves are not digested or absorbed normally, because fats and fat-soluble vitamins together are carried across the intestinal wall.

A second value of fats in the diet is to provide satiety value, preventing hunger from returning too soon after a meal. Because fats are digested more slowly than carbohydrates or proteins are, a meal high in fat stays in the stomach longer than a low-fat meal does. This is not to say that fats are not digested almost completely, as are other energy nutrients. Rather, the *time* required for this is comparatively long and as a result fats provide a relatively lasting sense of "fullness."

A third function of dietary fats is to provide flavor. Although pure fats in themselves are generally tasteless, they contain flavors absorbed from other components of foods; in particular, much of the flavor of meats is provided by the fat. A nondescript "meaty" flavor is common to the fat-free part of all meats; the *particular* flavor of a meat (beef, pork, chicken, or whatever) is obtained almost entirely from components in the fat. Meats specially treated to be as fat-free as possible may sound delicious, but they are actually almost inedible because of their lack of flavor as well as their dry texture.

The myth of no-calorie fats

Mineral oil is not, as the name might imply, a source of minerals, but is "mineral" only in the sense that it is not derived from any animal or plant. A by-product of oil refining, it is commonly used as a laxative. The body cannot digest it, so the oil passes through the digestive tract unaltered, lubricating the intestinal wastes so that they are more easily excreted. Because mineral oil is not digested or absorbed, it is not a source of energy.

Used occasionally as a laxative, mineral oil is probably harmless. However, some people routinely use mineral oil in place of vegetable oils in salad dressings in order to decrease their energy intake. Used often in this manner, mineral oil can result in significant losses of fat-soluble vitamins, because the vitamins in the intestinal tract dissolve in the mineral oil and are excreted along with it. The use of mineral oil as a substitute for other oils therefore is not recommended. Sad to say, there just are no good calorie-free fat substitutes available. Commercial low-calorie salad dressings are generally made with vinegar, tomato juice, lots of spices, and so on; it is the lack of salad oil, and not the presence of a low-energy oil, that accounts for their low energy values.

CARBOHYDRATES AND FATS IN THE BODY: SOURCES AND STORAGE

Neither the carbohydrate nor the fat molecules present in the body were necessarily present as carbohydrate or fat in the diet. As a quick review of the chapter on metabolism will show, body carbohydrate can be obtained from dietary carbohydrate as well as protein, and body fat can be produced from all classes of energy nutrients.

Stored carbohydrate, practically all of which is in the form of glycogen, is found in small amounts in all cells. Most of the total is found in muscle, simply because muscles constitute a larger portion of the body than do other cell types; the highest *concentration* of glycogen, however, is found in the liver. The total maximum capacity for stored carbohydrate in the human body is normally somewhat less than 1 pound.

In contrast to carbohydrate, stored fat is found mostly in specialized cells that make up the adipose tissue (Figure 14–3). Like all cells, adipose tissue cells contain protoplasm, a complex mixture of water, proteins, minerals, and other substances. However, the amount of protoplasm in a fat cell usually accounts for only about one-fifth of its total mass; the remaining four-fifths consist of an enormous globule of stored fat. The amount of fat in the human body can vary tremendously. As little as 3 percent or more than 50 percent of total body weight is compatible with survival, although not, obviously, with good health.

Differences in body fat content can be accounted for in two general ways. An individual can store excess body fat by packing more fat into already existing adipose tissue cells. Alternatively, new fat cells can be formed to hold fat. The timing appears to be a crucial factor in determining which of these storage methods is used. New fat cells are formed at only two stages of the human life cycle. The first stage is

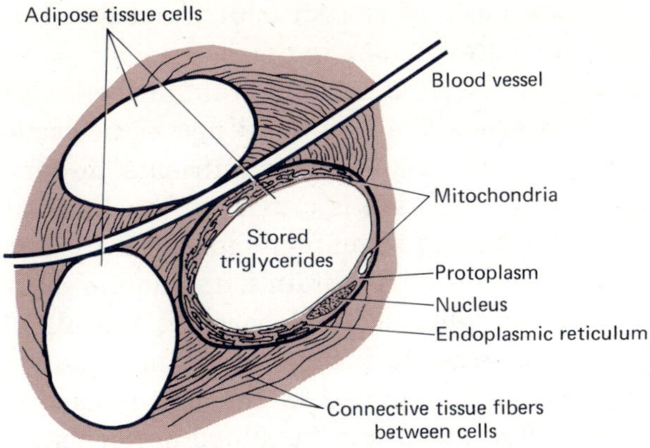

FIGURE 14–3. Adipose tissue, containing specialized cells that store most of the body's fat.

during the last few months before birth through the age of 1 year. The second burst of fat cell formation is believed to occur at around the age of 9–12 years. It is possible that overfeeding at these crucial times stimulates a person to produce excess numbers of fat cells. The individual may eventually produce twice or even three times the normal number of fat cells, which is estimated at some 25 billion in the average adult.

It might be asked what difference it makes whether a person's obesity is related to a normal number of overly stuffed fat cells or to an excess number of fat cells. The answer is that animals, including humans, appear to eat until their fat cells are reasonably filled up. Weight reduction in adults does not decrease the number of fat cells in the body; it merely brings about a drastic decrease in the amount of fat in each cell. It is believed that a decrease in size of an organism's fat cells somehow provokes a desire for increased food intake in an effort to restore the cells to their former size. How this effect on eating behavior is accomplished is not at all understood at present. However, those whose abesity had an onset early in life seem to have extreme difficulty in achieving permanent weight loss, compared to those who were normal in weight prior to adulthood. Prevention of obesity during the crucial periods of fat-cell formation may therefore be of extreme importance to the ease with which body weight can later be controlled. In this sense, an ounce of prevention may literally be worth a pound of cure.

Functions of stored carbohydrates and fats in the body

The relatively small amounts of carbohydrates and fats that form more or less permanent parts of cells are considered *structural components,* not stored nutrients. Stored carbohydrates and fats are those that are not necessary integral parts of cell structure, and which can therefore serve as a reserve to be drawn upon in times of need.

The sole function of stored carbohydrate in the body is to release glucose when it is needed. The brain and nerves in particular require glucose specifically, rather than energy nutrients in general, as fuel. Because the survival of the brain is crucial to the survival of the individual, the brain's fuel supply is guarded closely. If the level of glucose in the blood becomes too low, the brain's function is impaired. On the other hand, if the blood glucose level becomes too high, the kidneys cannot reabsorb the sugar into the bloodstream rapidly enough, and glucose is then wastefully excreted in the urine. Therefore, survival demands that the level of glucose in the blood be regulated rather carefully. This is accomplished largely by converting glucose to glycogen when the blood glucose level is high, and converting glycogen back to glucose when blood glucose is low. Several hormones—epinephrine, insulin, and others—help to insure that the blood glucose level remains within a normal range (Figure 14–4).

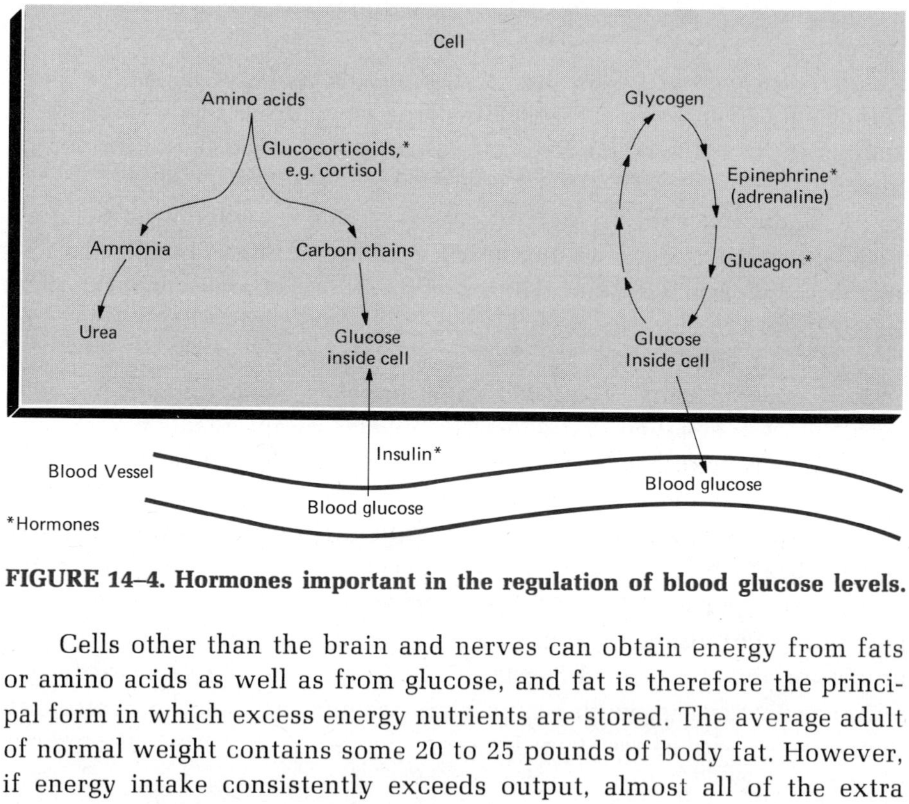

FIGURE 14–4. Hormones important in the regulation of blood glucose levels.

Cells other than the brain and nerves can obtain energy from fats or amino acids as well as from glucose, and fat is therefore the principal form in which excess energy nutrients are stored. The average adult of normal weight contains some 20 to 25 pounds of body fat. However, if energy intake consistently exceeds output, almost all of the extra energy nutrients are converted to fat, and an extra 100 pounds or more can be added to the body.

The advantage of storing energy as fat is that a given amount of energy can be stored much more compactly as fat than as protein or carbohydrate, just as a given amount of money is much less bulky in the form of ten-dollar bills than in the form of five-dollar bills. Because energy in the most compact form is not particularly important to organisms which do not move about, carbohydrate in the form of starch is a perfectly suitable reservoir of excess energy in plants. Among animals, however, storing the maximum amount of energy in the minimum bulk is very important in enabling the animal to move about without being encumbered by unnecessarily great mass. The few animals that store excess energy mostly as carbohydrate rather than as fat are organisms such as clams and oysters, which are hardly noted for their athletic ability.

FATS AND CARBOHYDRATES: FACTS AND MYTHS

Body fat and the sexes

The most striking sex difference with respect to body composition in humans is in the amount of body fat. Whereas some 14 percent of a well-nourished man's body consists of fat tissue, a normal woman's body generally contains 20–25 percent fat, or even more. The wide range of values for normal women results largely from the great variation in the amount of fat present in certain strategic sites, such as the breasts and buttocks.

Two main hypotheses have been offered to explain this sex difference. One is that the greater storage of fat in the female helps to insure the survival of a larger proportion of females during periods of severe food shortage. From the points of view of reproduction and survival of the species, a large number of females is more important than a large number of males. Any knowledgeable farmer knows this. Who ever saw a flock of chickens consisting of 50 percent hens and 50 percent roosters? One rooster will do nicely for a large number of hens. Our social conventions, not biological necessity, keep the same rule from applying to humans!

A second hypothesis is that body fat, distributed in certain ways on the female body, is of survival value because it acts as a sexual attractant to the male. Considering the great variation in what is considered sexually attractive from one society to another, one suspects that an enlarged muscle on the female's forehead could attract males as effectively as fatty breasts and buttocks could. However, this is a hypothesis that can neither be proved nor disproved.

There is no doubt, however, that body fat performs certain protective functions in both sexes. The subcutaneous fat layer, just beneath the skin, insulates the body and thereby prevents excessive heat loss. People who are very thin may for this reason find cold weather hard to bear, as those who are very fat may suffer in hot weather. Cushions of fat surrounding internal organs such as the heart and kidneys may serve a protective function, helping to prevent physical injury to these organs as a result of hard blows to the body.

Fats, carbohydrates, and exercise

It has been known for over a hundred years that the breakdown of body proteins and consequent catabolism of the amino acids are not increased by physical activity. Instead, muscle contraction uses energy derived from fat and carbohydrate. The relative contributions of these two can vary, depending on two main factors: the intensity of physical activity and the diet consumed prior to exercise.

It will be recalled that oxygen is necessary for the oxidation of both glucose and fatty acids. When oxygen is unavailable, fatty-acid oxidation halts completely, whereas glucose breakdown can continue, at least at a slow rate. This is because the hydrogen removed from glucose can be donated to pyruvic acid if oxygen is not present. Much less energy is released than would be if oxygen were present, but at least some energy can be obtained, as shown in Figure 14–5. During rest, or during exercise of mild or moderate intensity, breathing can keep up with the demands for oxygen needed to oxidize both glucose and fatty acids. Under these conditions, approximately half of the energy released is supplied by glucose and half from fatty acids.

As the intensity of exercise increases, however, it becomes more and more difficult to breathe rapidly enough to meet the demands for oxygen, and fewer and fewer fatty acids can be oxidized. Glucose then becomes the main, and finally the sole, energy source being used.

The diet prior to exercise also markedly affects the relative use of fat and carbohydrate as energy sources. A high-carbohydrate diet consumed for several days ahead of time increases the ability to perform long periods of heavy work. In particular, this effect is obtained if muscles are first depleted of glycogen by heavy exercise and a high-carbohydrate diet is then fed; resynthesis of glycogen is enhanced in muscles previously exhausted of their glycogen content. By appropriate schedules of exercise followed by high carbohydrate intake, the amount of glycogen stored in muscle can become over twice as great as that ordinarily present.

Although none of this information is new, it has had relatively little effect on the diets of many athletes or laborers engaged in heavy physical work. For many, the emotional association is still: protein = muscles = exercise. Extremely high protein diets, often supplemented with protein tablets, therefore continue to be favored by those who are convinced that exercise somehow "breaks down" muscle protein, thus necessitating enormous protein intakes to replace the "lost" muscle tissue.

Carbohydrates, fats, and weight control

Is it true that low-income people are commonly overweight because

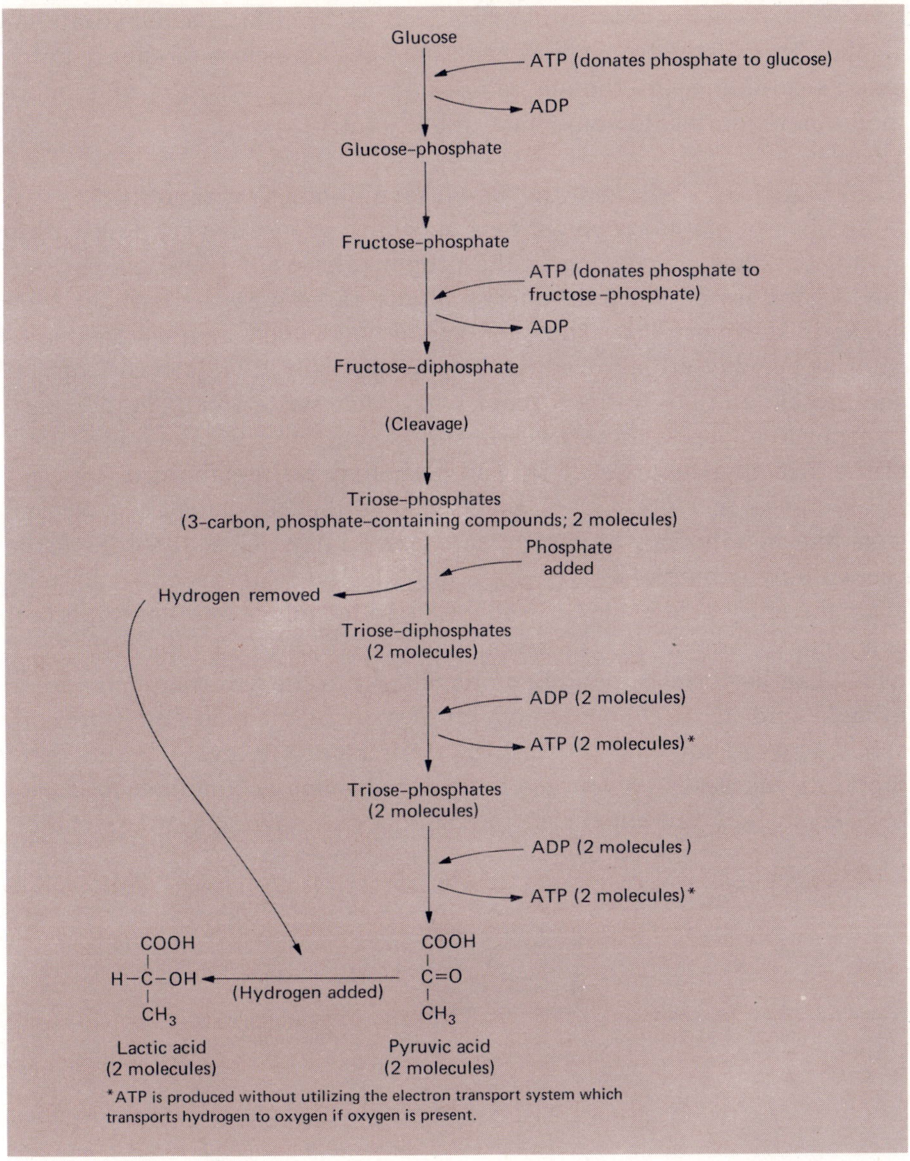

FIGURE 14–5. How glucose breakdown yields at least some energy even in the absence of oxygen.

they must subsist on "those cheap fattening carbohydrates"? Is it a fact that omitting fat from the diet will inevitably result in loss of fat from the body? In short, is it not true that particular amounts of carbohydrates or fats have specific effects on body fat? In short, no. The important point is the *total energy value of the diet.* If this exceeds energy output, body weight is gained, and if it is less than energy output, fat is lost.

Granted, it is easier to exceed energy needs by eating excess carbohydrate or fat than by eating excess protein. But obesity can result from excess energy from protein as well as from fat, carbohydrate, or alcohol. It is distinctly incorrect to brand any one class of energy nutrients as *fattening*—as though calories from this source are able, more than other calories, to contribute to body fat.

Those "low carbohydrate" diets: revolutionary or revolting? A number of popular weight-loss schemes advocate very low carbohydrate intakes. According to the proponents, weight will be lost rapidly regardless of the total energy intake as long as the carbohydrate intake is kept very low. Thus, intakes of 3000, 4000, or even 5000 kilocalories per day are allowed, as long as the energy is derived from fat and protein and not in the form of what some writers call "carbo-cals." In order to evaluate these programs, it is necessary to take a brief look at the principal features of fat and carbohydrate metabolism.

As seen in Figure 14–6, acetic acid is the key substance derived from the metabolism of both glucose and fatty acids. In order to be broken down completely to carbon dioxide and water, acetic acid must enter the citric acid cycle. It is now time to introduce another important compound. This is the 4-carbon compound called *oxaloacetic acid,* which can be formed by adding one carbon to the 3-carbon compound, pyruvic acid. If an adequate amount of oxaloacetic acid is not present, acetic acid cannot link to it to form citric acid; the level of acetic acid therefore increases. When acetic acid molecules accumulate to a very high level, they are converted to compounds known as *ketone bodies.*

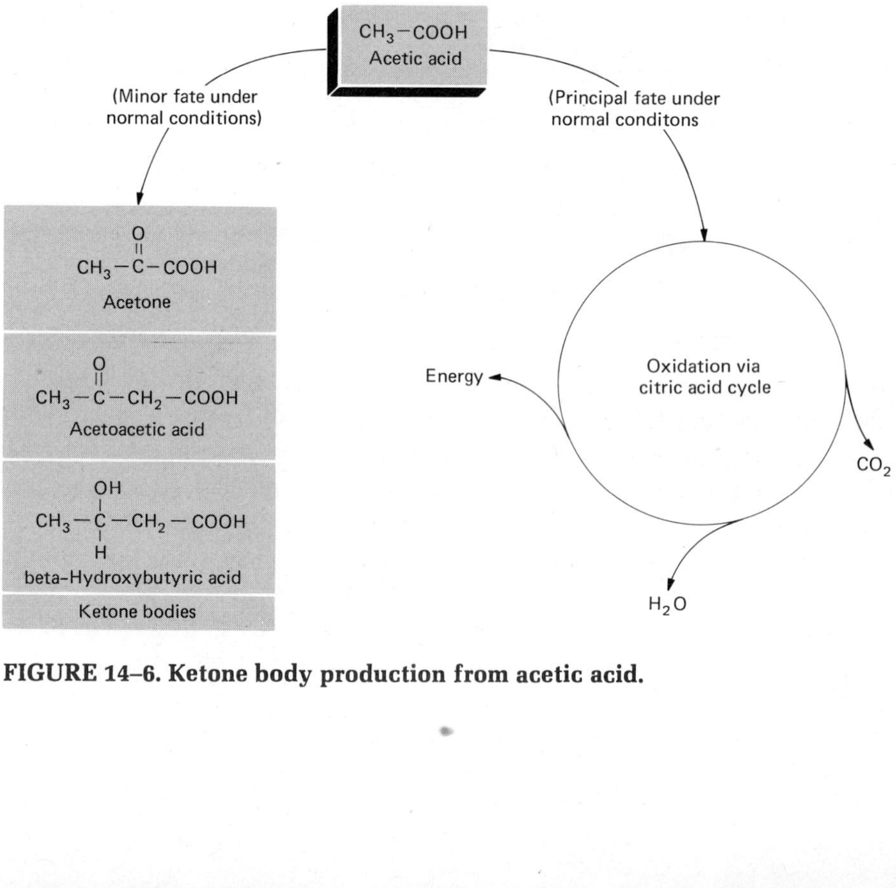

FIGURE 14–6. Ketone body production from acetic acid.

These compounds eventually can be excreted in the urine, and large volumes of water are therefore commonly recommended, supposedly to "wash out" these products of incomplete nutrient oxidation.

The line of reasoning behind the low-carbohydrate diets runs as follows:

> If carbohydrate is omitted from the diet, there will be no glucose in the cells.
> Without glucose, pyruvic acid cannot be produced.
> Without pyruvic acid, oxaloacetic acid cannot be produced.
> Without oxaloacetic acid, the citric acid cycle cannot operate.
> If the citric acid cycle is not operating, acetic acid formed from fat will be converted to ketone bodies.
> Ketone bodies are excreted in the urine, thereby ridding the body of enormous amounts of energy which otherwise could have been converted to fat.

The problem with this line of reasoning is that every statement in it is entirely erroneous.

First, a low-carbohydrate diet does not produce a correspondingly low level of glucose within the cells. As already seen, amino acids, whether recently derived from dietary proteins or obtained by breaking down cell proteins, are converted to glucose when necessary. As a result, a low-carbohydrate diet does not result in the absence of glucose, and hence of pyruvic acid, in cells.

Second, the amount of ketone bodies that can be excreted in the urine is ordinarily very small. Followers of low-carbohydrate diets are sometimes advised to test their own urine for the presence of ketone bodies, but the test kits available for this purpose are sensitive to extremely small amounts of ketone bodies. Thus a positive test result can be obtained even though the amount of energy lost as urinary ketone bodies is insignificant. Indeed, unusually high ketone body excretions represent the urinary loss of only a few hundred kilocalories daily. A loss of this magnitude cannot begin to counterbalance the enormous energy intakes—which these diets claim are compatible with losing weight.

Weight loss does, of course, commonly occur when dietary carbohydrates are restricted, but weight would also be lost if any other energy nutrients were similarly restricted. A diet very low in carbohydrates is almost certain to be very low in total energy value as well. The reason is the monotony of such diets, which almost inevitably causes a sharp decrease in total food intake, although the dieter may not even be conscious of this. If you are allowed unlimited amounts of meats, eggs, butter, margarine, salad dressings, and similar foods, you may be unaware that actual *intake* of these foods is self-limited. How many people really enjoy large servings of butter or margarine if there are no breads or potatoes to put them on? How appealing is salad dressing without the salad?

However, even if these low-carbohydrate diets worked as they are supposed to, they could not be recommended because too many essential nutrients are lacking. Milk, forbidden because of its lactose content, is an important source of calcium, complete proteins, riboflavin, and other nutrients. Breads and cereals, shunned because of their starch content, supply valuable amounts of iron and vitamins. Fruits and vegetables, restricted because they contain starch and sugars, are the main sources of vitamin A and vitamin C in American diets. Thus the intake of a large number of essential nutrients is sharply decreased on any diet that is extremely low in carbohydrate. All in all, then, it is probably a good thing that most people get too bored with these diets to stay with them for very long.

Hypoglycemia: dread disease or gross exaggeration?

Concern over hypoglycemia, or low blood sugar, has been stirred up by a rash of popular books and articles that have appeared in recent years. According to the writers of these, at least 5 million Americans suffer from hypoglycemia, with resulting symptoms of fatigue, nervousness, hunger, headaches, dizziness, insomnia, listlessness, childhood behavior problems, drug addiction, and sexual inadequacy.

Because glucose is indispensable to brain function, the body has developed more than one means of keeping the blood glucose concentration reasonably constant. Several hormones act to lower or raise the level as necessary. Insulin, secreted by the pancreas, acts at the membranes of various cells, facilitating the passage of glucose molecules into cells; this *decreases* the level of glucose in the blood. *Glucagon* (do not confuse this with the polysaccharide glycogen) is another hormone secreted by the pancreas, but with an effect exactly opposite to that of insulin; by stimulating an enzyme which breaks down glycogen to glucose, it *raises* the blood glucose. Adrenaline, or epinephrine, secreted by the inner portion, or medulla, of the adrenal glands, also activates the enzyme which converts glycogen to glucose. Epinephrine is commonly known as the "fight or flight" hormone, because increased amounts are secreted during times of acute fear. It provides a ready supply of glucose to furnish energy needed by the organism to flee or fight in response to danger. Finally, the glucocorticoids (which have already been discussed under the subject of proteins) bring about an increase in blood glucose, at the expense of amino acids.

Despite all of these control mechanisms, hypoglycemia is a condition that almost everybody experiences from time to time. Most commonly, it develops several hours after a meal rich in starches or sugars. Because carbohydrates are readily digested and absorbed, blood glucose rises rapidly; this stimulates the pancreas to secrete insulin, which facilitates the exit of glucose out of the blood into the cells. Commonly, the body overshoots its mark so that the blood sugar level temporarily reaches a below-average value. This is normal and short lived, for the *lowered* blood sugar signals the pancreas to secrete *less* insulin, and blood sugar levels are then restored to normal.

A relatively small number of people do in fact have hypoglycemia of a more serious nature. However, the hypoglycemia is not a disease itself, but merely a symptom of a disease. Tumors of the pancreas, for example, produce abnormally large amounts of insulin, and cirrhosis of the liver or disease of the adrenal glands can impair the ability of these organs to perform their normal roles in regulating blood glucose. Obviously, treatment of the underlying disease is indicated in these individuals.

According to many popular writers, however, hypoglycemia is a widespread disease that should be recognized as the cause of many symptoms that affect the American population. The treatment prescribed by these writers consists of a low-carbohydrate, high-protein diet, often in conjunction with a series of injections of material derived from the adrenal glands of animals. The material used in the injections is so ineffective that the rare individual who is truly hypoglycemic because of disease of the adrenal glands would need about $150 worth per day. This is in contrast to the medically approved and potent hormone preparations with which the person could be treated, for about 12 cents per day. Also, approved hormones can be taken orally rather than by injection, thereby saving the cost of frequent office visits.

Despite the facts, the success of the hypoglycemia movement is illustrated by the fact that one of the books on the subject is currently in its twenty-third printing. The explanation can probably be found in the eagerness of people to find some physical abnormality upon which their emotional disorders can be blamed, for, unfortunately, the stigma still attached to emotional illness is too great to be accepted by many. If people suffer from nervousness or depression, or if their children are addicted to drugs, how comforting to be told that these conditions are, after all, physical diseases, not mental or emotional problems.

Three organizations of physicians (the American Diabetes Association, the Endocrine Society, and the American Medical Association) have issued the following statement concerning hypoglycemia:

> **When it occurs, it is often attended by symptoms of sweating, shakiness, trembling, anxiety, fast heart action, headache, hunger sensations, brief feelings of weakness, and, occasionally, seizures and coma. However, the majority of people with these kinds of symptoms do not have hypoglycemia; a great many patients with anxiety reactions present with similar symptoms.**

SUGARS AND THE MOST COMMON DISEASE IN THE UNITED STATES

What is the most common disease in the American population, and indeed in most of the peoples of the world? The reason that few people can answer this question correctly is that the disease is so *very* common that many consider it an inevitable consequence of living, and not a disease at all. The most common disease is *dental decay*, or caries or cavities, which almost everybody suffers from to some degree.

What single dietary change would bring about the greatest reduction in tooth decay? A large number of people could give the correct answer to this question: Decrease the intake of sugar. Actually, however, dental decay is related to more than just the total amount of sugar eaten. In the *National Nutrition Survey*, the most significant correlation found between nutrition and dental health was the positive relationship between cavities and the frequency of eating high-carbohydrate foods between meals. Sugars that remain in the mouth are broken down by bacteria, producing acids which erode the surfaces of the teeth. By eating sugar frequently, people provide the bacteria with an almost continuous supply of sugar to work on.

The possibility of decreasing dental decay through diet modification was demonstrated very convincingly by a controlled study in Sweden. Diets of institutionalized patients were supplemented with various vitamins and minerals for the first year of the study. No differences were seen in the development of cavities as a result of the supplementation. The sugars of the diet were then changed as to form, amount, and frequency of use, and significant differences in caries appeared (Figure 14–7). The three most important conclusions of this study are:

1 Increased sugar intake causes increased tooth decay.
2 Sugar in foods which stick to the teeth causes more cavities than sugar in liquids or in foods which do not stick to teeth.
3 The more frequently sugar is eaten, the more tooth decay is seen.

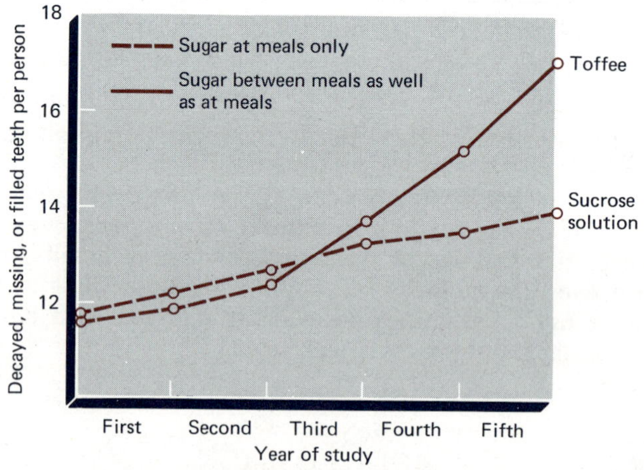

FIGURE 14–7. The effects of various forms of sugar on teeth. Results shown are similar to those of B. G. Bibby, "Cariogenicity of Foods," ***J. Amer. Med. Assoc. 177*****:316 (1961).**

Unfortunately, the knowledge that between-meal eating of sweets causes cavities has had little effect on diets. Parents sometimes take the line of least resistance and allow children to eat sweets at all times of the day, perhaps rationalizing that the child will have poor teeth anyway because it "runs in the family." Certainly it is true that genetic factors affect tooth development and the ability of the teeth to resist decay after they are formed. However, if genetics were the only important factor, all the teeth in a given individual would be expected to decay to about the same extent—which does not occur. Tooth surfaces that provide areas where food is retained, such as the biting surfaces of lower molars (grinding teeth), develop cavities several hundred times as frequently as do the smooth inner surfaces of the lower incisors (biting teeth). Because appetite, social factors, and advertising have far more effect on food intake than facts have, it would be unrealistic to expect people to avoid between-meal sweets altogether. A practical cavity-prevention must therefore concentrate on urging people (especially children) to brush their teeth after snacks, and on suggesting that the number of snacks be kept at least to a reasonable minimum.

The use of nonnutritive sweeteners in place of sugar is recommended by some dentists and nutritionists, but not by all. Sweeteners such as saccharine provide the flavor without providing the energy of sugar; they are therefore very useful to diabetics, who must restrict their carbohydrate intake, and are widely used by dieters who want the taste of sugar without the calories. Because they are not broken down by bacteria in the mouth, they cannot contribute to tooth decay, so some dentists recommend snacks such as sugarless gum and soft drinks. However, until the long-term effects of large amounts of nonnutritive sweeteners in the diets of children are known, unqualified approval must be withheld.

THE DIET-HEART DISEASE CONTROVERSY

Coronary heart disease is the most serious public health problem in most of the developed countries. In 1970, for example, approximately 666,000 Americans died of this disorder, and over one-fourth of these deaths occurred in people less than sixty-five years old. In addition, many more people who survived the disease were disabled by it.

A surprisingly large number of people believe that dietary fats have been proved beyond doubt to be the underlying cause of coronary heart disease. This belief is largely the result of very active advertising campaigns by the producers of foods high in unsaturated fats—liquid oils and products made from these, such as soft margarines.

The possibility of preventing heart attacks by manipulating the fat content of the diet can be assessed by examining the numerous *risk factors* that are associated with susceptibility to coronary heart disease:

TABLE 14–4
Cholesterol content of selected foods

Food	Cholesterol (milligrams)
Breads and cereals group	None (unless prepared with butter, milk, or other cholesterol-containing food)
Meat group	
2 ounces beef	40
2 ounces brains	>1100
2 ounces chicken	35
1 egg yolk (approximately ½ ounce)	250
2 ounces liver	170
2 ounces lobster	110
2 ounces pork	40
Milk group	
1 cup whole milk	25
1 cup skim milk	7
Vegetable–fruit group	None (unless prepared with butter, milk, or other cholesterol-containing food)
Miscellaneous	
1 tablespoon butter	35
1 tablespoon lard (animal fat)	15
1 tablespoon margarine (made from vegetable oil)	0
Sugars, syrups, jams, jellies, etc.	0
Vegetable oils	0

Note: Cholesterol is naturally present in foods of animal origin only, and the cholesterol of eggs is found entirely in the yolk.

Genetics
Sex
High blood pressure (hypertension)
Heavy cigarette smoking
Physical inactivity
Obesity
Elevated blood levels of liquids (cholesterol and triglycerides)

The first two risk factors, genetics and sex, obviously cannot be manipulated. The third, hypertension, can frequently be controlled by drugs; in addition, blood pressure can often be decreased by reducing the body weight. Heavy smoking, physical inactivity, and obesity can be corrected only if the individual is willing to modify his or her life style, a change which is very difficult for many people.

There is, then, only one risk factor which can be altered by changing the pattern of dietary fat: the level of lipids in the blood. Two different types of lipids need to be considered. Cholesterol, a fatlike substance known chemically as a *steroid,* will be considered first.

Judging from the publicity given in recent years to the dangers of "high cholesterol," one might conclude that people would be better off if all traces of this compound could be eradicated from the body. Actually, cholesterol is a normal body component with a number of important functions. In fact, cholesterol is the most abundant specific substance in the human brain other than water, accounting for 2 to 3 percent of the total weight of this organ. The steroid itself is an important structural part of certain organs, as, for example, in the insulating coverings, or *myelin sheaths,* of nerve fibers. In addition, cholesterol is the starting material used in synthesizing all the other steroids of the body: male and female sex hormones, the hormones of the adrenal cortex, and the bile acids which emulsify fat in the intestinal tract. Even one of the vitamins, vitamin D, is produced in the body from cholesterol. In fact, it is only in the absence of sufficient exposure to radiation that a dietary source of the vitamin is needed at all.

Why, then, is cholesterol so often considered an unmitigated evil? The answer is that nobody ever suffers from a cholesterol deficiency, whereas there is evidence that excess cholesterol in the blood is detrimental. However, excess cholesterol in the blood is not necessarily the result of a high cholesterol intake. Some people produce unusually large amounts within their own bodies, with the rate of synthesis depending upon a number of factors, including genes and hormones as well as a yet unknown number of dietary factors.

The dietary change that is most effective in reducing the level of blood cholesterol is replacement of at least part of the saturated fat with unsaturated fats, and especially with those rich in polyunsaturated fatty acids. This decreases the synthesis of cholesterol in the body itself. It is also suggested that cholesterol in foods be consumed in smaller amounts than those present in American diets. In practice, this means restricting the intake of certain high-cholesterol foods such as eggs and shellfish (Table 14–4).

A second aspect of blood lipid levels that is believed to be important is the level of triglycerides themselves. Elevated triglyceride levels in the blood appear to impose an increased risk of coronary heart disease, over and above that associated with increased cholesterol production from fats.

Although a great deal remains to be learned about the extent to which coronary heart disease can be prevented by dietary changes, the evidence at present has prompted the following joint policy statement from the American Medical Association and the National Academy of Sciences:

> Measurement of plasma lipids should become a routine part of all health maintenance physical examinations.
> Persons with undesirably high lipid levels should be advised to decrease substantially their intake of saturated fats and of cholesterol.
> People should be advised to achieve and maintain a normal body weight by appropriately altering physical activity and total energy intake.

The dietary advice should insure that blood lipid reduction and weight reduction does not occur at the expense of inadequate intake of essential nutrients.

A final recommendation is that foods needed to achieve these goals be readily available, reasonably priced, and labeled so as to be easily identified.

It is not known how effective the foregoing recommendations will be in preventing heart disease, and may not be known for decades. It is important to recognize that available evidence strongly suggests that increasing the intake of polyunsaturated fats and decreasing the intake of saturated fats, and perhaps of cholesterol, may be of benefit. It is equally important to recognize that diet alone will probably have little success in protecting the heart of the overweight, chain-smoking, sedentary person found too often in the American population.

Sex, eggs, cholesterol and nonsense

The egg industry is battling for its economic life; per capita consumption has declined to the lowest point since the economic depression of the 1930s. A good deal of psychological hypothesizing has been done in an effort to explain this change in eating habits. It has been solemnly suggested, for example, that adolescent girls and women avoid eggs because of "subconscious fantasies of oral impregnation." Eggs are, of course, a symbol of fertility in many cultures, including our own; Americans color eggs at Easter (the time of resurrection which, like reproduction, produces new life). Children are told that the dyed eggs were brought by—what else?—a rabbit, the sexuality of which is, of course, legendary. In fact, a whole business enterprise is built around the supposed sexual activities of young women dressed as "bunnies." However, it is hardly necessary to invoke fear of pregnancy as a cause of decreased egg consumption by females. More likely, eggs are not eaten because breakfast is not eaten; this may be related to the hope of losing weight by skipping a meal, the rush of getting ready for work or school in the morning, or the large number of "instant" convenience foods designed to replace the morning meal.

The most recent threat to the egg industry is the publicity linking cholesterol to possible heart disease. Massive advertising campaigns have therefore been designed to reassure consumers that fears of dietary cholesterol are unfounded. One proposed advertisement even implied that the cholesterol in eggs is positively beneficial, featured the "sexy" egg, and noted that "cholesterol is the building block of sex hormones." Unfounded statements abound, obviously, on both sides of the cholesterol-heart disease debate. Until more facts are available, it would seem prudent to accept the egg as it has always been accepted—as a nutritious food that makes valuable contributions to the diet. Let's not expect it, or anything else, to be a "wonder food" which can insure our health or happiness—or our sexiness.

SUGGESTED READINGS

Bergstrom, J. and E. Hultman. "Nutrition for Maximal Sports Performance." *Journal of the American Medical Association* 221 (1972):999.

Björntorp, P. "Effects of Age, Sex, and Clinical Conditions on Adipose Tissue Cellularity in Man." *Metabolism* 23 (1974):1091.

Council on Foods and Nutrition. "A Critique of Low-Carbohydrate Ketogenic Weight Reduction Regimens." *Journal of the American Medical Association* 224 (1973):1415.

Food and Nutrition Board, NAS-NRC, and the Council on Foods and Nutrition, American Medical Association. "Diet and Coronary Heart Disease." *Nutrition Reviews* 30 (1972):223.

Hersh, T. "Lactose Intolerance in Health and Disease." *Nutrition News* 35 (1972):5.

Inter-Society Commission for Heart Disease. Report of the Inter-Society Commission for Heart Disease Resources (revised). *Circulation* 42 (1972):1.

Levine, R. "Hypoglycemia." *Journal of the American Medical Association* 230 (1974):462.

Lewis, S. and B. Gutin. "Nutrition and Endurance." *American Journal of Clinical Nutrition* 26 (1973):1011.

Nizel, A. E. The Science of Nutrition and Its Application in Clinical Dentistry, second edition. Philadelphia: Saunders, 1966.

Reiser, R. "The Roles of Cholesterol in Normal Metabolism." *Nutrition News* 35 (1972):13.

Sipple, H. L. and K. W. McNutt, eds. *Sugars in Nutrition.* New York: Academic, 1974.

15

the vitamins

The concealed curriculum of advertising has done much to "educate" the public on the subject of vitamins. As a result, millions of well fed or even overfed Americans swallow a daily multivitamin pill "to be sure"; sales of vitamins constitute a business of over a billion dollars per year, second only to antibiotics among all drug sales. And a large segment of the public uncritically accepts vitamins as minor miracle drugs, entirely safe and effective in the prevention and treatment of a variety of human ills (Table 15–1).

In point of fact, vitamins are simply *organic compounds which are required in the diet in extremely small amounts.* This definition distinguishes vitamins from other organic compounds (such as essential fatty acids and essential amino acids, which are required in relatively large amounts); from minerals (which are inorganic); and from water (which is both inorganic and required in very large amounts).

The most recently discovered class of nutrients, vitamins have all been identified as dietary essentials only since the beginning of the twentieth century.

In contrast to the very minute amounts in which vitamins exist both in foods and in the human body, their importance to all cells is enormous. Their outstanding function is to regulate biological processes, particularly by acting in partnership with enzymes in biochemical reactions (Figure 15–1). Thus, although *vitamins themselves are not energy nutrients,* they are vital parts of the biological machinery whereby energy is released from fats, carbohydrates, and proteins; and although vitamins do not constitute an appreciable proportion of the whole body, they make it possible for the body to transform other nutrients into the living material produced in growth, renewal, and reproduction.

By long-standing tradition, vitamins are classed in two broad categories. Vitamins A, D, E, and K are called *fat-soluble* because they dissolve in fat solvents such as ether and chloroform as well as in fats. All other vitamins are designated as *water-soluble.* However, because this classification has very little relationship to food sources of vitamins, it should be recognized that this was merely a convenient way for chemists to describe the solubility of these compounds as they isolated and studied them.

Although people commonly refer to "vitamin B," no such thing actually exists. Vitamin B was the name first given to a water-soluble material thought to be a single compound. Later it was found that this material consists of a group of vitamins, each with its own distinctive properties. However, these vitamins tend to be found together, occurring in small amounts in a wide variety of foods, in contrast to certain other vitamins which are found in relatively high concentrations in a

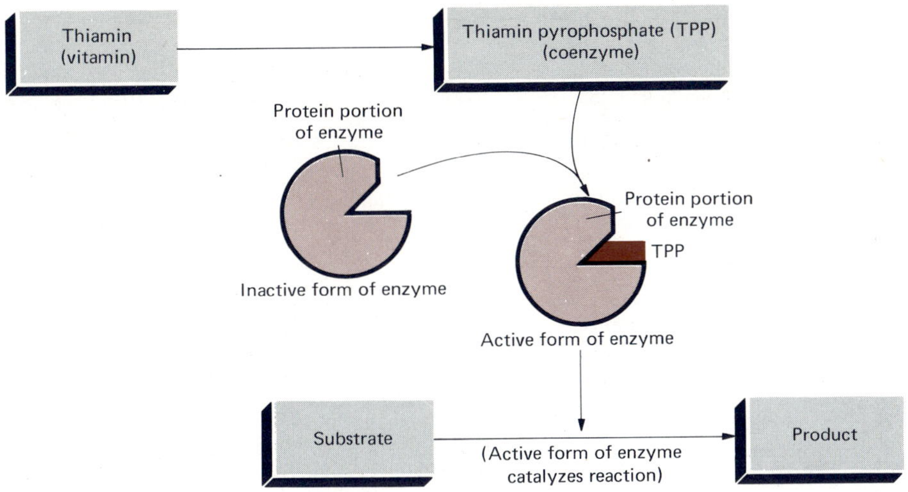

FIGURE 15–1. A vitamin acting in partnership with an enzyme.

narrow range of foods. The term *vitamin B complex* is therefore sometimes used for the group which includes all water-soluble vitamins other than ascorbic acid. However, the preferred system is to call each vitamin by its correct name: thiamin, riboflavin, niacin, and so on.

VITAMINS AND DISEASES

A deficiency of any vitamin would eventually result in a corresponding deficiency disease. In practice, however, some vitamin deficiencies are very serious world health problems, whereas others are very rarely seen in humans. This is not because some vitamins are less important than others, but rather because some are so easily obtained from a wide range of foods that the likelihood of deficiency is almost nil. In fact, a major problem in studying some vitamin deficiencies in humans is that it is so difficult to find deficient humans to observe.

It is extremely important to recognize that *a vitamin will correct a disease or disorder if, and only if, the condition was caused by a lack of that vitamin in the first place.* For example, a child whose growth has been impaired by deficiency of a particular vitamin will grow normally when adequate amounts are given, whereas a child with growth failure caused by any other problem will be unaffected by increased vitamin intake; a person who bruises easily because of vitamin C deficiency will be helped by vitamin C, but the vitamin will have no effect on those who bruise readily for reasons unrelated to vitamin C deficiency, and so on.

Although some of the symptoms of vitamin deficiencies are very specific, many others are vague and general. Fatigue and decreased appetite, for example, are caused by a variety of deficiencies as well by

TABLE 15–1

Vitamins: facts and fallacies

Vitamin	Some known functions	Some unsupported claims
Ascorbic acid (Vitamin C)	Necessary for synthesis of connective tissue protein and for steroid metabolism	Prevents colds and other infections; decreases blood cholesterol
Vitamin A	Involved in vision; important in maintaining health of many tissues, especially skin and mucous membranes	Cures acne and other skin disorders; protects against air pollution and certain toxins; specifically prevents many infections
Vitamin D	Necessary for normal bone mineralization	In massive doses, promotes "miraculous" healing of fractures and sprains; treats "hot flashes" and other symptoms of menopause
Thiamin (vitamin B_1)	Important in the metabolism of energy nutrients, especially glucose	Raises morale; cures alcoholism and drug addiction; reduces anxiety and "nervousness"
Riboflavin (vitamin B_2)	Important in the metabolism of energy nutrients, especially amino acids	Cures cataracts; prevents birth defects if given in large doses to pregnant women
Niacin	Important in the metabolism of energy nutrients	Cures mental disorders, including schizophrenia
Vitamin B_6	Necessary in various reactions of amino acids	Relieves nervous disorders, including Parkinson's disease; prevents convulsions in conditions such as epilepsy
Vitamin B_{12}	Necessary for DNA synthesis, hence for division and functioning of all cells	Cures neuritis, psoriasis; relieves pain; cures "general debility"
Folacin	Acts with vitamin B_{12} in DNA synthesis; transfers small C-containing fragments from one compound to another	Treats dizziness, fatigue and depression; prevents birth defects; treats skin blemishes and many infections
Vitamin E	Acts as an antioxidant to protect certain components in cells from destruction by oxygen	Prevents heart attacks; treats muscular dystrophy; cures impotence; prevents spontaneous abortion; improves appearance of skin and hair when applied externally; cures anemia by "strengthening" red blood cells
Vitamin K	Necessary for normal blood clotting	Quickly stops bleeding after childbirth, surgery, tooth extractions, and injuries
Pantothenic acid	Involved in the metabolism of energy nutrients	Restores color to gray hair; treats diseases of the adrenal glands; prevents neuritis and ulcers
Biotin	"Fixes" carbon dioxide molecules into certain compounds	Cures eczema and other skin disorders; restores color to gray hair; prevents baldness, mental depression, and cancer

infections, emotional disorders, and many other conditions not related to nutrients at all. For this reason, discussion of deficiency symptoms can be greatly condensed by confining it to those most specifically related to the particular vitamin being considered.

The amount of each vitamin required by a given individual can vary, depending upon genetics, hormones, and various extrinsic factors, including other constituents of the diet. For example, fat-soluble vitamins are absorbed along with fat; absorption of these can therefore be impaired if either bile or dietary fat is absent.

Any vitamin can be toxic and produce a disease of excess if taken in great enough amounts. In practice, however, excesses of fat-soluble vitamins are more likely to be toxic than are excesses of water-soluble vitamins. This is because water-soluble vitamins over and above actual needs are largely excreted in the urine, whereas excess fat soluble vitamins can accumulate in huge amounts in the body, particularly in the liver (Figure 15–2).

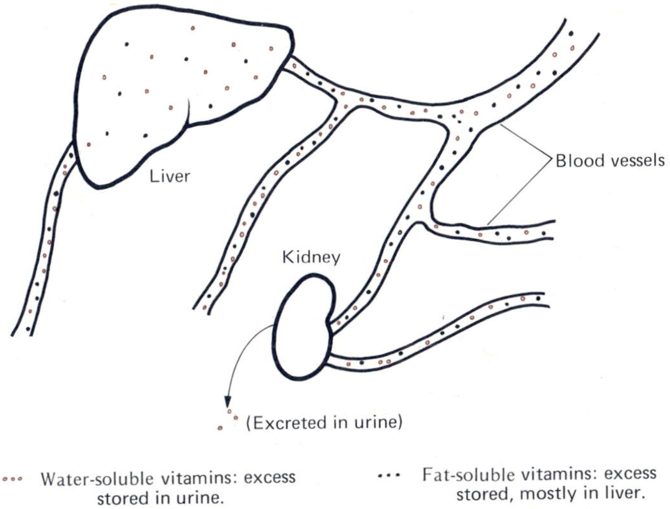

FIGURE 15–2. The different fates of excess fat-soluble and water-soluble vitamins.

LOSING VITAMINS FROM FOODS

The concentration of a vitamin present in a particular food at harvest is largely a matter of the genetics of the plant or animal from which the food was obtained, rather than the animal's diet, the fertilizer used on the soil, or other external factors.

However, storage, processing, or food preparation techniques can decrease the amounts of vitamins after food is harvested. This can occur in three principal ways:

1 **Solubility.** Water-soluble vitamins can be dissolved or leached out into the water in which foods are cooked or soaked. If this liquid is discarded, the dissolved vitamins are thrown away along with it.

TABLE 15–2
Vitamin C content of some common foods

Food	Vitamin C (milligrams)
Bread and cereal group	
Breads and cereals, all types, 1 serving	0 – trace
Meat group	
Muscle meats (beef, pork, chicken, fish, etc.), 2 ounces	0
Liver (beef), fried, 2 ounces	15
Cooked dry beans, 1 cup	0
Milk group	
Whole or skim milk, 1 cup	2
Cheese (all types), 1½ ounces	0
Ice cream, 2 cups	2
Vegetable and fruit group	
Apple, 1 medium	3
Asparagus, ½ cup cooked	19
Banana, 1 medium	12
Beets, ½ cup cooked	4
Broccoli, ½ cup cooked	70
Brussels sprouts, ½ cup cooked	70
Cabbage, ½ cup raw, shredded	20
Cantaloupe, ½ medium	32
Carrots, ½ cup, raw or cooked	4
Cauliflower, ½ cup cooked	33
Collards, ½ cup cooked	44
Green beans, ½ cup cooked	8
Green peas, ½ cup cooked	16
Orange, 1 medium	66
Orange juice, ½ cup	62
Peach, 1 medium	7
Spinach, ½ cup cooked	25
Tomato juice, ½ cup	20

Note: Vitamin C is very narrowly distributed in nature, confined almost exclusively to the vegetable and fruit group. Within this group, foods vary greatly in vitamin C content.
From "Home and Garden Bulletin No. 72," *USDA*, Washington, D.C., 1970.

2 **Lability.** Many vitamins are labile, or unstable, in that they readily undergo actual chemical changes which convert them to inactive substances. Heat, light, and oxygen are examples of agents that can diminish the ability of certain vitamins to perform their usual roles by changing the normal structure of the vitamin molecule.

3 **Deliberate removal of parts of the food.** An example of this is seen in the refining of grains, in which the outer coats are removed. Because most of the iron and vitamins are in these outer layers, refined grain has less of these nutrients than the original whole grain had. Enrichment of refined grain products replaces the nutrients which, if not replaced, might well result in practical health problems.

Of the enormous number of facts available, perhaps the most useful information about each vitamin is that which attempts to answer the following questions:

1. What are the important ordinary foods which can supply significant amounts of the vitamin?
2. Are the common opinions about the vitamin based on fact or on fancy?

ASCORBIC ACID, ALSO KNOWN AS VITAMIN C

"Limey" has been the name for a British sailor since it was shown that a ration of citrus fruit juice could prevent the disease scurvy, which we now know to be caused by ascorbic acid deficiency. A look at the ascorbic acid content of common foods (Table 15–2) readily explains why this disease occurred most commonly on long sea voyages. The good and fair vitamin C sources contain large amounts; other vegetables and fruits supply at least some; but most foods outside of the vegetable-fruit group contain very little ascorbic acid. During the great age of exploration, from the sixteenth through the eighteenth century, food-processing methods such as canning and freezing were unknown. The sailor's diet therefore consisted mostly of hard biscuits, dried meat, cheese, beer, and rum; the only fruits or vegetables taken along were those which had been preserved by drying. Because vitamin C is the most labile of all the vitamins, readily destroyed by agents such as oxygen, excessive heat, and certain metal ions, dried fruits and vegetables supplied far too little of the vitamin to prevent scurvy.

The animals which were sometimes taken along on sea voyages to provide fresh meat never suffered from scurvy as the sailors did. This is because most species can produce the ascorbic acid they need in their own cells. Vitamin C is therefore really a vitamin only for the few species which have lost the ability to synthesize it: the human and other primates, the guinea pig, the Indian fruit bat, and the bulbul bird.

A major function of ascorbic acid is as a cofactor in one step in synthesizing the connective tissue protein, collagen. Collagen is, in a sense, Nature's "glue," holding groups of cells together. Ascorbic acid deficiency therefore results in a defect in wound healing, which requires the formation of new connective tissue to fill the gap. In the days of the swashbuckling, sword-fighting seafarer, impaired wound healing would have been a serious matter indeed. Decreased ability to synthesize collagen in the walls of blood vessels causes the vessels to break easily so that hemorrhages occur readily: this is particularly obvious in the gums, which are subjected to a good deal of physical stress. However, additional vitamin C is useless in treating bleeding gums unless the condition has resulted from vitamin C deficiency rather than from any of the numerous other possible causes. Holding the teeth in their sockets is another role of collagen; in previous centuries the smiling young sailor who left port with gleaming white teeth might return months later with no teeth left. Loosening or falling out of teeth can be caused by many other factors, however, and professional dental treatment, not vitamin C, is the solution in these cases.

In addition to its role in collagen synthesis, ascorbic acid has several other functions; it enhances the absorption of iron and calcium in the intestine, and acts as a coenzyme in the synthesis of hormones of the adrenal glands, and in the interconversions of certain amino acids. However, perhaps the statement most widely believed about ascorbic acid, despite the lack of scientific evidence, is its supposed ability to combat the common cold.

Vitamin C and the common cold

Recommended allowances for ascorbic acid are already far above the levels (about 10 milligrams in adults) needed to prevent scurvy, thereby affording a wide safety margin above actual minimum needs. Nevertheless, a large number of people have been persuaded that an even greater ascorbic acid intake will confer additional benefits; in particular, they believe that enormous doses will prevent or cure the common cold. By "enormous" is meant 20 to 25 times the RDA, or even more—sometimes over 5000 milligrams daily. Because it is virtually impossible to obtain these amounts even from the richest food sources, the vitamin C–common cold debate has been a boon for the pharmaceutical firms which produce vitamin C tablets. Briefly, the claims made for vitamin C are that:

1. It is effective in reducing the number of colds, or at least reducing their severity and duration, or relieving some of the symptoms.
2. It is entirely safe at the high doses advocated.

The claim for effectiveness has very little support. Controlled studies on human subjects indicate that if there is any relief of symptoms, it is because of a drug-like action rather than the result of the vitamin acting in its usual biological role. As for any effect on the number of colds, a decrease is reported as often for the control subjects as for those receiving large doses of vitamin C.

The second claim—safety at any dose—can certainly be questioned. Unpleasant side effects such as nausea and diarrhea are commonly seen soon after ingestion of large doses of vitamin C. It is not yet known whether more serious effects of long-term excess intakes will be evident later. For example, vitamin C is known to be converted in the body to a substance which forms a major part of many kidney stones. Thus, although vitamin C, being water-soluble, is *less* toxic than equal excesses of fat-soluble vitamins, the claim that it is "safe in any amount" may prove to be too good to be true.

VITAMIN A

"Of course it's good for your eyes; did you ever see a rabbit wearing glasses?" Obviously many people are aware of at least two facts about vitamin A: It has something to do with the eyes, and something to do with foods such as carrots.

Actually, though, vitamin A itself is *not* found in carrots or in any other foods of plant origin. Two components of the diet contribute vitamin A:

"Preformed" vitamin A, found only in certain foods of animal origin such as egg yolk, liver, kidney, and the fat of milk, is the vitamin itself, useful to the body just as it is.

Carotenes, the "pro-vitamin A" or "vitamin A precursors" of the diet, are certain deep yellow or orange pigments found in large amounts in dark green and deep yellow vegetables and fruits. In the cells lining the intestine, these compounds can be *converted* to vitamin A, which the body can use.

Therefore, although carrots and other foods in the dark green-deep yellow subgroup of the Basic Four Plan really do not contain vitamin A itself, they are important sources of a diet's total "vitamin A activity" or "vitamin A value"—the sum of performed vitamin A *plus* the potential vitamin A of carotenes.

Because vitamin A and carotenes are not water-soluble, very little vitamin A value is lost in the water in which foods are cooked. In addition, these substances are very stable to agents such as heat and light, which readily destroy some of the other vitamins. In fact, the only agent to which vitamin A is labile is oxygen, so that prolonged exposure to oxygen, as in the slow drying of fruits, is the one process which can significantly decrease the vitamin A value of foods.

Although the Basic Four Plan recommends dark green and deep yellow vegetables and fruits as the main sources of vitamin A value, not all people choose to eat many of these. For these individuals, other foods such as dairy products may well be the most significant vitamin A sources (Table 15–3). It is for this reason that margarine, which is produced from vegetable oils containing very little vitamin A compared to the cream from which butter is made, is fortified with vitamin A. Otherwise, it would not be a satisfactory substitute for those who would otherwise obtain much of their vitamin A from butter.

Pills, polar bears, and poisoning

A *moderate* excess of vitamin A results when people habitually consume larger than necessary amounts of ordinary food sources. Far from being detrimental, this results in the storage of a useful reserve of the vitamin in the liver.

The problem of toxicity arises when intake is *far* in excess of needs. Most commonly this is caused by overuse of vitamin A supplements. People may take 50,000 to 100,000 International Units of vitamin

TABLE 15–3
Vitamin A activity of some common foods

Food	**Vitamin A activity (IU)**
Bread and cereal group	
Enriched white bread, 1 slice	trace
Whole wheat bread, 1 slice	trace
Meat group	
Beef, all types, 2 ounces	trace–50
Chicken, flesh only, 2 ounces	50
Liver (beef), fried, 2 ounces	30,000+
*Kidney (beef), cooked, 2 ounces	660
Pork (chops, roasts, etc.), 2 ounces	0
Eggs, 2 large	1180
Cooked dry beans, 1 cup	0
Milk group	
Milk, whole, 1 cup	350
Milk, unfortified skim, 1 cup	10
Cheese (American, cheddar, etc.), 1½ ounces	500–550
Ice cream, regular, 2 cups	1180
Ice cream, rich (16% fat), 2 cups	1960
Vegetable and fruit group	
Apple, 1 medium	50
Banana, 1 medium	230
Beet greens, ½ cup cooked	3700
Beets, ½ cup cooked	15
Broccoli, ½ cup cooked	3880
Brussels sprouts, ½ cup cooked	400
Cabbage, shredded raw, ½ cup	60
Cantaloupe, ½ medium	6540
Carrot, ½ cup cooked or raw	7600
Collards, ½ cup cooked	5100
Green beans, ½ cup cooked	340
Green peas, ½ cup cooked	430
Orange, 1 medium	260
Spinach, ½ cup cooked	7200
Tomato, 1 medium	1600
Miscellaneous	
Butter, 1 tablespoon	470
Margarine, 1 tablespoon	470
Vegetable oils	0
Sugar, syrup, etc.	0–trace

* Calculated from data in "Agricultural Handbook No. 8," *USDA*, Washington, D.C. 1963.
From "Home and Garden Bulletin No. 72," *USDA*, Washington, D.C., 1970.

A daily—many times the 4000 to 5000 units recommended. Adolescents in particular may do this in an attempt to treat the acne which plagues so many young people. Although it is true that vitamin A is very important in maintaining healthy epithelial tissue, and that vitamin A deficiency causes a particular type of dermatitis, common acne is an outcome of the action of male sex hormones on glands in the skin, and acne therefore does not respond to vitamin A supplements. Overdoses of vitamin A can lead to headaches, nausea, and a variety of other unpleasant or dangerous consequences, without having any beneficial effect on the skin disorders or other problems which the person is trying to treat.

A second practice that can lead to vitamin A toxicity is the eating of certain very unusual, even bizarre, diets. Arctic explorers, for example, have suffered extreme toxicity as the result of eating polar bear liver. The livers of all animals are rich in vitamin A, but polar bears store such astonishing amounts of the vitamin in their livers that humans who eat the liver may become poisoned. Vitamin A toxicity is also seen in people who are so convinced of the health value of carrot juice that they may drink as much as two quarts or more daily. Because the carotene intake exceeds the intestine's ability to convert the pigments to the colorless vitamin, carotenes may be absorbed into the body until the skin and even the eyes become bright yellow or orange. The color will fade and the toxicity disappear only if these people can be persuaded to decrease their carrot juice intake to a reasonable level.

Vitamin A deficiency: the most devastating world wide vitamin deficiency

Because previously well nourished people have stored up reserves that can be drawn upon, deficiency of vitamin A does not ordinarily result in symptoms until after several months have passed. Eventually, however, reserves are exhausted and changes then occur in various cells and organs. The most obvious changes are seen in two types of structures: epithelium (the skin and mucous membranes) and the eyes.

The skin of a vitamin A deficient person becomes rough, dry, and hardened, and hair follicles become raised so that the skin acquires a "goose-pimple" appearance. Degeneration of cells of the mucous membranes may be even more serious, causing decreased resistance to infections of the lungs, ears, genitourinary tract, and nasal passages. This fact has led to the inaccurate description of vitamin A as "the anti-infection vitamin." Certainly adequate amounts of vitamins, including vitamin A, are necessary for normal resistance to infection. However, excess amounts will *not* produce above-normal resistance as the "anti-infection" label might imply.

Vitamin A deficiency affects the eyes in two entirely different ways, depending upon the part which is affected. If the degree of deficiency is mild, it is the retina, which corresponds to the film in a camera, which suffers. If the deficiency is severe and prolonged enough, an entirely different kind of damage occurs in the cornea, or clear outer part of the eye.

FIGURE 15–3

A Vietnamese girl blinded by vitamin A deficiency. The amount of vitamin A costing about 10 cents per year could have saved her sight. (UNICEF, photo by Jacques Danois.)

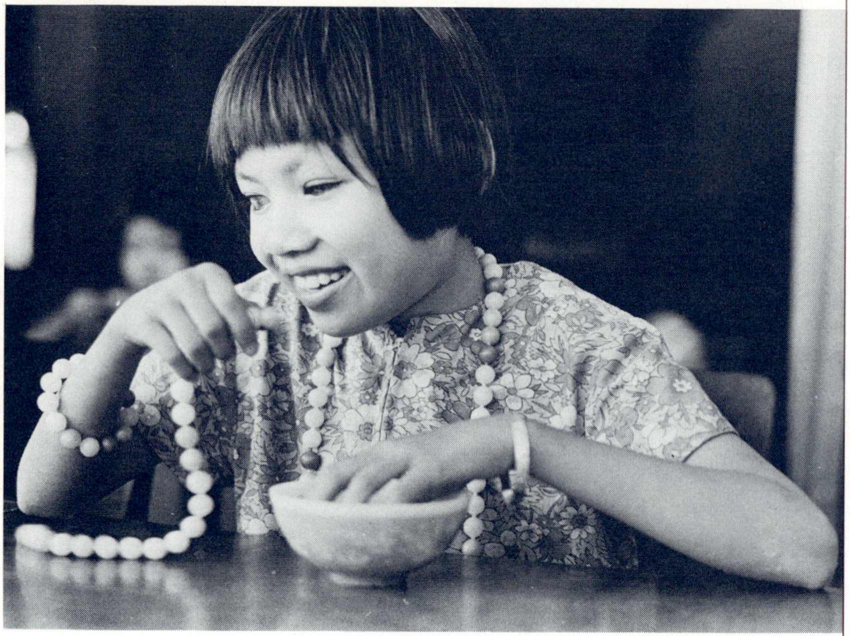

Light, sight, and the changeable colors of eyes

Cells in the retina contain "visual pigments" which consist of vitamin A linked to specific proteins. Although they do not inspire poetry, as the outwardly visible eye colors do, these pigments are the ones that are really important in the process of sight. Their ability to function in vision is the result of an unusual characteristic: they bleach in the presence of light, and return to normal color when light is absent. The alternate bleaching and recoloring of these pigments stimulates nerves, which carry impulses to the brain. It is in the brain that these impulses are sorted out, and are experienced by the person as something that is seen. The bleaching occurs because light causes the colored complex to split into its colorless components, vitamin A and protein; the regeneration of color occurs when the complex is re-formed. However, the vitamin A needed to re-form the complex must be obtained continuously from the blood. Deficiency of vitamin A therefore slows down the rate of regeneration of visual pigment and results in "night blindness," a greatly impaired ability to adapt to dim light.

Vitamin A deficiency does *not* impair the ability to respond to bright light. This is because the retina contains two distinct types of cells, called rods and cones because of their shapes. These cells differ greatly in their sensitivity to changes in the vitamin A supply; the rods, which function in dim-light vision, are far more sensitive to decreased vitamin A availability than are the cones, which are responsible for bright-light vision.

The cornea and vitamin A deficiency

If vitamin A deficiency is very severe and prolonged, the cornea becomes extremely dry as the result of blocking of the tear ducts. The cells of the cornea may then undergo a series of degenerative changes until the cornea eventually becomes opaque. At the most advanced stage, known as *xerophthalmia,* total and irreversible blindness is a common result. Although this is virtually never a cause of blindness in developed countries, many thousands of people, mostly children, become irreversibly blind each year because of vitamin A deficiency, in India, countries of the Near East, and other parts of the world (Figure 15–3).

In developed countries, severe vitamin A deficiency has occurred as a result of unusual conditions, such as those seen during war. For example, during World War II, most of the butter and other dairy products were exported from Denmark by the occupation government in order to buy war materials, thus effectively removing a major vitamin A source from the Danish population. Vitamin A deficiency, including cases of xerophthalmia, became very prevalent in children as a result, although previously this disease had been unseen in Denmark. "Guns and butter" is the expression used to this day to describe the conflict between demands for war materials and the needs of life for a nation's people.

VITAMIN D: A VITAMIN OR A HORMONE?

Perhaps vitamin D should not be considered a vitamin at all, but a hormone. Certainly for many years humanity managed to survive without having it in the diet. This is because, in the presence of an adequate supply of sunlight, the skin itself can use a *sterol* to produce adequate amounts of vitamin D. It was not until the time of the industrial revolution that vitamin D deficiency became widespread, as vast numbers of people migrated into cities. There the crowded, smoky environment effectively prevented them from gaining access to sunlight, and vitamin D, previously manufactured in adequate amounts endogenously, then became a dietary essential.

The problem of getting an adequate dietary supply is that *no common food is naturally rich in vitamin D.* People must therefore obtain vitamin D from one or more of the following sources:

1 *Endogenous vitamin D,* produced by irradiation of a steroid produced in the skin, is adequate for most adults upon casual exposure to sunlight. Hence there is no RDA for vitamin D for adults except during pregnancy and lactation.

2 *Vitamin D-fortified milk* is recommended particularly for those who, because of growth, pregnancy, or lactation, may need more than the amount produced in the body. Milk actually contains very little

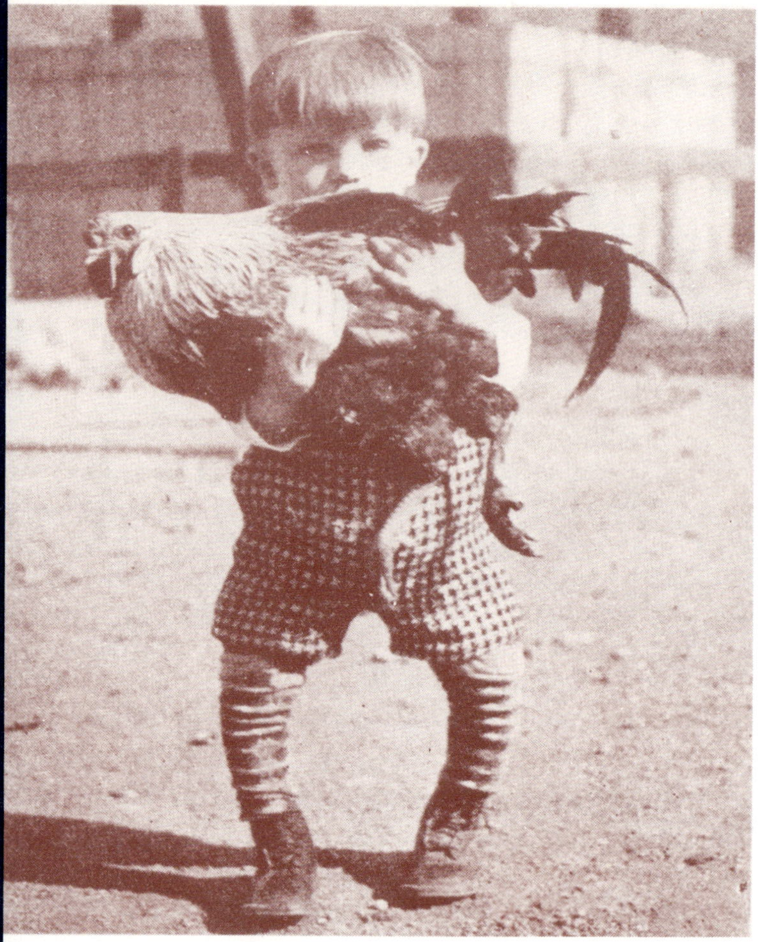

FIGURE 15–4
A little boy with all the signs of rickets: misshapen head, bowlegs, flat feet, and abnormal bone formation as seen by the swelling at the wrists. This photograph was taken in 1936, when rickets was far from rare in the United States. (Photograph courtesy National Library of Medicine, Bethesda, Maryland, 20014.)

vitamin D as it comes from a cow or human or any other mammal, but it has been selected as an ideal food to be fortified with vitamin D. Although foods other than milk are also sometimes fortified with the vitamin, the use of these is not recommended because undesirably high intakes can result.

3 *Supplements,* formerly cod liver oil but now usually drops, pills, or capsules containing vitamin D, are recommended if vitamin D-fortified foods are not used *and* exposure to sunlight is inadequate.

Rickets: A Disease of Civilization

The outstanding role of vitamin D in the body is in enhancing the absorption of calcium in the intestine; deficient individuals may absorb as little as 10 percent of the calcium in their diets, compared to 30 to 40 percent in those with an adequate vitamin D intake. A second function is to remove phosphate from certain phosphate-containing compounds in the body. These combined effects serve to insure that the blood contains suitable levels of calcium and phosphate for the formation of normally mineralized bones.

In the absence of adequate vitamin D, infants and children develop the deficiency disease *rickets,* in which the bones remain soft and poorly mineralized rather than becoming strong and rigid. When the child begins to walk, the legs become severely bowed and "knock-kneed" because the bones are subjected to weight which they are not equipped to bear (Figure 15–4). Because the skull bones do not fuse together at the normal rate, the head of a child with rickets may be larger than normal. Interestingly, the combination of delayed walking and head enlargement was formerly believed to indicate that these unfortunate children were unusually intelligent; "all the energy goes to the brain instead of into walking." Little did the parents realize that their children were suffering deformities which could have been prevented at no cost, merely by exposing the bare skin to sunlight.

Overdosing with vitamin D

In most developed countries today, the main concern in relation to vitamin D is not rickets, but the disease of toxicity caused by excess. This is never caused by excess vitamin D from ordinary foods or by excess synthesis in the body, but from the practices of overzealous people who reason that, if one daily dose of a supplement is good, ten doses must be ten times as good. Permanent damage can be done to the heart, kidney, and other organs because, as more and more calcium is absorbed, it is eventually deposited in soft tissues—which were never meant to be mineralized. Clearly, major problems related to vitamin D today are in educating people regarding the danger of overuse of supplements, and persuading food processors to stop adding vitamin D to breakfast cereals, bread, milk flavorings, and the many other foods which are currently fortified.

THIAMIN (VITAMIN B_1)

The "morale vitamin" and the "appetite vitamin" are but two of the erroneous names given to thiamin. It is true, however, that this compound is particularly important in nerve function, because of its roles in carbohydrate metabolism (Figure 15–5).

Beriberi, the disease resulting from severe thiamin deficiency, clearly reflects the results of impaired carbohydrate metabolism on nervous system function. The victim becomes irritable, confused, and depressed, and appetite virtually disappears. These changes, which are the basis of the "morale vitamin" and "appetite vitamin" misnomers, are of course seen in many forms of emotional as well as physical diseases. When caused by thiamin deficiency, however, they are accompanied by many other symptoms: the muscles become wasted and weakened, and the heart beat becomes abnormally rapid. In "wet"

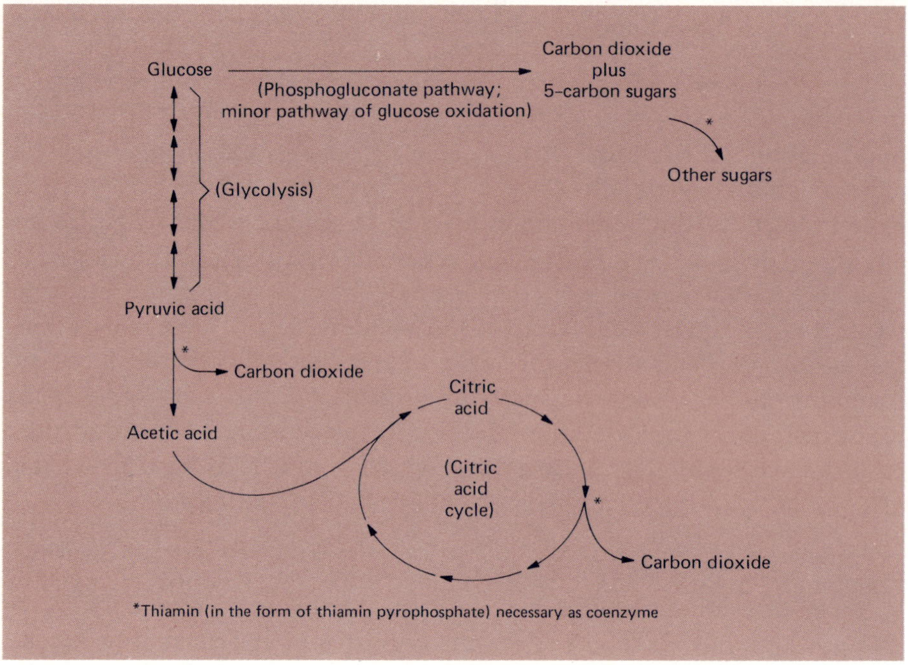

FIGURE 15–5. Some important roles of thiamin in carbohydrate catabolism.

beriberi, massive fluid accumulation is seen; in others, edema is absent and the emaciation as the result of muscle wasting is therefore very obvious.

Beriberi, like rickets, is an example of a "disease of civilization." It was rarely seen until about 1850, when refined grains largely replaced whole, unpolished grains in the diets of many people. Most of the thiamin in grains is found in the outer coats removed by refining. For people with few alternate sources of thiamin, replacement of whole grains with refined grains created a serious shortage of the vitamin. In particular, peoples of the Far East were affected because a grain (rice) commonly constituted a disproportionate part of the total diet. For populations with more varied diets, refining of grains had much less effect on total thiamin intake.

Beriberi could be prevented merely by enriching refined grains, but because this knowledge is often not practiced, beriberi continues to be one of the leading causes of death in some parts of the world. In the Philippines, for example, the American habit of refining grains was adopted enthusiastically when the islands became an American protectorate; however, the American practice of enriching refined grains was not widely adopted. The American custom of getting thiamin from a wide variety of other foods is economically impossible for many of the people of the Philippines. As long as this combination of problems exists, people will continue to die of thiamin deficiency while in the midst of unrefined rice which, if consumed in that state, could prevent the disease.

Food sources of thiamin

Pork is an outstandingly rich source of thiamin, but most people do not eat pork every day. The average person therefore obtains thiamin by getting small amounts here and there from the many common foods which provide small but useful amounts (Table 15–4). Enriched and whole grain breads and cereals are particularly useful and reliable daily sources, and people who avoid grain products as "fattening" or "nothing but starch" should be aware that the four servings of enriched or whole grain breads and cereals recommended daily supply a significant proportion of the RDA for thiamin. Because thiamin is quite unstable to heat and other agents, some degree of planning is necessary to insure an adequate intake.

RIBOFLAVIN

Riboflavin is particularly important as part of a cofactor involved in amino acid breakdown (Figure 15–6), and as a vital part of one of the carriers which transport hydrogen from all classes of energy nutrients to oxygen (Figure 15–6). In view of these roles in metabolism, one

FIGURE 15–6. Some important roles of riboflavin in metabolism.

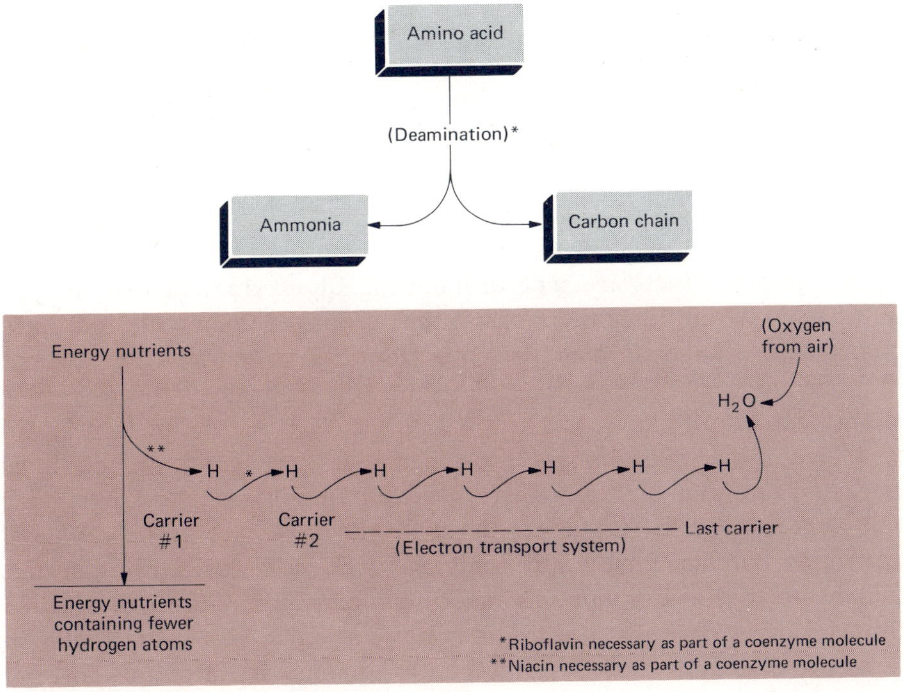

TABLE 15–4
Thiamin content of some common foods

Foods	Thiamin (milligrams)
Bread and cereal group	
Enriched white bread, 1 slice	0.07
Whole wheat bread, 1 slice	0.09
Meat group	
Beef (hamburger), cooked, 2 ounces	0.05
Chicken, flesh only, fried, 2 ounces	0.03
Liver (beef), fried, 2 ounces	0.15
Pork, lean only, roast, 2 ounces	0.60
Eggs, 2	0.10
Cooked dry beans, 1 cup	0.13
Milk group	
Milk, whole, 1 cup	0.07
Cheese (American, cheddar, etc.), 1½ ounces	0.01
Ice cream, regular, 2 cups	0.10
Vegetable and fruit group	
Apple, 1 medium	0.04
Banana, 1 medium	0.06
Carrots, cooked, ½ cup	0.04
Corn, cooked, ½ cup	0.04
Green beans, cooked, ½ cup	0.05
Green peas, cooked, ½ cup	0.22
Orange, 1 medium	0.13
Orange juice, ½ cup	0.11
Potato, boiled, 1 medium	0.12
Miscellaneous	
Unenriched white bread, 1 slice	0.02
Bacon, 2 slices, cooked	0.08
Fats and oils	0
White sugar, 1 tablespoon	0
Honey, 1 tablespoon	trace

From "Home and Garden Bulletin No. 72," *USDA*, Washington, D.C., 1970.

might anticipate spectacular deficiency symptoms, but curiously, no such dramatic effects are seen in humans. Riboflavin deficiency causes a dry scaly dermatitis and cracks at the corners of the mouth, but these changes are similar to those resulting from many other causes. Further, there is no hard-to-remember name for the deficiency disease: it is simply called *ariboflavinosis*.

Two effects seen in severely deficient experimental animals have attracted a great deal of attention. In developing rat embryos, deficiency causes a variety of congenital defects including harelip, cleft palate, and bone defects. Postnatally, deficiency in rats results in cataracts, which are the most common cause of human blindness in the United States. However, there appears to be no relationship between riboflavin and either birth defects or cataracts in humans, and attempts to treat or prevent these conditions with large doses of riboflavin are therefore futile.

Although riboflavin is widely distributed in foods, the outstandingly useful common sources are in the milk group (Table 15–5). Two cups of milk alone provide over one-half of the RDA for riboflavin for adults.

Riboflavin is a rather stable vitamin, resisting destruction by heat, acid, or oxygen, and is only slightly unstable to bases. In fact, the most extensive losses occur upon prolonged exposure to light. Nevertheless, packaging of milk in brown bottles or opaque paper or plastic cartons, which protect riboflavin from destruction by light, has been resisted by some consumers. For some reason, people who readily accept beer or soft drinks in colored bottles somehow feel that milk is less acceptable in the same kind of packaging. It should be recognized, however, that very little riboflavin is destroyed by *brief* exposure to light, so it is hardly necessary to gulp milk down immediately after it is poured into the glass in order to protect its riboflavin content.

NIACIN

The only vitamin deficiency disease that has ever been a widespread public health problem in the United States is *pellagra,* resulting from niacin deficiency. Particularly among the poor in the South, pellagra once caused thousands of deaths each year, many cases of mental illness, and hundreds of thousands of cases of serious physical illness. Although niacin deficiency was established as the cause of the disease in the late 1930s, deaths from pellagra continued to occur well into the 1940s, when the rising economy of the World War II era finally made a better diet possible for many.

Pellagra has been called "the disease of the three Ms" because it was associated with a diet of "meat," "meal," and molasses. The "meat" was not really meat at all; in fact, meats are good niacin sources which could have prevented pellagra. Rather, "meat" for the Southern poor was fatback or salt pork—mostly fat with only a very thin streak of lean. The "meal" was cornmeal, and of all grains corn is the poorest niacin source. Molasses, of course, is not a rich source of any vitamin.

Pellagra has also been called "the disease of the four Ds": *dermatitis* (a particularly severe skin disorder); *diarrhea* (presumably caused by degeneration of intestinal cells); *dementia* (mental illness); and finally *death.* The finding that mental illness can be caused by niacin deficiency has generated a good many misconceptions, culminating in so-called "megavitamin therapy" which utilizes large doses of niacin, plus other vitamins and often minerals as well, in the treatment of mental illness, regardless of cause. Proponents of megavitamin therapy have even suggested that the food supply should be enriched so as to provide over 50 times the RDA for niacin. However, a task force of the

TABLE 15–5
Riboflavin content of some common foods

Foods	Riboflavin (milligrams)
Bread and cereal group	
Enriched white bread, 1 slice	0.06
Whote wheat bread, 1 slice	0.03
Meat group	
Beef (hamburger), cooked, 2 ounces	0.12
Chicken, (flesh only), broiled, 2 ounces	0.10
Eggs, 2 large	0.30
Cooked dry beans, 1 cup	0.26
Milk group	
Whole milk, 1 cup	0.41
Skim milk, 1 cup	0.44
2% milk, 1 cup	0.52
Cheese (cheddar, American, etc.), 1½ ounces	0.20
Cottage cheese, 1⅓ cups	0.75
Ice cream, regular, 2 cups	0.56
Vegetable and fruit group	
Apple, 1 medium	0.02
Green beans, cooked, ½ cup	0.05
Green peas, cooked, ½ cup	0.08
Orange, 1 medium	0.05
Orange juice, ½ cup	0.03
Potato, boiled, 1 medium	0.04

From "Home and Garden Bulletin No. 72," *USDA*, Washington, D.C., 1970.

TABLE 15–6
Total Niacin obtained from one cup of milk

	Milligrams
Tryptophan	120*
A. Tryptophan milligrams ÷ 60	2
B. Preformed niacin	0.2**
Total niacin (A plus B)	2.2

* From "Amino Acid Content of Foods and Biological Data on Proteins," *FAO Report No. 24*, Rome, 1970.
** From "Home and Garden Bulletin No. 72," *USDA*, Washington, D.C., 1970.

American Psychiatric Association has examined the literature of the megavitamin proponents and concluded that their credibility is very low:

> **Under these circumstances, this Task Force considers the massive publicity which they promulgate via radio, the lay press and popular books, using catch phrases which are really misnomers like "megavitamin therapy" and "orthomolecular treatment," to be deplorable.**

Sources of niacin: internal, external

Niacin is found as such in foods, but the amount actually obtainable from a food may be far greater than the amount existing in the preformed state. This is because cells can synthesize niacin from the essential amino acid, *tryptophan.* In the various proteins in foods, tryptophan ordinarily constitutes at least 1 percent of the total amino acids. Of this tryptophan, $\frac{1}{60}$ is converted to niacin on the average; the other $\frac{59}{60}$ are of course used for other purposes, such as protein synthesis. The total amount of niacin obtainable from 1 cup of milk, for example, is calculated as shown in Table 15–6. Because foods which contain complete proteins contain the precursor tryptophan, many foods are good niacin sources even though they may not contain the preformed vitamin itself. In fact, all four food groups are good niacin sources. In addition, very little of the vitamin is lost during food processing or preparation, because niacin is stable to heat, oxygen, acid, base, light, and other agents to which other vitamins may be labile.

VITAMIN B_6

As part of a cofactor, *pyridoxal phosphate,* vitamin B_6 functions in many reactions. However, its best-known roles are related to amino acid metabolism. *Transamination,* the transfer of an amino group from an amino acid to another compound, requires vitamin B_6, as does the conversion of certain amino acids to other substances, such as tryptophan to niacin and phenylalanine to adrenaline (epinephrine).

In general, diets that are adequate in other nutrients will be adequate in vitamin B_6, and deficiency of this vitamin is therefore rare in humans. Attempts to use it in treating a variety of disorders, ranging from the nausea of pregnancy to Parkinson's disease and muscular dystrophy, have been very disappointing. However, that the vitamin is essential to humans is unquestioned. During the 1950s a formula used in feeding infants caused irritability and convulsions, later shown to be the result of improper processing which had destroyed most of the vitamin B_6 in the formula.

VITAMIN B_{12}

The name "red vitamin," as vitamin B_{12} is sometimes called in advertising of supplements, is accurate in that the vitamin is indeed red. The name is somewhat misleading, however, in that it may imply that vitamin B_{12} deficiency is a common cause of anemia; to some, the association of vitamin B_{12} and red blood seems clear. Actually, vitamin B_{12} deficiency is a *rare* cause of anemia, occurring as the result of two distinctly different conditions: a disease (usually genetic), or a strict vegetarian diet (Figure 15–7).

Pernicious anemia is the name of the disease caused by vitamin B_{12} deficiency. Until the 1920s, there was no known treatment for the disease. *Pernicious,* in fact, means deadly or fatal. Then it was discovered that people with this disease could be restored to health by feeding

TABLE 15–7
Vitamin B_{12} content of some common foods

Foods	Approximate vitamin B_{12} content (micrograms)
Bread and cereal group	
All items	0 or very low*
Meat group	
Beef (hamburger), 2 ounces	1
Eggs, 2 medium	3
Liver (beef), 2 ounces	65
Liverwurst, 2 ounces	8
Milk group	
Milk, whole, 1 cup	0.9
Cheese, cheddar, 1½ ounces	0.4
Vegetable and fruit group	
All Items	0 or very low*

* As they are harvested, foods of plant origin are devoid of vitamin B_{12}. However, the vitamin is often added, at least in small amounts, during food preparation. Examples are the use of milk as an ingredient in bread, and the inclusion of eggs, milk, or cheese in cream sauces served with vegetables.
From H. Lichtenstein, A. Beloian, and E. W. Murphy, "Home Economics Research Report No. 13," *USDA,* Washington, D.C., 1961.

them either one of two things: up to a pound of raw or very rare liver daily, or stomach juice obtained from normal people. Needless to say, neither of these treatments was acceptable to many people; however, the alternative was progressive nerve damage, extreme anemia, and eventual death.

The discovery that liver could be used to treat pernicious anemia led to the concept that there was some *extrinsic factor* involved; this turned out to be vitamin B_{12}. Gastric juice must, therefore, contain an *intrinsic factor*—something produced inside the body itself and necessary for utilizing vitamin B_{12}. This proved to be a specific protein,

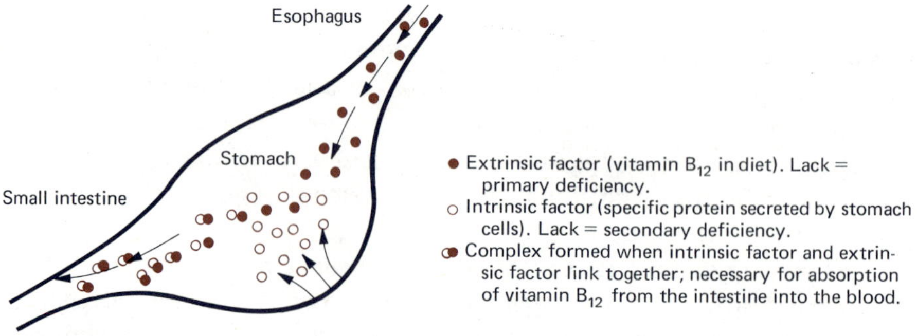

FIGURE 15–7. The two possible causes of vitamin B_{12} deficiency.

secreted by the cells of the stomach, which links to the vitamin and carries it across the intestinal wall.

People who lack the intrinsic factor genetically, or as the result of diseases or surgical removal of the stomach, can be treated in two ways:

1 Vitamin B_{12} can be injected, thereby getting around the problem of absorption from the intestine.
2 Alternatively, the vitamin can be given by mouth in *huge* doses; absorption of even a small proportion of the very large dose results in delivery of the small amount needed to the cells.

Vitamin B_{12} is found only in foods of animal origin, not in foods of plant origin (Table 15–7). For this reason, those on strict vegetarian diets may develop vitamin B_{12} deficiency even though they produce normal amounts of the intrinsic factor. This statement is denied by some, who insist that a strict vegetarian diet can support health. However, there are several possible explanations for the fact that people sometimes remain healthy on supposedly strict vegetarian diets. One is the presence of inadvertent foods of animal origin, such as insects which commonly infest grain. Another is the feces (animal or human) used as fertilizer in many parts of the world. Bacteria produce vitamin B_{12} and, in fact, sewage sludge, rat feces in foods, and feces on unwashed vegetable crops may provide adequate vitamin B_{12} produced by the bacteria in feces. It is thus possible that low standards of sanitation actually help to prevent vitamin B_{12} deficiency in some populations. Obviously, people who are more fastidious about sanitation will not be protected in this manner.

FOLACIN

Folacin (folic acid) comes from the same root word as *foliage*, because the vitamin is found in large amounts in certain green leafy vegetables. However, many other common foods are also good sources, and the milk group is the only food group which is actually low in folacin content.

Folacin is related to several important medical problems. Because the vitamin is part of a cofactor needed for synthesizing one of the subunits of DNA, folacin deficiency causes decreased cell division. This results in the appearance in the blood stream of large immature blood cells, which are unable to complete, by further cell division, their maturation. The condition is called *megaloblastic anemia* (megalo: large; blast: immature). Large doses of folacin can of course correct the megaloblastic anemia of folacin deficiency. Unfortunately, it may also correct the megaloblastic anemia caused by deficiency of another nutrient, vitamin B_{12}. If this occurs, a person may have normal-appearing blood but continue to suffer progressive nerve damage as the result of undiagnosed vitamin B_{12} deficiency. In order to avoid the possi-

TABLE 15-8
Vitamin E content of some common foods

Foods	Approximate vitamin E content (milligrams)*
Bread and cereal group	
Enriched white bread, 1 slice	0.06
Whole wheat bread, 1 slice	0.6
Meat group	
Beef (hamburger), cooked, 2 ounces	0.35
Eggs, 2 medium	1.4
Pork sausage, fried, 2 ounces	0.18
Milk group	
Whole milk, 1 cup	0.24
Ice cream, vanilla, 2 cups	1.1
Vegetable and fruit group	
Apple, 1 medium	0.7
Green beans, cooked frozen, ½ cup	0.3
Green peas, cooked frozen, ½ cup	0.7
Potato, baked, 1 medium	0.06
Miscellaneous	
Bacon, fried, 2 slices	0.09
Butter, 1 tablespoon	0.14
Margarine (made from vegetable oil), 1 tablespoon	7.4

* Several closely related compounds possess vitamin E activity, although to varying degrees. An international unit (IU) of vitamin E is defined as the activity of 1 milligram of one of these compounds: dl-alpha-tocopherol acetate.
Figures calculated from data of R. H. Bunnell, J. Keating, A. Quaresimo, and G. K. Parman, "Alpha-tocopherol Content of Foods," *American Journal of Chemical Nutrition, 17*:1 (1965).

bility of this masking effect, the amount of folacin in nonprescription vitamin supplements is limited by law.

Another medical aspect of folacin is the use of antifolacin compounds, or *folacin antagonists,* in the treatment of certain types of cancer. These drugs resemble folacin so closely that enzymes link to them rather than to folacin; the resulting complex is unable to catalyze the usual reactions. Consequently, the rate of DNA synthesis, and hence of cell division, is slowed. Thus, although many food faddists insist that cancer can be "cured" by a variety of diets or nutrient supplements, the only relationship between nutrition and cancer that has been established is that a relative folacin *deficiency,* induced by folacin-antagonizing drugs, can slow the growth of cancer cells.

VITAMIN E

The "sex vitamin" and the "fertility factor" are names that have been given, erroneously, to vitamin E. Although it is true that animals made severely deficient in vitamin E are unable to reproduce, reproductive failures can be caused by many factors, and vitamin E is ineffective in the treatment of human reproductive problems. Nevertheless, it continues to be sold on the basis of its supposed effectiveness in cases of inability to conceive, repeated spontaneous abortion, and even frigidity and impotence. Advertisements generally imply, rather than stating explicitly, that vitamin E has a particularly satisfactory rejuvenating effect on aging males.

Although much remains to be learned about the functions of vitamin E, it is known to prevent destruction of certain other nutrients by oxygen; vitamin A, ascorbic acid, and unsaturated fatty acids, in the cells as well as in foods, are protected in this manner. In addition, vitamin E appears to function as a cofactor in the release of energy from glucose and fatty acids, particularly in the heart and other muscles. Because of this, athletes sometimes take enormous doses of vitamin E in a useless attempt at improving muscle performance. Results of studies that have sought to establish a link between vitamin E and human diseases such as heart disease and muscular dystrophy have been disappointing, to say the least. Because these diseases were not caused by vitamin E deficiency, they obviously cannot be treated by giving the vitamin. Among humans, only premature newborn babies commonly show signs of vitamin E deficiency: their red blood cells are abnormally fragile. This conditions *can* be corrected by administration of the vitamin.

Adequate amounts of vitamin E are rather easy to obtain because useful amounts are present in many common foods, although the most outstandingly rich sources are vegetable oils and foods made with these oils (Table 15–8). Whole grain products are richer sources than enriched refined grain products because of the oil in the germ of whole grains. However, the difference is insignificant compared to the vitamin E intake obtainable from other sources, and the choice of whole grain or refined grain products can therefore be made on the basis of taste, without any risk of vitamin E shortage.

One interesting factor in the need for vitamin E is the amount of polyunsaturated fat in the diet; the higher the polyunsaturated fat intake, the greater the need for vitamin E, presumably because of its role in protecting the fatty acids from destruction by oxygen. Fortunately, polyunsaturated fats themselves are generally accompanied by large amounts of vitamin E, so that the increased vitamin requirement is likely to be met automatically.

VITAMIN K

K stands for *koagulation,* the Danish spelling used by the discoverer of this vitamin. The name reflects the fact that vitamin K is necessary for the synthesis of a specific protein, *prothrombin,* which is a vital part of the blood's mechanism for clotting, or coagulation (Figure 15–8).

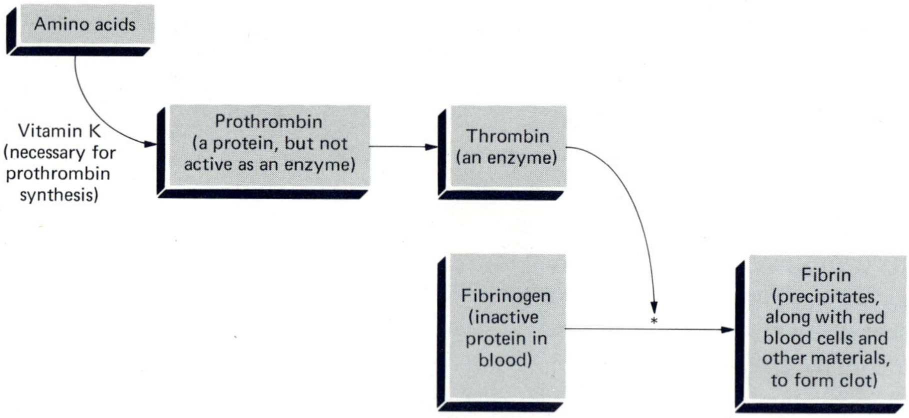

*Thrombin is an enzyme that catalyzes the conversion of fibrinogen to fibrin.

FIGURE 15–8. The role of vitamin K in blood clotting.

Vitamin K is supplied in two ways: In the diet, vitamin K is obtained from a variety of foods; green vegetables are especially good sources, and milk supplies significant amounts.

Bacteria in the intestine also produce large amounts of the vitamin, which can then be absorbed. For this reason, even a diet devoid of vitamin K would not necessarily produce a state of deficiency. When deficiency does occur, therefore, it is generally the result of impaired synthesis by the intestinal microorganisms or of defective absorption of the vitamin. Occasionally this happens in people who have taken antibiotics, by mouth, over a long period of time, thereby killing many of the bacteria in the intestinal tract, or in people whose absorption of fats is defective. However, despite the unliklihood of vitamin K deficiency in humans, health-food store proprietors find a ready market for alfalfa, sold as a source of vitamin K.

The only group of people commonly found to be vitamin K deficient are newborn infants, because the intestinal tract is normally sterile at birth. Several days must elapse before intestinal bacteria become established and synthesize adequate amounts of vitamin K. Because of the danger of uncontrolled hemorrhage, newborn infants are routinely given vitamin K by injection, providing protection until the intestinal bacteria are well established.

In many parts of the world, however, the need for vitamin K in the newborn is not met, and consequently a certain number of babies die of blood loss soon after birth. It is interesting that the ancient Hebrews specified that circumcision be performed on the eighth day of life, by which time intestinal microorganisms have synthesized the vitamin K needed to protect against the extensive blood loss which could occur if this surgery were performed in the first few days of life.

PANTOTHENIC ACID

According to the label on one brand of hair spray, *pantothenic acid* is "the hair-absorbable vitamin B!" Apparently some people do not know that hair is dead, and therefore cannot be nourished by pantothenic acid or by any other nutrient.

Pantothenic acid is, however, extremely important in the metabolism of living cells, because it is part of coenzyme A (A for acetic acid). In previous sections, acetic acid has been discussed as an important intermediate in the metabolism of energy nutrients. Actually, it is not the free acid, but a complex formed by linking acetic acid to the coenzyme, which participates in cellular reactions.

However, there is little concern about pantothenic acid deficiency, because *pantothenic* means *found everywhere,* and this describes its distribution in foods. In black rats, graying of the hair is seen when pantothenic acid deficiency is induced by feeding specially treated diets. This has no relationship to the gray hair seen as a normal part of the aging process in humans, and the diets fed to the experimental rats are totally unlike diets consumed by humans. Nevertheless, pantothenic acid is often included in vitamin supplements, hair sprays, and other products, although this addition is of no real use to the buyers.

BIOTIN

Biotin deficiency is extremely unlikely, although it can be induced in volunteer subjects by feeding them 20 or 25 raw egg whites daily. Egg whites contain a protein, *avidin,* which binds biotin to form an unabsorbable complex in the digestive tract. Cooking destroys avidin, so cooked egg whites, or *reasonable* amounts of raw egg whites, have no effect on biotin absorption.

Metabolically, biotin is very important as a cofactor in transferring carbon dioxide to and from certain compounds. An example given previously is the addition of CO_2 to pyruvic acid, thereby forming the oxaloacetic acid necessary to keep the citric acid cycle going. From the point of view of practical nutrition, any reasonably well-balanced diet can provide adequate biotin, and the dietary intake is further supplemented by an undetermined amount produced by intestinal bacteria. The inclusion of biotin in multivitamin pills is therefore of absolutely no value to consumers.

OTHER VITAMINS

It is impossible either to prove or disprove the contention that yet-undiscovered vitamins exist. Choline, for example, is a dietary essential for certain animals, and is an important material synthesized at least to some extent in the human body. The problem in deciding whether a compound such as this is essential in the diets of humans is that it is found in such abundance in so many common foods that deficient humans simply are not available to study. Thus although there may be certain factors which the human body cannot synthesize in quantities sufficient to meet its needs, these must be required in such small amounts compared to those present in foods that anybody eating anything can be assured of getting enough.

POSTULATED ADDITIONAL VITAMINS: AN UNFINISHED SYMPHONY IN B?

Most nutritionists agree that the 13 vitamins discussed in this chapter probably constitute a complete list of the vitamins needed by humans. Some would at least tentatively accept *choline* as an additional vitamin, because it is required in the diets of rats, dogs, pigs, and monkeys. However, there is no evidence that choline deficiency occurs in humans, probably because of two factors:

1 Humans apparently synthesize it readily in their cells.
2 Choline is so widespread in nature that it would be difficult to avoid getting enough dietary choline, even if it were not synthesized in the body.

However, despite the impressive body of evidence which indicates that there probably are no remaining undiscovered vitamins, substances purported to be "vital factors which are undoubtedly vitamins" abound. *Rutin,* for example, is called *Vitamin P* by those who insist that it is specifically needed to "restore fragile capillaries to normal" in those unfortunates who have supposedly failed to obtain enough of it. *Bioflavinoids,* said to be found in the pulp and white rind (but, curiously, not in the juice) of citrus fruits, are sold to those who hope to reduce inflammation, speed up the healing of injuries, and somehow "make vitamin C more effective." Because neither rutin nor bioflavinoids are normal constituents of human tissues, the rationale for these claims is a mystery.

In contrast, two other compounds—*inositol* and *lipoic acid—are* normal components of human cells. However, the cells' facility in producing these substances automatically precludes their being considered vitamins. Inositol has been claimed to be effective in treating gray hair, aiding the functioning of the brain, skeletal muscles, and heart, and "increasing the elimination of cholesterol from the body." Lipoic acid, it is claimed, somehow helps to "hold the organs of the body in place," as well as aiding in the absorption of vitamins. One could hardly fail to be impressed with such credentials were it not for the fact that there is not a shred of evidence to support them.

One "vitamin," called "vitamin B_{17}" or *laetrile* is worth particular mention because of the potential danger associated with its use. In the body, this substance breaks down and releases, among other things, cyanide. Several people have actually died as a result of taking "vitamin B_{17}," or of eating fruit pits such as apricot kernels, which contain high concentrations of this "vitamin." The reason given by people who take this dangerous substance is, "Vitamin B_{17} is supposed to prevent cancer, and how do you know it won't help?" With respect to this or to any other untested substance which is "supposed" to be a vitamin or treat a disease there is, of course, a good retort: How do you know it won't *hurt*? Without doubt, in the case of a substance such as "vitamin B_{17}," it can.

SUGGESTED READINGS

American Academy of Pediatrics Committee on Drugs. "Vitamin C and the Common Cold." *Newsletter of the American Academy of Pediatrics* 22 (November 1, 1971).

American Academy of Pediatrics Committees on Drugs and on Nutrition. "The Use and Abuse of Vitamin A." *Pediatrics* 48 (1971):655.

American Psychiatric Task Force Report No. 7. "Megavitamin and Orthomolecular Therapy in Psychiatry." Washington, D.C., American Psychiatric Association, 1973.

"Vitamin E—Miracle or Myth?" FDA Consumer, U.S. Dept. of Health, Education and Welfare, July–August, 1973.

Committee on Nutrition. "The Prophylactic Requirement and the Toxicity of Vitamin D." *Pediatrics* 31 (1963):512.

Food and Nutrition Board–National Research Council. "Supplementation of Human Diets with Vitamin E." Washington, D.C., National Academy of Sciences, 1975.

"Handbook on Human Nutritional Requirements." FAO/WHO. Rome, 1974.

Kamil, A. "How Natural Are Those 'Natural' Vitamins?" *Nutrition Reviews* 32, Supplement No. 1 (1974):34.

Mariam, T. W. and G. Sterky. "Severe Rickets in Infancy and Childhood in Ethiopia." *Journal of Pediatrics* 82 (1973):876.

16

the minerals: from soil to cells to soil...

Minerals, the nutrient class which includes all inorganic substances needed in the diet other than water, perform vital functions of two general types. As *structural* materials, they make up approximately 4 to 5 percent of the total weight of the human body. As *regulators,* many play indispensable roles in numerous biological functions, serving, as vitamins do, as cofactors in biochemical reactions.

One method of classifying minerals is based upon the amounts needed (Table 16–1).

A FEW GENERALIZATIONS ABOUT MINERALS

Although it is common to speak of minerals as if they exist as ordinary, uncharged elements in foods and in living things, uncharged elements such as sodium, chlorine, phosphorus, and so on are actually highly toxic. So when these are mentioned, it is understood that it is the *charged* forms that are meant: sodium ion, chloride ion, phosphate ion.

Compared to many other nutrients, minerals are commonly quite incompletely absorbed; the efficiency of absorption may be as low as 10 percent or less, as in the case of iron. This means that the amount needed *in the diet* may be much greater than the amount needed *by the body,* since only the proportion actually absorbed is available to meet the body's demands; the unabsorbed portion is excreted by the intestine.

After absorption, minerals may exit from the body by several means. For most minerals, the urine is the principal route of excretion; for others, losses in sweat account for a significant proportion of the total excreted. For iron, and perhaps for zinc as well, blood loss may be an extremely important means whereby the mineral leaves the body.

Like certain vitamins, minerals can be lost by dissolving in the water used to soak or cook foods. Unlike vitamins, however, minerals are not *labile* to agents such as heat, light, or oxygen. This is because minerals are atoms rather than molecules, and atoms are not broken down in chemical reactions in living systems, any more than they are in chemical reactions in the nonliving world.

Recommended allowances have been set for six minerals: calcium, phosphorus, iodine, iron, magnesium, and zinc. A seventh mineral, fluoride, is lacking frequently enough to merit concern. Other minerals, although by no means less important, are necessarily considered in much less detail than those listed above.

CALCIUM

Calcium as a structural material

Humans, like other vertebrates, contain a rather large proportion of calcium because it is a major constituent of bones. In fact, calcium is the most abundant mineral in the human body, accounting for approximately 1.5 to 2 percent of body weight, or around one-third of the total minerals present.

However, the presence of large amounts of calcium in bones and teeth should not obscure the fact that these structures are living organs, not merely inert blocks of inanimate material like sticks of chalk. Bones develop by first forming a flexible *matrix* (framework) of the connective tissue protein, collagen, imbedded in soft material known as *ground substance*. Teeth develop somewhat analogously, although the protein of the hardest part of the teeth, the enamel, is keratin rather than collagen. During fetal life, the bones contain relatively little calcium, perhaps as a means of facilitating the birth process by insuring that the bones bend easily rather than fracturing, as more rigid bones would.

Crystals of minerals are deposited in the matrix, a process commonly called *calcification*. However, *mineralization* is really the more accurate term because more than just calcium is involved. Phosphorus, in the form of negatively charged phosphate irons, and other ions such as magnesium, fluoride, and chloride are also deposited. The resulting crystalline material is called *hydroxyapatite*.

If mineralization occurs normally, the bones of the legs become rigid enough to support the infant's weight by the time he or she begins to walk and stand. However, minerals once deposited in bones do not stay there for the rest of the individual's life. New bone is constantly being formed as previously formed bone is constantly being broken down. In this manner, bones are reshaped as the demands on them change; a bone can therefore become thicker at one site or another if this is the form most compatible with the size, shape, and physical activities of the body. If the stress on bones is greatly decreased, as during enforced inactivity in the ill or the elderly, the breakdown of bone material may greatly exceed the building processes, and a net loss of total bone material can result. Astronauts, unable to move about freely, and freed even from the force of gravity, commonly suffer a slight but definite loss of bone minerals during space flight.

Regulatory functions of calcium

Although approximately 99 percent of the total body calcium is found in the bones and teeth, the remaining 1 percent, distributed throughout the body fluids and the cells of soft tissues, is necessary for a variety of important regulatory roles. For example, calcium helps to regulate the contraction of muscles and the transmission of impulses along

TABLE 16–1
Four classes of minerals

Class	Minerals	
Macronutrients essential at levels of 100 milligrams or more per day for adult humans *Macronutrient* mineral elements are those needed in relatively large amounts, hundreds of milligrams daily, and constituting a relatively large proportion of body weight.	Calcium Phosphorus Magnesium	Sodium Potassium Chloride
Micronutrients essential at levels no higher than a few milligrams per day for adult humans *Micronutrient* mineral elements are those needed in small or "trace" amounts, ranging from a small fraction of one milligram to a few milligrams.	Iron Iodine Zinc	Chromium Fluoride
Minerals known or suspected to be essential for humans, but in amounts that cannot even be estimated at present This category includes those minerals known or assumed to be necessary, but about which too little is known to make any reliable estimate of the amounts needed.	Manganese Molybdenum Selenium Nickel	Tin Vanadium Silicon
Minerals present in the human body but with no known function The fourth group consists of minerals which may or may not serve any useful biological function. For example, the body contains traces of elements such as gold, silver, platinum, and lead. Are these necessary for some purpose, or are they merely useless contaminants obtained incidentally from the environment? The answer is unknown, and indeed may never be determined. The need for such elements could be demonstrated only by showing that their *absence* causes some significant biological effect. This would require that organisms be raised in an environment strictly free of these materials—a state of purity difficult and perhaps impossible to attain.	Aluminum Arsenic Barium Cadmium	Gold Lead Silver Others

nerves. If the level of calcium in the blood decreases below a certain critical level, muscles go into uncontrolled contraction known as *tetany*. This occurs, however, only as the result of unusual circumstances such as certain diseases, which cause impaired control of blood calcium levels. Sheer lack of dietary calcium does not in itself cause seriously decreased blood levels of the mineral, because it normally can be withdrawn from the bones as necessary.

Calcium must be present in minute amounts in blood in order for normal clotting to occur (Figure 16–1). It is for this reason that blood

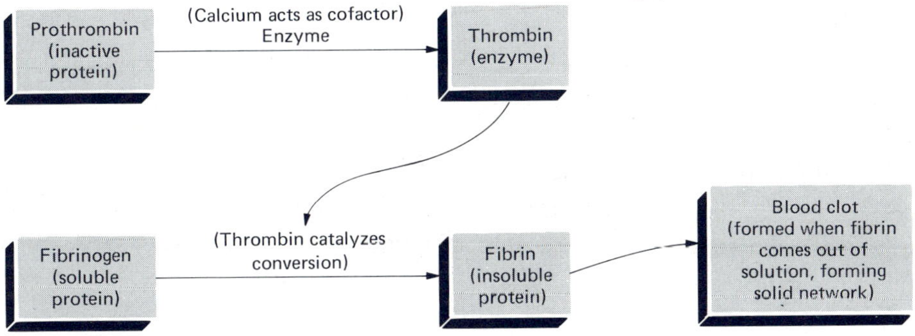

FIGURE 16–1. The role of calcium in blood clotting.

collected for donation to others is collected in specially treated containers. In these containers are small amounts of substances that react with calcium. Citric acid or oxalic acid, for example, are commonly used anticlotting agents which act by binding calcium, thereby making it unable to perform its usual role in coagulation.

In considering the roles of a nutrient, it is very important to recognize that the amount necessary for one function may be very different from the amount needed for another. For example, in view of the importance of calcium in blood clotting, one might assume that calcium deficiency would result in impaired clotting, or that perhaps calcium supplements might be useful in increasing the ability of blood to clot. In fact, however, lowered blood calcium levels stimulate the mobilization of calcium from the bones in order to restore the blood level to normal. Although the bones may eventually become so softened that no further calcium can be removed, even at that point the blood level of calcium would never become so low that the blood would fail to clot. The reason is that the person would die of tetany, which prevents the normal contraction of muscles involved in respiration, long before the blood calcium level could fall below the very minute concentration necessary for normal blood clotting.

Absorption of calcium

Normal people may absorb as little as 10 percent or as much as 40 percent of the amount ingested; on the average, probably no more than 30 percent of the calcium in the diet ever actually gets into the body. In addition to this individual variation, numerous other factors can modify the absorption of calcium. Some of the most important are the following:

Vitamin D. Calcium is transported across the intestinal wall by a specific carrier, and vitamin D is necessary for the production of this carrier in the cells lining the intestine.

Dietary sugars. Various sugars improve the efficiency of calcium absorption, with lactose having the most marked effect. Milk is therefore an excellent calcium source, not only because of its high calcium content, but because of its content of the sugar which increases the proportion of the mineral absorbed.

Dietary fats. Fat may have two completely opposite effects. By slowing down the rate at which food moves along the intestinal tract, fat can increase the time available for absorption of many nutrients, including calcium. Counteracting this, however, is the tendency of certain fatty acids to form insoluble compounds with calcium—just as the fatty acids of soaps react with calcium in hard water to form a bathtub ring. The insoluble calcium compounds formed in the intestinal tract are excreted in the feces rather than being absorbed.

Oxalic acid. The naturally occurring compound, oxalic acid, is found in many foods of plant origin; rhubarb, chocolate, and spinach contain unusually high concentrations. This acid reacts with calcium to form an insoluble compound which cannot be absorbed. Unfortunately, this fact has led to the misconception that spinach "robs the body of calcium." Although it is true that the oxalic acid in spinach prevents the absorption of the calcium *present in spinach,* it is not true that the calcium in other foods is similarly affected by the oxalic acid in spinach. Similarly, the amount of oxalic acid in chocolate is far too small to cause a significant decrease in the absorption of the calcium present in the total diet. Therefore, parents who are reluctant to allow their children to drink chocolate milk because they have heard that chocolate decreases the use of calcium in the body are showing an unnecessary degree of concern. Actually, the amount of chocolate necessary to bring about a serious reduction in the absorption of calcium in the chocolate milk would be so great as to cause nausea, making this a self-limiting problem.

Phytic acid. Found mostly in the outer layers of whole grains, phytic acid is another food component that can depress calcium absorption by forming an insoluble compound. From a practical point of view this is a problem only when diets are simultaneously very low in calcium and very high in phytic acid, as may be the case in developing countries where populations live mostly on grains and where very little milk is available. In a country such as the United States, nobody need worry about the possibility of impairing calcium absorption by serving the breakfast milk with whole grain cereal.

Phosphorus. In the form of phosphate ions, dietary phosphorus is important in calcium absorption because the ratio of one mineral to the other affects the absorption of each. Absorption is most efficient when the two minerals are present in approximately equal amounts. However, deviations from this ideal one-to-one ratio, which commonly occur in American diets, generally have little or no significance. An exception may be seen in the case of infants, who may develop tetany caused by seriously decreased blood calcium levels if the diet is very high in phosphates relative to calcium. In practice, this is possible only if very young infants are fed excessive amounts of phosphate-rich, calcium-poor foods (such as cereals and meats) at the expense of the milk they need.

Protein. As the level of dietary protein increases, the efficiency of calcium absorption decreases. This is no problem with milk, which contains abundant amounts of both calcium *and* protein. It may well become a problem, however, when diets include large amounts of meat and very little milk, for meat is rich in protein as well as phosphate but contains practically no calcium.

Adaptation to varying calcium intakes. Of all the factors that can influence calcium absorption, the marvelous ability of the organism to adapt is the one which most confounds the attempts to determine human requirements for calcium. This is how it works:

In studying calcium requirements, the loss of calcium in the feces, urine, and sweat is determined; this total loss is then subtracted from the known calcium intake. If there is no difference between intake and loss, the individual is said to be in calcium balance, which means that there is neither a net loss nor gain of calcium by the body. If, on the other hand, calcium losses *exceed* intake, the person is in negative balance, and it is assumed that this will eventually result in a significantly decreased calcium content of the body.

Many balance studies have been done on college students whose diets generally provide some 800 milligrams of calcium daily—an amount commonly provided by ordinary American diets. These subjects go into negative calcium balance on intakes considerably less than 800 milligrams of calcium daily; that is, they continue to excrete as much calcium as they did previously, even though their intake has been decreased drastically. As a result, many nutritionists in developed countries such as the United States assume that a calcium intake of 800 milligrams per day for adults is necessary to avoid negative calcium balance.

However, there is a good deal of evidence that far lower calcium intakes may be adequate. Studies of populations in other parts of the world show that people may have very healthy bones and teeth even on calcium intakes less than half that recommended in the United States. The explanation is that the proportion of calcium absorbed varies according to the amount in the diet. However, this adaptation requires time, and short-term balance experiments do not allow time for the individual to respond by absorbing calcium more efficiently. Hence the negative calcium balance seen when intake is *suddenly* reduced does not necessarily prove that the same negative balance would continue if low intakes were fed for weeks, months, or years.

What, then, is the justification for the high calcium intakes recommended in countries such as the United States? One important factor is availability; the existence of a large dairy industry in this country makes it feasible for people to meet the RDA for calcium quite easily. Of course, the other valuable nutrients provided along with the calcium in milk also influence the high reputation of milk as a nutritionally valuable food.

However, it would be ridiculous to assume that people who do not drink milk, and therefore probably do not meet the RDA for calcium, are necessarily suffering from calcium deficiency. To propose an international standard that could not be reached in the many areas of the world where milk is not available, and where, despite calcium intakes which are low by American standards, no sign of calcium deficiency is seen, is therefore questionable. The inconsistency between the RDA for calcium in the United States and the standards recommended by the United Nations for use in developing countries does not necessarily mean that an inferior diet is being recommended for people in other parts of the world; the ability to adapt to low intakes may well offset differences in intakes from one population to another.

Calcium and diseases

High or low calcium intakes in themselves do not cause any of the following conditions; rather the diseases reflect abnormalities of the *metabolism* of calcium or related substances.

Some people believe that kidney stones can be caused by high calcium intakes. Actually, kidney stones are composed of a large number of substances; some stones contain no calcium at all, and in no case does a stone consist of pure calcium. Calcification of soft tissues in general—not only the kidneys but other organs such as the heart and blood vessels—is likely only when the blood level of calcium is abnormally elevated, as can occur with excess vitamin D intake or in a variety of nonnutritional diseases. Obviously, treatment of the underlying cause of the elevated blood calcium, rather than decreasing the calcium intake, is the rational approach to treatment.

Osteoporosis, seen more and more frequently as life expectancy increases, is a condition in which the rate of breakdown of bone material exceeds the rate at which new bone material is formed. The eventual result is that bones become porous—honeycombed with minute holes—and fracture easily; bone pain is also common, particularly in the spine. Both the causes and the recommended treatments are matters of considerable controversy. Inadequate calcium intakes over a period of many years may be *one* factor in the occurrence or severity of this disease, but it is obviously not the only factor. Sex hormones are involved, as seen from the fact that the disease develops most commonly in women after the menopause. The treatment of osteoporosis therefore involves not only a high calcium intake in order to replace the lost bone mass, but also the administration of other agents: vitamin D, fluoride, sex hormones, and sometimes other substances as well. Certainly the idea that bones, once built, can be expected to last forever must be discarded. Maintenance of bones throughout life, and not just growth of bones in the young, requires a complex interplay of nutrients and the internal factors which govern nutrient utilization.

Food sources of calcium

Although it is possible to meet the RDA for calcium without the use of foods in the milk group, it is very difficult. Of the 800 milligrams of calcium recommended, almost 600 are provided by the equivalent of two cups of milk (Table 16–2). Many people, however, do not drink milk, or drink very little. In some, this is a matter of personal taste; others are allergic to the proteins of milk; still others cannot tolerate milk because they lack the enzyme needed to digest milk sugar. Alternate ways to meet the RDA for calcium include the following:

1. **Milk group foods other than milk.** For those who dislike milk, calcium can be obtained from foods such as cheese, cottage cheese, and ice cream. The disadvantages of this approach are the monotony of eating large amounts of these every day, and the high energy values of some of them. One pint of ice cream, for example, supplies the calcium of 1 cup of milk—but also furnishes over 500 kilocalories, as opposed to the 90 in skim or 170 in whole milk.

2. **Foods other than milk group foods.** A person could obtain the calcium of 1 cup of milk by eating 6 ounces of sardines (the calcium is in the bones, not the flesh); 6 oranges, $2\frac{1}{2}$ cups of broccoli, or 10 eggs would do as well. The limitations of this approach are obvious.

3. **Calcium supplements.** Pregnant women in particular often feel that they probably should drink more milk than they really enjoy drinking, and decide that calcium pills offer the ideal solution. There are several disadvantages to this approach. One is that calcium pills are not really the nutritional equivalent of milk because they do not contain the proteins, riboflavin, and other nutrients of milk. Another disadvantage is the number of pills that must be taken in order to make a significant contribution to calcium intake; the sheer bulk of 800 milligrams of calcium, combined with the necessary phosphate or other anion, is far too great to be put into one tablet. A further problem arises from a peculiar practice in the manufacture of supplements; for example, a pill containing only 5–10 percent of the RDA for calcium may contain fully 100 percent of the RDA for vitamin D. Taking this type of supplement makes it impossible to meet the RDA for calcium without greatly exceeding the RDA for vitamin D.

TABLE 16–2

Approximate calcium content of some common foods

	Calcium (milligrams)
Bread and cereal group	
Enriched white bread, 1 slice	25
Whole wheat bread, 1 slice	25
Meat group	
Beef, pork, poultry, fish, etc. (flesh only), cooked, 2 ounces	5–15
Clams, crabmeat, oysters, cooked, 2 ounces	25–55
*Salmon, canned, 2 ounces	110
*Sardines, canned, 2 ounces	250
Eggs, 2 large	55
Cooked dry beans, 1 cup	90
Peanut butter, 4 tablespoons	35
Milk group	
Whole milk, 1 cup	290
Skim milk, 1 cup	295
2% milk, 1 cup	350
Cheese (American, cheddar, etc.), 1½ ounces	300–400
Cottage cheese, 1⅓ cups	250–300
Ice cream, regular, 2 cups	390
Ice cream, rich, 2 cups	230
Vegetable and fruit group	
Apple, 1 medium	10
Broccoli, chopped, cooked, ½ cup	50
Carrot, raw, 1 medium	20
Collards, cooked, ½ cup	145
Green beans, cooked, ½ cup	30
Green peas, cooked, ½ cup	20
Orange, 1 medium	55
Orange juice, ½ cup	15
Potato, baked or boiled, 1 medium	10
**Rhubarb, cooked, ½ cup	105
**Spinach, cooked, ½ cup	85
Tomato juice, ½ cup	10

*Calcium content because of bones. If pieces of bone in canned salmon are discarded, calcium content will be greatly decreased.
** Calcium largely unavailable because of oxalic acid in rhubarb and spinach.
From "Home and Garden Bulletin No. 72," *USDA*, Washington, D.C., 1970.

PHOSPHORUS

The concern over pollution of water with excess phosphates from detergents or fertilizers emphasizes the importance of phosphate as a nutrient necessary for life. High phosphate levels in water are not in themselves harmful; on the contrary, they are so beneficial to growth that small aquatic plants, algae, multiply prodigously in phosphate-rich water, even to the point of crowding out other forms of life. Algae can eventually convert a body of water to a stagnant bog if enough phosphate and other nutrients are available to support their prolific growth.

Compared to calcium, phosphate is much more widely distributed, in the human body as well as in the bodies of the plants and animals we use as foods. Of the $1\frac{1}{2}$ pounds or so of phosphate present in the average adult, about 85 percent is in the calcium phosphate crystals in the bones and teeth. The other 15 percent is distributed throughout all of the cells and fluids of the body, where it performs a number of important metabolic roles. For example, ATP, the unit of energy exchange in cells, contains phosphorus; many proteins contain phosphate linked to the amino acids of which the protein chain is composed; the nucleic acids, DNA and RNA, contain phosphate as a major part of their structure. Phospholipids in cell membranes, various intermediates of carbohydrate metabolism, and numerous other phosphate-containing substances are important in the functioning of living organisms.

It is not surprising then that foods, which are all derived from living things, are generally good phosphorus sources. Meats in particular are much richer in phosphorus than in calcium. In fact it is a fairly reliable rule of thumb that any diet rich in protein will also be rich in phosphate, although by no means necessarily in calcium. The ease with which the RDA for phosphorus is met can be seen from Table 16–3.

Phosphorus deficiency sometimes occurs in grazing animals, especially dairy cattle, which lose enormous amounts of the mineral in their milk. In humans, however, low phosphorus levels in the body are generally secondary to conditions that interfere with normal utilization of the mineral, such as prolonged use of certain antacids. The wide distribution of the mineral, plus the fact that almost three-fourths of the amount ingested in normally absorbed, make the possibility of primary deficiency caused by sheer lack of dietary phosphate remote indeed.

IRON

Advertisers of iron-containing supplements have accomplished at least this much in the way of public education: Almost everybody knows that iron is the one nutrient needed in larger amounts by women than by men!

Although the average normal adult human contains only some 3 to 5 grams (a fraction of a teaspoon) of iron, the small amount present is completely out of proportion to the importance of this mineral in the body. For example, *myoglobin*, an iron-containing protein in muscles, holds oxygen temporarily until needed, and a number of enzymes require iron as a cofactor. The most widely studied roles of iron, however, are in relation to two processes related to the metabolism of energy nutrients. Although they are completely different, the two processes are commonly confused because of the similarity of the names: *oxidation*, and *oxygen transport*.

TABLE 16–3

Approximate phosphorus content of some common foods

	Phosphorus (milligrams)
Bread and cereal group	
Enriched white bread, 1 slice	30
Whole wheat bread, 1 slice	65
Meat group	
Beef (hamburger), cooked, 2 ounces	65
Chicken (flesh only), broiled, 2 ounces	55
Eggs, 2 large	205
Cooked dry beans, 1 cup	170
Milk group	
Whole milk, 1 cup	225
Skim milk, 1 cup	235
2% milk, 1 cup	275
Cheese (American, cheddar,etc.), 1½ ounces	210
Vegetable and fruit group	
Apple, 1 medium	15
Carrot, 1 medium	20
Green beans, cooked, ½ cup	25
Green peas, cooked, ½ cup	55
Orange, 1 medium	35
Potato, baked or boiled, 1 medium	75

From "Composition of Foods," Agriculture Handbook No. 8, *USDA*, Washington, D.C., 1963.

Iron and the metabolism of energy nutrients

Oxidation of energy nutrients, it will be recalled, is a process in which hydrogen, with electrons attached, is removed and passed along a chain of proteins which act as carriers (Figure 16–2). Some of these carriers contain the vitamins niacin or riboflavin as parts of their structures. The final components of the chain, however, are iron-containing proteins called *cytochromes*. In fact, the entire electron-transport chain is sometimes called the *cytochrome system;* the iron in these proteins makes them colored (*chrome* indicates color), which resulted in their being noticed and studied earlier than were some of the other components of the chain.

When hydrogen reaches the end of the transport chain, it must be accepted by some other substance; otherwise, the entire chain could become jammed up with hydrogen and cease to function further. It is here that iron plays a second vital role in energy release. Oxygen is the ultimate acceptor of the hydrogen and electrons removed from energy nutrients, and it is the iron-containing protein hemoglobin which transports a continuous supply of oxygen to the cells (Figure 16–2). If the supply of oxygen is inadequate, hydrogen atoms cannot continue to move along the electron-transport system as they normally do. Because biologically useful energy is *trapped* in ATP as hydrogen and electrons

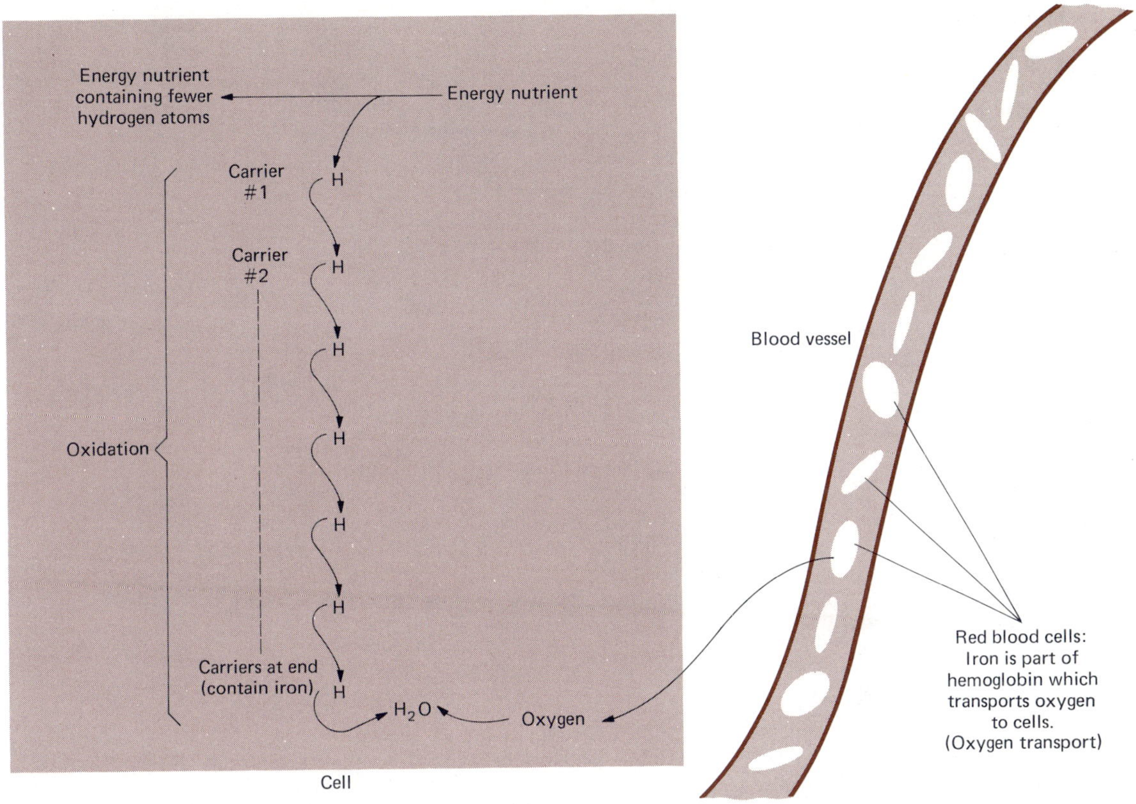

FIGURE 16–2. The action of iron in oxygen transport and in the oxidation of energy nutrients.

flow along the chain, energy harnessing ceases and the organism suffers irreversible damage and dies unless the lack of oxygen is reversed fairly rapidly.

The association of iron-blood-energy therefore obviously has some basis in biological reality. However, the association is greatly exaggerated or even distorted in the minds of many. For example, people often assume that one who is easily fatigued (or in popular terminology "lacks energy") must need iron supplements to cure the assumed anemia. Actually, fatigue can result from so many causes, emotional as well as physical, that there is no justification for indiscriminate self-prescribing of iron-containing supplements. Still, the advertising of such products is persuasive enough to convince millions of people, especially women, that life would somehow be bright if they used the supplement in question. Yet, "I'm tired all the time!" remains one of the commonest complaints, especially of women of childbearing age, regardless of whether or not they take iron supplements. Therefore, the lingering suspicion remains that in many cases it is anxiety or boredom, rather than any blood factor, which underlies the fatigue so common in modern society.

TABLE 16–4

Effect of menstrual losses on iron requirements

Iron content of blood: 0.4–0.5 milligram per milliliter (figures typical of women and men respectively)	**Estimated iron loss*, milligrams/per/day**
1. Normal women who do not menstruate, and normal men:	0.5–1
2. Average menstruating women: Blood loss/menstrual period: 42 milliliters** Iron loss/menstrual period: 17 milligrams (43 × 0.4) Iron loss/day as result of menses: 0.5 milligrams (17 ÷ 30 days) **Total:** sum of 0.5 (lower end of range for Group 1 above) and 0.5 (menstrual loss of average women):	1
3. Women with unusually high menstrual losses*** Blood loss/menstrual period: 100 milliliters Iron loss/menstrual period: 40 milligrams (100 × 0.4) Iron loss/day as result of menses: 1.3 milligrams (40 ÷ 30 days) **Total:** sum of 0.5 (lower end of range for Group 1 above) and 1.3 (unusually high menstrual loss):	1.8

* Iron requirement is approximately 10 times as great as iron loss, assuming 10 percent absorption of ingested iron.
** Approximately 1½ ounces—much less than many people would guess.
*** Note that the RDA for iron for women (18 milligrams) is based on this group's iron loss, which equals or exceeds iron loss of 95 percent of normal women.
From "Iron Deficiency in the United States," Committee on Iron Deficiency, *Journal of the American Medical Association,* 203:119 (1968).

The absorption of iron and its subsequent fates

Iron absorption is very incomplete; on the average, only about 10 percent of the iron in the diet ever leaves the intestine to enter the body itself. However, once absorbed, iron is guarded rather jealously compared to the casual way in which other minerals are allowed to leave via such routes as the urine and sweat.

Of the total iron which is absorbed and subsequently becomes part of a person's body, about 70 percent is designated as *functional* iron, because it is part of working molecules such as hemoglobin or cytochromes. The remaining 30 percent is *stored* iron, not currently in use but reserved in sites such as the liver, spleen, and bone marrow, to be drawn upon as needed for future use. The figures given can, of course, vary greatly; in fact, a person whose diet has provided barely enough iron for synthesizing functional iron-containing molecules may have virtually no storage iron.

Where is the highest concentration of iron found in the body?

Most people would probably guess that it is in the liver; this is understandable, because liver has a well-deserved reputation as an exceptionally rich iron source compared to meats obtained from the muscles or other organs of an animal's body. Actually, however, the most iron-rich part of the body is not the liver, but the blood. The significance of this to nutrition is twofold.

First, most people do not use blood as a food. Therefore, unlike animals which eat the blood as well as the other parts of their prey, humans discard the most valuable iron source obtainable from the animals they use as food.

Second, blood loss results in a significant loss of iron from the body. No other nutrient, such as proteins, vitamins, or minerals other than iron and possibly zinc, could be lost in serious amounts through blood loss; the person would die of shock before the body became depleted of these through losses in the blood. However, because such a large proportion of the body's total iron supply is in the red blood cells, blood loss is a major route of departure of iron from the body.

Blood can be lost as the result of a variety of experiences, such as surgery, accidents, childbirth, or blood donations. For most people, however, these are not common occurrences. The most common way in which blood loss affects iron nutriture significantly is through menstruation. In human females, as in the females of other primate species, menstrual periods are part of the reproductive process. (The loss of blood during *estrus,* or "heat," in nonprimates such as dogs and cats is not menstruation, as many people believe.) The effect of menstrual losses on the RDA for iron is shown in Table 16–4. Because many women lose more than the average amount of blood through menstruation, the RDA for iron is set high enough to cover the needs of most. However, some women experience average daily menstrual losses that are simply too high to be considered in setting the RDA for iron. About 5 percent of women, for example, lose an average of over 1.4 milligrams of iron daily in the menses. Covering their needs would bring the RDA to 24 milligrams (14 milligrams, of which 1.4 would be absorbed, plus the 10 milligrams to replace iron lost by routes other than menstruation). The needs of these women must therefore be met through iron supplements or by medical treatment to correct their abnormally great menstrual losses.

Foods as iron sources: the realities

For years, nutritionists have attempted to persuade people to eat liver and the few other foods which are naturally rich in iron. Many now concede that there is not much point in continuing such efforts, because too many people simply do not like these foods well enough to eat them regularly. In fact, no common, everyday, well-liked food is outstandingly iron-rich, unless it has been highly fortified, as are certain breakfast cereals.

TABLE 16–5

Approximate iron content of some common foods

	Iron (milligrams)
Bread and cereal group	
Enriched white bread, 1 slice	0.7
Whole wheat bread, 1 slice	0.8
Meat group	
Beef (hamburger), cooked, 2 ounces	2.0
Chicken (flesh only), broiled, 2 ounces	1.0
* Liver (beef), fried, 2 ounces	5.0
Liver sausage (braunschweiger), 2 ounces	1.7
Eggs, 2 large	2.2
Cooked dry beans, 1 cup	4.9
Peanut butter, 4 tablespoons	1.2
Milk group	
Milk (whole, skim, or 2 percent), 1 cup	0.1
Cheese (American, cheddar, etc.), 1½ ounces	0.2–0.5
Ice cream, regular, 2 cups	0.2
Vegetable and fruit group	
Apple, 1 medium	0.4
Broccoli, chopped cooked, ½ cup	0.6
Green beans, cooked, ½ cup	0.4
Green peas, cooked, ½ cup	1.5
Orange, 1 medium	0.5
Orange juice, ½ cup	0.3
Potato, boiled or baked, 1 medium	0.7
** Raisins, 1 ounce	1.0
Miscellaneous	
Unenriched white bread, 1 slice	0.2
Bacon, 2 slices	0.5
Honey, 1 tablespoon	0.1
Chocolate (bitter or baking), 1 ounce	1.9
Molasses, light, 1 tablespoon	0.9
Yeast (baker's), 1 tablespoon	1.1
Yeast (brewers), 1 tablespoon	1.4
Fats and oils, all types	0

* Livers from all animals are rich in iron, but figures vary from species to species, and with age. For example, calf liver is more than 50 percent richer in iron than beef liver because the calf, like all young mammals, accumulated a store of iron in the liver before birth. This store is drawn upon while the calf is on a low-iron diet of milk.

** One ounce of dried fruit represents approximately ½ cup of the original fresh fruit.

From "Home and Garden Bulletin No. 72," *USDA,* Washington, D.C., 1970.

However, as shown in Table 16–5, many *fairly* good iron sources are found in all of the food groups *except* the milk group, which is very low in iron. Meats and meat alternates supply useful amounts, as do enriched or whole grain cereal products and many fruits and vegetables. Dried fruits such as raisins are particularly concentrated iron sources, but this is merely because most of the water has been removed. Thus one cup of raisins contains as much iron as the 4 or 5 cups of grapes from which the raisins were made—but unfortunately the energy value of raisins compared to grapes is correspondingly increased!

Balanced, varied diets in the United States generally furnish approximately 6 milligrams of iron per 1000 calories. Therefore most men can meet the RDA for iron simply by including ordinary amounts of moderately good iron sources. Most women, however, cannot meet the RDA for iron in this way, for the recommendation is so high that most women could meet it only at the cost of exceeding the energy intake compatible with normal weight. Thus iron is an exception to the general rule that a diet planned around the Basic Four provides recommended amounts of essential nutrients.

How, then, can a woman meet the RDA for iron? Some of the suggested solutions are as follows:

The amount of iron added to enriched breads and cereals could be increased. Opponents to this idea point out that this could result in an undesirably high intake for men. It is well known that excess iron can be toxic; among the Bantu people of Africa, for example, disease is caused by the enormous iron intake resulting from drinking beer brewed in iron pots.

Highly fortified foods such as breakfast cereals, containing perhaps 10 milligrams of iron in a single serving, are available, but nutritionists are divided on their use. Some feel that these are nothing more than "an iron pill in flaked form"; others believe that they offer a sensible, pleasant way of increasing iron intake.

Iron supplements, or multivitamin supplements with iron added, are of course used by many, but most nutritionists agree that such routine self-medication should not be encouraged.

Although certain rather strange foods are offered in health food stores as very rich iron sources, few would care to resort to them. Blackstrap molasses, the dregs of the sugar-refining process, is too bitter to appeal to most people, and dried liver tablets offer no advantage over more ordinary supplements.

There is, of course, one approach other than meeting the RDA for iron, and this is to recognize the fact that many who do not meet the RDA are nevertheless healthy. Thus, although the RDA represents a desirable goal, the idea that anemia is inevitable in those who do not meet it obviously should not be accepted uncritically.

IODINE

Iodine is a unique nutrient in several respects. First, it is the one nutrient with only a single known function. Second, severe early iodine deficiency is the *only* form of malnutrition definitely known to cause mental retardation in humans. Third, low iodine content of soils is the only known example in which deficiency of a nutrient in the soil causes a specific deficiency disease in humans.

The function of iodine

The function of iodine is to become an integral part of thyroid hormones, mostly thyroxine; thus the need for iodine can be equated with the need for thyroid hormone production. Of the 30 milligrams or so of iodine in the body, about three-fourths is concentrated in the thyroid gland, from which thyroid hormones are secreted into the blood stream.

One important function of thyroid hormones is in the regulation of basal metabolism; consequently, deficiency of iodine leads to decreased thyroid hormone production (*hypothyroidism*) and consequently decreased basal metabolic rate. The pituitary gland responds by sending out more and more thyroid-stimulating hormone in an attempt to force the thyroid gland to produce more thyroxine. This stimulation can cause the thyroid gland to enlarge until it becomes a goiter, a condition so common in parts of the world that it may be considered normal, or even a sign of beauty. Iodine deficiency is not the only cause of goiter; in fact, goiter can be associated with *hyperthyroidism* (excessive thyroid hormone synthesis) as well as hypothyroidism, or with the presence of goiter-causing toxins in certain foods. However, the majority of goiters seen worldwide are "simple" goiters, caused by lack of iodine in the diet.

It might seem reasonable to assume that if iodine deficiency decreases the BMR, excessive iodine might increase the BMR. Indeed, at least one popular fad diet recommends eating kelp (a type of iodine-rich seaweed) in order to "burn up body fat" more rapidly by "stepping up the body's metabolism." In fact, the normal thyroid gland produces the amount of thyroxine needed and no more; excess iodine, from kelp or any other source, is excreted in the urine.

In women who are *severely* iodine-deficient, reproduction may be impaired; *amenorrhea*, or cessation of menstrual periods, may occur and the woman could become sterile for as long as the deficiency continues. In some women, however, conception is possible despite severe iodine deficiency. If this occurs, a *cretin*, or dwarfed and mentally retarded infant, may be born as the result. Unless the infant is treated starting soon after birth, permanent mental retardation is the usual result.

Prevention of iodine deficiency

In many areas, the iodine content of the soil is high enough so that adequate iodine can be obtained from crops grown on these soils; in other areas, however, very little iodine is present in soils. If iodine were a mineral needed by plants, plants would grow poorly in iodine-deficient soils, and although total crop size would be greatly decreased, the iodine concentration of each *individual* plant would be essentially normal. However, iodine is not an essential nutrient for a plant, because plants do not have thyroid glands. Therefore, plants grown on iodine-deficient soils produce crops of normal composition, except for their very low iodine content. This is in distinct contrast to the results seen when plants are grown on soils deficient in minerals such as iron, phosphorus, magnesium, or other elements needed by the plant itself. In these cases, *total* crop size is decreased, but the mineral concentration of each individual plant is affected little or not at all.

Although iodine deficiency could be prevented or treated by adding the mineral to soils or to water, adding it to salt is such an effective method that it is the method used in most countries today. Almost all people use salt, and as little as a fraction of a teaspoon of iodized salt daily provides an adequate iodine intake. Those who do not use salt and who live in areas where the soil is low in iodine must find some other iodine source. Because few common foods are rich iodine sources, an iodine-containing supplement may be the most practical choice. Large amounts of sea foods (not freshwater fish), and odd items such as kelp and sea salt offered in health food stores, are rich in iodine; however, these are hardly acceptable as everyday fare for most people.

MAGNESIUM

A number of popular publications, especially women's magazines, contain various strange statements about magnesium. For example, magnesium deficiency is claimed to be a very common cause of fatigue, cramps, weakness, irritability, impaired sexual responsiveness, and a multitude of other symptoms.

Magnesium performs very important roles in metabolism, acting as a cofactor in numerous enzymatic reactions and affecting protein synthesis through its effects on RNA and on ribosomes. Needless to say, then, an actual deficiency of magnesium in cells would be serious indeed. However, and fortunately, magnesium deficiency is also highly unlikely in normal people. All four food groups contribute some magnesium; green leafy vegetables are particularly good sources because magnesium is part of the chlorophyll molecule.

Magnesium deficiency, characterized by tetany similar to that caused by low blood calcium, is sometimes seen, but only in unusual circumstances. Alcoholics can suffer from magnesium deficiency (in addition, of course, to many other deficiencies); apparently, alcohol increases the rate of excretion of the mineral in the urine. Prolonged vomiting or diarrhea can also lead to deficiency because of loss of the mineral from the digestive tract. In cases such as these, however, treatment of the underlying disorder, not merely increasing the magnesium intake, is obviously indicated.

In cases of fatigue, irritability, and similar symptoms, attempts at self-treatment with magnesium as a purported "natural tranquillizer" are to be deplored. The likelihood that magnesium deficiency is the cause is virtually nil, and the suffering person will therefore not be relieved by supplements of this mineral.

FLUORIDE

No nutrient has aroused more emotional debate than fluoride has, despite the scientific evidence of its benefits. It has been amply demonstrated that the incidence of dental caries, or decay, can be decreased by about 50 percent by the simple presence of optimal levels of fluoride in public water supplies. The water in some areas already contains sufficient fluoride. In fact, it was the presence of *excessive* fluoride which first pointed out the relationship of fluoride to dental health; very excessive fluoride intake causes teeth to become susceptible to mottling, or discoloration. However undesirable this is cosmetically, the mottled teeth are remarkably resistant to decay. Repeated controlled studies have shown that water containing 1 part per million of fluoride can decrease the incidence of tooth decay *without* causing the mottling seen at much higher fluoride levels. (One part per million means 1 milligram per liter of water, or approximately 0.00004 ounces per quart).

Fluoride acts by replacing a minute amount of the material in the hydroxyapatite crystals deposited during formation of teeth, resulting in a denser type of crystal. For this reason fluoride is most beneficial to infants, children, and adolescents, but has very little effect on adults' teeth. The younger the age at which fluoride is provided, the greater the benefits.

An adequate fluoride intake is possible by means other than drinking fluoridated water; drops or tablets containing fluoride, with or without added vitamins, can be obtained by prescription. And topical application, in which a fluoride-containing substance is painted on tooth surfaces, is also of some value. Fluoride-containing toothpastes are probably of trivial benefit, however, because the amount of fluoride, and the time during which the toothpaste is in contact with the teeth, are insufficient. The most effective means of insuring regularly adequate intakes for the maximum number of people is therefore through fluoridation of water supplies. Yet opposition to this practice continues, based largely on the following claims:

It is said to constitute "compulsory medication," forcing people to buy unfluoridated bottled water if they wish to avoid this "infringement on their freedom of choice."

Some insist that it is dangerous; "poisons in our water" is the usual expression. Studies are cited to "prove" that fluoride is toxic; the fact that the studies used fluoride levels 10, 100, or even 1000 times higher than intakes possible from fluoridated water is obscured.

It is ineffective, others claim; invariably these individuals point to the lack of benefits to the teeth of *older* people—a lack which proponents of fluoridation readily acknowledge, although there is evidence that fluoride may benefit the bones, if not the teeth, of elderly people.

Finally, it is branded as "unnatural": "If Nature had wanted fluoride in the water, she would have put it there." Why, one must wonder, did "Nature" decide to put adequate fluoride in the water of some areas but not others?

Arguments such as those against fluoridation offer an unusually good example of the techniques used by faddists, appealing as they do to fear and ignorance rather than to reason. Unfortunately these arguments have proved to be so effective that the public has often rejected fluoridation when it has been put to a vote through referendum (and what other nutrient has ever been put to a vote?). Confused because they believe that the controversy reflects a genuine conflict between different factions of the scientific community, rather than a conflict between science and nonscience, voters often decide to avoid the supposed possible dangers of fluoride. Thereby they lose the benefits they could so easily and inexpensively obtain.

ZINC

Zinc deficiency is so rare that it is only since the early 1960s that it has been demonstrated in any human population. In Egypt and other parts of the Near East, where the diets of the poor consist mostly of whole wheat, growth retardation and delayed sexual development have been associated with zinc deficiency. However, the underlying cause may be impaired absorption or utilization of zinc, rather than an uncomplicated dietary deficiency, because whole wheat contains a high concentration of zinc compared to many other foods.

In the United States, zinc deficiency has been found to coexist with certain diseases, especially those in which blood loss is extensive. The symptoms include *hypogeusia* (decreased sense of taste) and *dysgeusia* (distorted taste sensation). Because these can be corrected by zinc supplements, it is assumed that zinc deficiency caused the symptoms—although not, of course, the accompanying diseases.

The first RDA for zinc was not set until 1973, because of the lack of data on which to base a recommendation before then. No particular effort appears to be necessary to meet the recommendation, because zinc is found in a wide variety of common foods. In fact, toxicity caused by *excess* zinc is a more serious problem than deficiency in the United States, and generally is the result of using galvanized pans in preparing acid foods.

Because zinc is a cofactor for many metabolic reactions, and is necessary for the activity of insulin, it is sometimes claimed to be uniquely effective in weight reduction by "stimulating carbohydrate metabolism." This is entirely incorrect, and zinc supplements, for weight reduction or any other purpose, are totally unnecessary except for people with unusual diseases which increase their requirement for zinc.

A BRIEF LOOK AT OTHER MINERALS

The minerals discussed so far are those for which official recommended allowances have been set, plus fluoride which is lacking often enough to justify its being considered in some detail.

However, other minerals are also known or believed to be essential to humans, and may play roles equally as vital as those of the minerals already discussed. It is only because they are so seldom related to practical problems in normal human nutrition that they will be covered much more briefly than the others were.

Sodium is the most abundant positively charged mineral in the body fluids outside of cells. An important factor in sodium intake is taste, because the amount of table salt (sodium chloride) used as seasoning can result in tremendous individual variations. Although toxic in large amounts, sodium is nevertheless not ingested in dangerous quantities by most people because such large amounts would make food inedible. Sodium *can* be detrimental to those with certain diseases, such as high blood pressure and kidney disease, and these individuals must therefore restrict their sodium intake to a level far below that of the usual American diet.

Because large amounts of sodium can be lost through sweating, extra salt is recommended if sweating is profuse. However, the additional amount needed is equivalent to only about $\frac{1}{5}$ teaspoon of salt per quart of water lost as sweat. Taking salt tablets by the handful, as athletes sometimes do, is therefore rarely necessary.

Aldosterone, a steroid hormone secreted by the adrenal cortex, is important in regulating the salt content of the body, stimulating the kidney to reabsorb sodium rather than excreting it in the urine. Decreased aldosterone secretion, which may result from disease of the adrenal glands, can therefore lead to the loss of enormous amounts of sodium in the urine. This condition, known as *Addison's disease,* can partially be controlled by increasing the salt intake.

When excess salt accumulates in the body, water is retained along with it. *Edema,* as this accumulation of excess fluid is called, can therefore be treated by decreasing the salt intake rather than the water intake. Diuretics, drugs which flush excess fluid from the tissues, are also sometimes used to relieve edema. Many of them act by counteracting the effects of aldosterone, thereby causing sodium to be excreted rather than reabsorbed by the kidney.

Potassium is the most abundant positively charged mineral in the fluid *inside* cells, as sodium is outside the cells. In fact, measurement of the naturally occurring radioactive potassium in the body can be used to estimate the body's lean-cell mass.

Potassium excess or deficiency in the body generally occurs as a result of impaired function of the body rather than of excess or inadequate dietary intake. Vomiting or diarrhea is a common cause of potassium depletion, especially in infants and children, and prompt replacement of lost potassium is important if depletion is severe. Salt substitutes, used by those who must restrict their sodium intake, often consist of potassium chloride; they taste similar to salt without promoting the retention of fluid in the body as sodium does in some people. Certain diuretics, although taken for the purpose of increasing the urinary excretion of sodium, can concomitantly increase the loss of potassium, sometimes to an undesirably large degree.

Chloride is a very abundant anion in foods as they are obtained from nature, and the amount in the diet is further increased through the addition of sodium chloride to foods. When large amounts of sodium are lost in urine or sweat, parallel amounts of chloride are also lost. However, when sodium is replaced by increasing the salt intake, as is generally done, chloride is also automatically replaced.

Combined with hydrogen, chloride forms the hydrochloric acid secreted by the stomach and important in digestion. Some individuals lack the ability to produce normal amounts of this acid. However, in these people the problem lies in the functioning of the stomach cells themselves, and never in a lack of the necessary chloride.

Copper, in minute amounts, is necessary for hemoglobin synthesis even though it does not become an integral part of the completed hemoglobin molecule. Because milk is very low in copper content, infants fed exclusively on milk for prolonged periods of time may become anemic as the result of copper deficiency, as well as iron deficiency. Otherwise, deficiency in humans is very rare.

In addition to its role as a cofactor in hemoglobin synthesis, copper acts as a cofactor in a variety of other reactions whereby important biochemicals are produced. One of these is *melanin,* the pigment of skin and hair. However, *albinism,* the lack of coloring matter, is never caused by copper deficiency; it is a genetic disease in which an enzyme involved in melanin synthesis is lacking.

In *Wilson's disease,* another genetic disorder, *excessive* amounts of copper accumulate in the liver, brain, and other organs; even the eyes may accumulate copper until visible colored rings can be seen in the cornea. Although a low copper diet has been used in attempts to control the disease, the widespread occurrence of the mineral makes this approach relatively unsuccessful. Fortunately, drugs are now available which bind copper to form a complex which is then readily excreted by the kidneys. Thus increased output, rather than decreased intake, can be used to control the accumulation of copper in this disease.

Chromium helps to regulate glucose metabolism, possibly by increasing the ability of cells to respond to insulin. However, chromium is by no means effective in the treatment of diabetes, as has been claimed. In some individuals, chromium has been reported to correct abnormal glucose metabolism related to old age, pregnancy, and protein deficiency. These findings may suggest that chromium deficiency in humans, although rare, does occasionally occur.

Manganese, among its other roles, acts as a cofactor in reactions of fatty acid synthesis and urea formation. Deficiency has never been observed in a human. In poultry, however, manganese deficiency is the cause of severe bone abnormalities; the disease, called *perosis,* was a serious source of economic loss to the poultry industry until the value of manganese supplements was discovered.

Molybdenum may or may not be essential for humans. It acts as a cofactor for certain enzymes, but the reactions catalyzed by these enzymes may not really be vital to human cells. Molybdenum is important in nutrition primarily because of the danger of toxicity to grazing animals; plants grown on soils high in this mineral can accumulate such high levels that they poison the animals feeding upon them.

Selenium is somewhat of an embarrassment to those who insist on banning any substance which causes any form of cancer in any type of animal under any conditions; large doses of selenium *can* cause cancer in experimental animals, yet small amounts of selenium are essential to life.

Selenium is also interesting in that variations in the amount of the mineral in the soil can produce tremendous variations in the amounts in plants, to the extent that animals may develop either toxicity or deficiency, depending upon the soil on which their food grows.

Selenium has the ability to protect certain compounds from destruction by oxygen, although vitamin E and selenium can replace each other in this respect. In addition, the mineral has some functions which are unique to it, and for which it cannot be replaced by any other nutrient.

Cobalt in and of itself is not really an essential nutrient for humans. It is part of the vitamin B_{12} molecule, and is therefore of no value to human cells, which cannot synthesize vitamin B_{12}. However, the microorganisms in the digestive tracts of many animals *can* utilize cobalt for producing vitamin B_{12}, which the animal then absorbs and which humans eventually obtain from the flesh, milk, and eggs of the animals.

Sulfur, like cobalt, is not an essential element in itself, but only as part of other substances which are essential. It is part of two vitamins—biotin and thiamin. However, most of the dietary sulfur is part of the 3 sulfur-containing amino acids, cysteine, cystine, and methionine. These amino acids are found in unusually great concentrations in the protein keratin, which is present in hair, skin, hoofs, and nails. Thus the animal tissues richest in sulfur are discarded rather than used for food. Nevertheless, diets that provide adequate amounts of all other amino acids can be counted upon to supply adequate amounts of the sulphur-containing ones as well.

Nickel, tin, vanadium and *silicon* deficiencies have recently been produced in experimental animals, but only by raising the animals in an environment made as free as possible of these minerals. This suggests that humans, like the experimental animals, may require these elements. It also points out the very low probability that any human diet would fail to supply adequate amounts of them.

Multimineral supplements: a word of caution

Although mineral supplements are not as widely sold and advertised as vitamin supplements are, they are available enough to warrant a few points of caution. If a mineral is required in relatively large amounts, a significant proportion of the requirement simply cannot fit into a pill or tablet. If a mineral is required in very small amounts, there is a very good chance that it will be present in adequate amounts in the diet. What, then, is the justification for such products? The answer is found in the prices. One typical brand costs $20.75 for 100 tablets, with 6 tablets per day needed to provide the nutrients described in the accompanying advertising. A consumer using this product would receive insignificant amounts of minerals needed in large amounts, and adequate amounts of most of those needed in such small amounts as to make supplementation absurd. Who benefits from such a product? The answer, of course, is the seller.

SUGGESTED READINGS

Council on Foods and Nutrition. "Iron Deficiency in the United States." *Journal of the American Medical Association* 203 (1968):119.

"Essential Inorganic Elements in Nutrition: Functions and Interrelationships." *Dairy Council Digest* 39 (1968):25.

Food and Nutrition Board, National Research Council–National Academy of Sciences. *Recommended Dietary Allowances*, eighth edition. Washington, D.C., 1974.

Piomelli, S. "Diagnostic Approaches to Anemia." *Pediatric Clinics of North America* 18 (1971):3.

Smith, E. H. "Fluoridation of Water Supply." *Journal of the American Medical Association* 230 (1974):1569.

Webb, T. E. and F. A. Oski. "Iron Deficiency Anemia and Scholastic Achievement in Young Adolescents." *Journal of Pediatrics* 82 (1973):827.

17

nutrition in growth and development: in the beginning

Human life, like all life, is a continuum (Figure 17–1). Through the processes of growth and development, successive stages of the life cycle are attained. The resulting adults may reproduce, and inevitably undergo changes collectively known as aging. This brings about the eventual death of the individual, whose life, however, has been passed on to the next generation. In fact, biological success has been defined as the ability to eat and to avoid being eaten until reproduction has been achieved, thus insuring the continuation of the species.

A few generalizations regarding growth and development are necessary, for although these two words are often used as if they were synonyms, they can be distinguished from each other in several important ways.

Growth is a net increase in the amount of protoplasm in an organism. It can be of two types. *Hyperplasia,* an increase in cell number through cell division, is the means whereby the early growth of an individual or of an organ mostly occurs. *Hypertrophy,* an increase in the *size* of individual cells, accounts mostly for further growth and is in fact responsible for all growth after maximum cell number is achieved. It is particularly important for certain cell types such as muscle cells.

Growth, generally measured in terms of height (or length) and weight, can be dramatically impaired by detrimental factors such as severe prolonged undernutrition. In general, weight is more sensitive to undernutrition than is height. Overnutrition has no ability to accelerate growth in terms of height, and actually has little effect on growth as measured by weight gain. This is because weight gained as a result of excess energy intake represents fat tissue, rather than the added protoplasm characteristic of true growth.

Although each organ system within an individual has a distinctive growth rate, the four *major* patterns of growth, and an example of an organ system or tissue type which each pattern typifies, are shown in Figure 17–2. It can be seen that the nervous system approaches adult size much earlier than does the skeleton, which grows in a pattern similar to the body as a whole; lymphoid tissue grows so rapidly in the child that it actually exceeds the adult size, after which involution, or "atrophy," brings it down to adult size; and reproductive tissue grows very slowly until reproductive age is approached.

Development, in contrast to growth, refers to an increase in complexity of structure or function of cells, organs, or individuals (Figure 17–3). At the level of the cell, the term *differentiation* is commonly used because in development cells become remarkably different from each other with respect to structure and function. When discussing

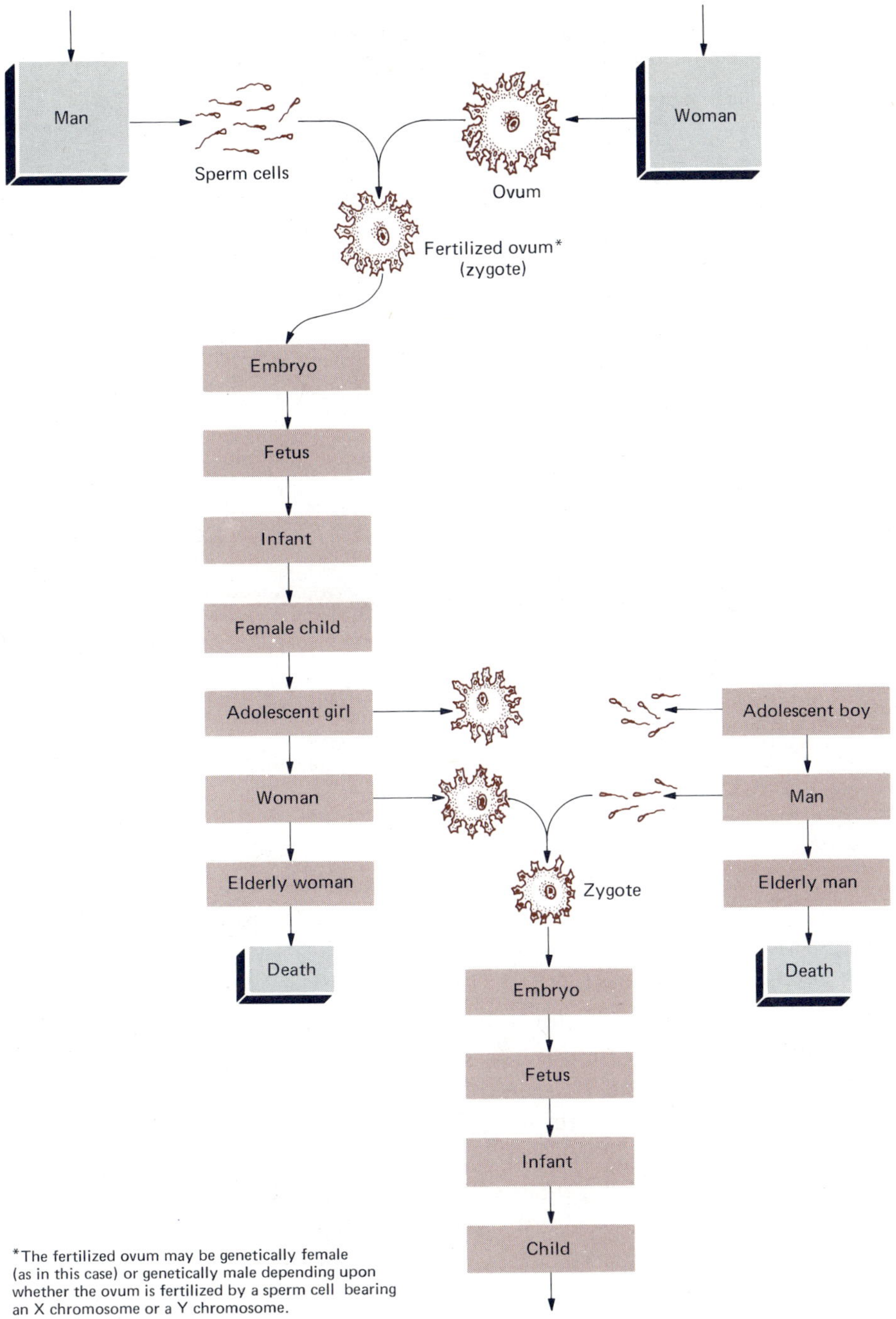

*The fertilized ovum may be genetically female (as in this case) or genetically male depending upon whether the ovum is fertilized by a sperm cell bearing an X chromosome or a Y chromosome.

FIGURE 17–1. The continuum of life.

organs or whole individuals, the term *maturation* is often used to describe the developmental changes seen.

Because growth and development often occur together, they are commonly assumed to be identical. However, there are many examples

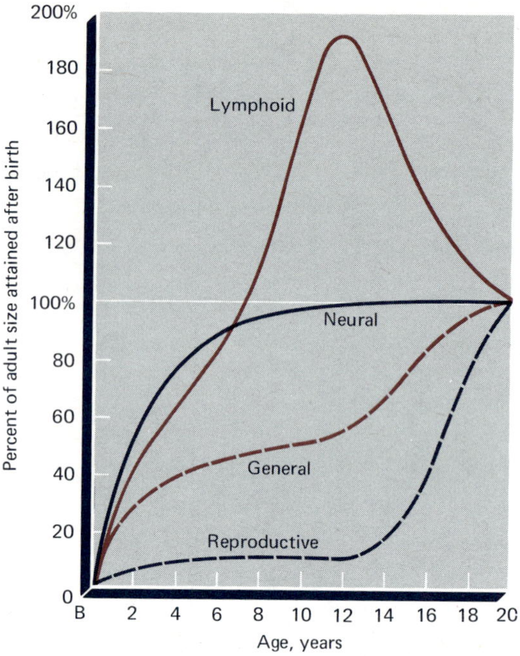

FIGURE 17–2. The four main patterns of growth, with an example of a tissue type for each pattern. "General" growth includes the body as a whole, skeleton, respiratory and digestive systems, muscles, blood.

in which increased size and increased complexity are not parallel. The newborn female infant is smaller but more mature than the male; the newborn black baby is smaller but more advanced in development than the white; during adolescence, growth is less rapid but maturation earlier in girls than in boys. These examples show that growth and development are separable and are therefore two different processes.

The result of a person's physical growth and development is a given body type, or *somatotype,* which is largely determined by genetics. Three chief physical components can be distinguished: endomorphy, mesomorphy, and ectomorphy. Although each individual has a combination of these three components, one or the other often predominates. Endomorphs, people in whom the endomorphic component predominates, have a generally soft and fatty body build; mesomorphs are characteristically muscular; and ectomorphs tend to be lean and linear. It was once believed that certain personality types were closely associated with these different body types: mesomorphs were supposed to be aggressive and active by nature, endomorphs naturally slothful and indolent, and ectomorphs sensitive and "high strung." Modern psychologists, however, believe that personality development is much more related to social and psychological environmental factors than to genetically fixed body build.

Superimposed upon your genetic heritage are other factors that can modify growth and development. Essentially these are the same factors that affect health, such as hormones, nutrients, drugs, toxins, radiation, infection. As a general rule, a given degree of an unfavorable influence (such as malnutrition) will be more likely to impair growth than to impair development. Timing, however, is crucially important. During the development of each organ, there is a particular time during which changes in structure and function occur most rapidly. This *critical* or *vulnerable period,* as it is called, is the time of most rapid cell division, for it is during division that cells change to form new daughter cells, which are structurally and functionally different from the parent cells. Therefore, while this relatively short period of very marked development lasts, an organ is far more susceptible to abnormal development than when cell division is less rapid. Further, if the abnormality is extreme, it will be permanent, for a body part which once develops in a grossly abnormal manner can never repair the damage and become normal at a later time.

By contrast, growth can be considerably impaired at *any* point before final adult size is reached; however, whether the damage is permanent or not depends upon the kind, degree, and timing of the damaging agent. For example, if malnutrition is severe, prolonged, and

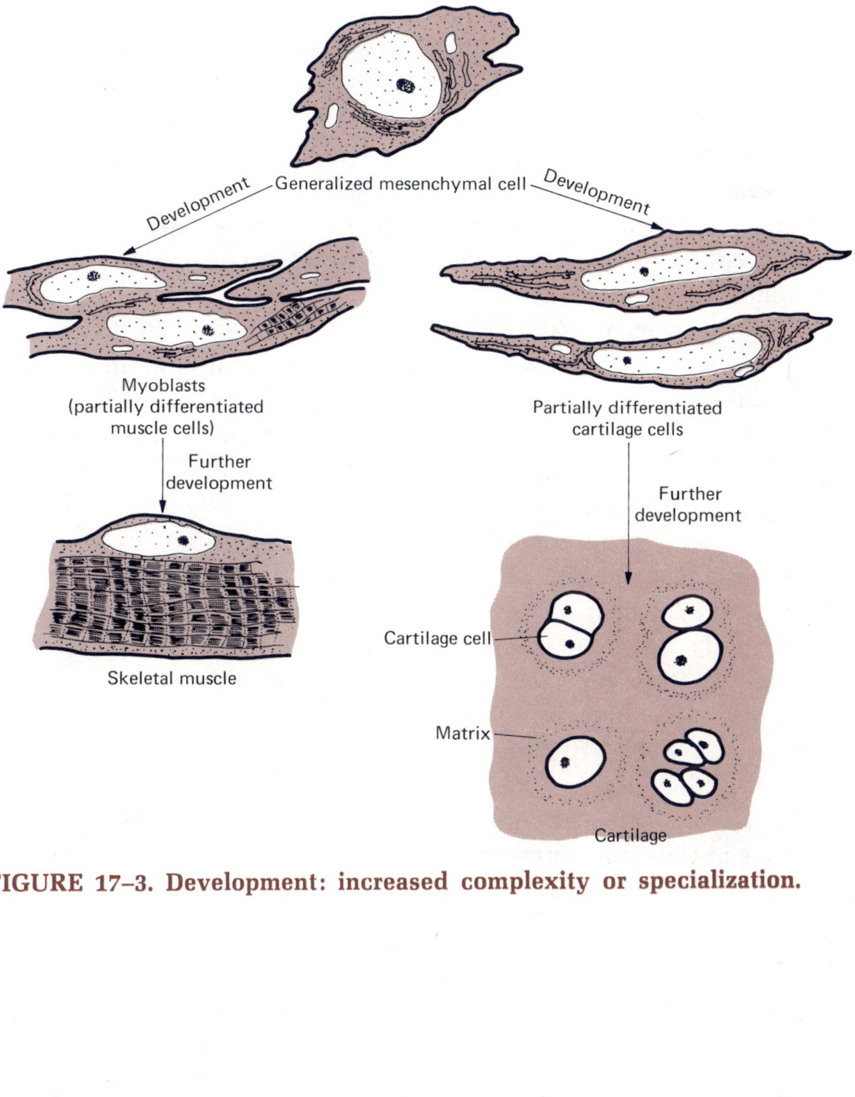

FIGURE 17–3. Development: increased complexity or specialization.

early enough, the individual may never attain the potential size which was his or her genetic heritage. In less extreme circumstances, however, "catch-up" growth is possible, as when a previously malnourished child is given an adequate diet.

As Figure 17–1 shows, the adult's life flows in either of two directions: through reproduction the next generation arrives onstage, and through aging the former generation passes from the scene. Because no particular event can be designated as the moment at which human life begins, a discussion can start at any arbitrarily chosen point. The nutritional aspects of reproduction is as good a place to begin as any.

NUTRITION AND CONCEPTION

Although malnutrition with respect to a variety of nutrients can cause reproductive disorders in animals, the applicability of this observation to humans is largely unknown. Very briefly, the effects of nutrition on the successive stages of human reproduction can be summarized as follows:

The formation of germ cells, largely under the control of hormones, can be impaired by general undernutrition only if the degree of deprivation is severe. Further, this effect is seen only in females, and the sterility caused by starvation or semistarvation is readily reversible when the diet improves. Mild or moderate general undernutrition does not appear to impair human fertility significantly, as is apparent from the birth rates in developing countries. Of all deficiencies of *specific* nutrients, iodine deficiency is the only one known to result in failure of the female to produce ova. Zinc deficiency, which delays sexual development and causes hypogonadism in the rare type of dwarfism seen in Egypt, is the only specific deficiency known to affect males in this manner.

As nearly everyone knows, *fertilization* of the human ovum ordinarily requires sexual intercourse. One could postulate that an extremely underweight or overweight individual might find it impossible to attract a mate, or that extreme anemia might make sexual activity difficult because of the exertion. In fact, however, only severe undernutrition, again of a general type rather than with respect to a specific nutrient, appears to have a significant effect on the tendency of men and women (and hence sperm cells and ova) to get together.

The fertilized egg, or *zygote,* divides to form a mass of smaller cells. The only nutrients available to support this activity are those present in the fertilized ovum itself. Therefore, although the number of cells increases, there is no increase in the total mass of cells.

About one week after fertilization, the cell mass begins to invade the lining of the uterus. The invading cells produce enzymes which break down the cells lining the uterus, thereby releasing nutrients which the embryo-to-be absorbs and uses. The cell mass nestles into the space produced, a process known as *implantation.* This is actually a second conception; the placenta "takes in" the zygote, just as the egg "takes in" the sperm cell during the first conception known as fertilization.

The placenta then forms. This remarkable organ transfers substances back and forth between the bloodstream of the pregnant woman and that of the developing embryo or fetus. The cells which invaded the uterine lining grow rapidly, forming folds known as *villi*, similar to the villi found in the digestive tract. By this means the surface area across which materials are transferred is enormously increased, until near the end of pregnancy the placenta has a total surface area of approximately 160 square feet.

Implantation and the formation of the placenta do not always occur normally, and failures at these points are a common cause of very early spontaneous abortion. Indeed, many biologists do not even use the term *abortion* to describe failure at any stage prior to the development of a functioning placenta, and many women never realize that they have harbored a fertilized ovum. The reasons for the frequent failures at these early stages are not completely known, but no form of malnutrition has ever been shown to be a cause in humans.

NUTRITION OF THE OVUM, THE EMBRYO, AND THE FETUS

During the first two weeks following fertilization, it is customary to call the cell mass an *ovum*, even though it actually consists of many cells which have differentiated into several distinct types. From two to eight weeks, the term *embryo* is generally used. During this time all of the organs develop, although of course in very rudimentary forms incapable of mature function. After eight weeks and until birth, the term *fetus* is employed. However, there is not complete agreement as to how these terms should be used; some would extend the embryo stage to 12 weeks or so. For this reason, many prefer to use the single term *fetus* for all stages from implantation until birth.

The health and survival of the fetus depends upon three major factors. The first is the metabolism of the fetus itself, which is largely controlled by the genetic endowment of the fetus. However, a number of nongenetic factors can interfere with normal fetal metabolism. Infectious diseases such as *rubella*, *syphilis*, and *toxoplasmosis* can cause fetal malformations: heart defects, mental retardation, and deafness in the infant have, in many cases, been traced to infection of the mother during pregnancy. The fetus is also susceptible to many toxins and drugs. During the period of most rapid development, extreme fetal damage can result from doses of drugs harmless to the maternal organism, and cigarette smoking by pregnant women appears to retard fetal growth.

The second factor in fetal health is the functioning of the placenta. In a set of identical twins, one baby may actually weigh twice as much

TABLE 17–1

Human prenatal growth

Time after conception (weeks)	Approximate weight
0	0.7 microgram
8	*3–5 grams
20	0.5 to 1 pound
28	2 to 2.5 pounds
32	4 to 4.5 pounds
40	7 to 7.5 pounds

* Note the very small amount of material required during the first eight weeks, when organogenesis is essentially completed. Three grams equals roughly one-tenth of an ounce.

TABLE 17–2

Two classes of low birth-weight infants

Prematurity
Associated with:
Lower socioeconomic status
Age of woman (less than 17 or more than 40 years)
Hypertension
Toxemia of pregnancy
Maternal heart disease
Other

*** Prenatal growth retardation**
Associated with:
Maternal heart disease
Toxemia of pregnancy
Maternal rubella (German measles) during first trimester
Heavy cigarette smoking
Alcoholism
Fetal genetic abnormalities
Severe maternal undernutrition
Other

* Approximately one-third of all infants of low-birth weight are in this category.

at birth as the other depending upon differences in the placentae via which the twins were nourished.

The third factor in fetal health is the nutritional status of the pregnant woman. The unique feature of this factor is that, compared to fetal metabolism and placental functioning, maternal nutrition can be rather readily manipulated and improved.

Of the many aspects of fetal health that have been studied, the following have been investigated most intensively with respect to relationships to maternal nutrition.

MALFORMATIONS (BIRTH DEFECTS)

For many centuries, fetal malformations or defects were believed to be caused by the pregnant woman's fears, cravings, and other emotions.

With the rise of the science of genetics in the early part of the twentieth century, opinion swung to the opposite view that *all* congenital malformations were caused by gene mutations and that the prenatal environment therefore could not alter development. However, in the early 1930s, a pregnant sow, which had inadvertently been fed a vitamin A-deficient diet, gave birth to a litter of eleven pigs, all of which completely lacked eyes. The title of the paper published as the result of this accidental experiment, "Pigs Born Without Eye Balls," stands as a model of straightforward description. Since that time, other severe fetal malformations have been induced experimentally by malnutrition in laboratory animals; for example, riboflavin deficiency in rats causes cleft palate, abnormally short limbs, absence of ribs, and other defects resembling those sometimes seen in human infants.

These findings naturally led to the hope that the answer to human birth defects had been found. However, attempts to show that malnutrition in humans is *teratogenic* (literally, monster-producing) have been disappointing. This is probably because only very small amounts of nutrients are needed during organ development in the human fetus (Table 17–1). By the time that *organogenesis* is essentially completed (during the first eight weeks of pregnancy) the human fetus weighs only a fraction of an ounce. It is extremely unlikely that a human female would be so undernourished as to be unable to supply these small needs. By contrast, the organs of the rat fetus undergo rapid development during more than three-quarters of the entire gestation period, by which time the total litter weight may be over one-fifth of the pregnant rat's weight. Therefore, compared to a woman, there is a great possibility that the pregnant rat, deliberately made deficient for experimental purposes, will be unable to supply enough materials to meet the demands of fetal development.

PREMATURITY AND FETAL GROWTH RETARDATION

In the past, all newborn babies weighing less than 2500 grams (5½ pounds) were arbitrarily called *premature.* This unsatisfactory system has now been largely replaced by a system that attempts to differentiate low-birth-weight babies into two classes (Table 17–2). Truly premature infants are those born less than 37 weeks after the mother's last menstrual period, at which time the average weight is approximately 5½ pounds. However, about one-third of all babies weighing less than 5½ pounds at birth are not actually premature, but have suffered fetal growth retardation.

It can be seen from Table 17–2 that many factors other than nutrition can influence both the duration of pregnancy and the fetal growth rate. Nevertheless, numerous overly enthusiastic hypotheses have in the past attempted to relate *all* cases of low birth weight to maternal malnutrition. For example, it has been suggested that low birth weight associated with small maternal size is actually an indirect result of former malnutrition which stunted the growth of the mother. The reasoning is specious, and the fact remains that the causes of low birth weight are many, and are incompletely understood.

A good deal of confusion exists with regard to the question: Does the fetus or the pregnant woman suffer more as the result of maternal malnutrition? In general, a fetus will grow normally at the expense of the pregnant woman even if she is mildly undernourished herself. In cases of *severe* maternal malnutrition, however, fetal growth can be impaired because even an efficient parasite cannot obtain what is not there.

However, it is commonly stated that the opposite is true: that with an inadequate diet the fetus is more affected than is the mother. This conclusion is largely the result of misinterpretation of data, such as those shown in Figure 17–4. Because *most* babies are born in good

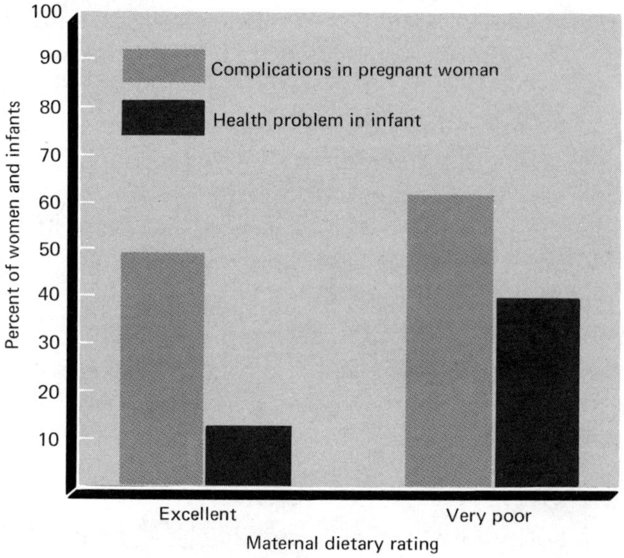

FIGURE 17–4. An example of how diet during pregnancy could be *associated* with the health of the woman and of the baby.

condition, it is possible to increase several-fold the proportion of babies *not* born in good condition. On the other hand, because many women have one or more complications of pregnancy regardless of diet, it is simply not possible to increase this already large number by very much. The situation is similar to that which would be seen if food prices suddenly tripled. A wealthy family might then spend 15 percent rather than 5 percent of its total income for food, but a very poor family that previously spent 50 percent on food obviously could not spend over 100 percent of its income. It would be absurd, however, to conclude that, because inflation increases food expenditures threefold for the rich and only twofold for the poor, the rich suffer more from inflation than do the poor.

Both prematurity and fetal growth retardation are established as antecedents of death in infants, and of later mental retardation and other serious disorders in many who survive. Severe maternal undernutrition during mid and late pregnancy, when most of fetal growth occurs, can result in an infant of low birth weight, and it is assumed that most of these infants are growth-retarded rather than truly premature. However, it should be recognized that the duration of pregnancy is not always easy to determine accurately. Many women are not sure of the time at which an infant was conceived, and some would prefer not to give this information. (The 8-pound baby born after seven months of marriage *might* be premature. Then again, maybe it was not that the baby was early but that the wedding was late.)

MEETING NUTRITIONAL NEEDS DURING PREGNANCY

It might seem that energy and nutrient needs of a pregnant woman could be easily determined by estimating the nutrient needs of the fetus and superimposing them upon the needs of the nonpregnant woman. Actually it is not this simple, because a woman undergoes marked metabolic adjustments during pregnancy. As a result, some nutrients are absorbed or utilized in a more efficient manner than in the nonpregnant woman. The combined nutrient needs of the fetus plus the pregnant woman may therefore be considerably less than might be expected.

Figure 17–5 shows how the RDA are changed during pregnancy. The figures represent the estimated increased needs during the second and third trimesters only, because the small proportion of fetal growth that occurs during the first trimester demands essentially no more than what is adequate for nonpregnant women. The following generalizations can be noted:

The degree to which recommendations are increased varies. The increase is 15 percent for energy and for niacin, 65 percent for protein, 100 percent for folacin, and 25 to 50 percent for most nutrients (vitamins A and E, ascorbic acid, riboflavin, thiamin, vitamins B_6 and B_{12}, calcium, phosphorus, magnesium, and zinc).

The RDA for vitamin D is 400 IU (International Units) for the pregnant woman, which is the same as for those 22 years old or younger; for most people over this age there is no RDA for this vitamin.

Because there is no practical dietary means for most women to obtain the increased iron needed during pregnancy, the use of supplemental iron is recommended.

The increase in the RDA for niacin is smaller than for other vitamins; however, because cells produce niacin from the amino acid tryptophan, the vitamin is available in larger amounts when the increased RDA for protein is met.

The greatest percentage increase is for folacin. This is because growth in the fetus is largely a matter of increased cell number, in contrast to the increase in cell size which becomes more significant after birth. Also, the pregnant woman produces more red blood cells than usual. Cell division requires DNA synthesis, and large amounts of folacin, a cofactor for DNA synthesis, are therefore needed during pregnancy to meet the demands of the fetus as well as the increased maternal red blood cell number.

Vitamin B_{12}, as well as folacin, is a cofactor in DNA synthesis. However, the reserves in the liver of a normal woman are so great that fetal needs can be met by releasing stored vitamin B_{12}. There is therefore no need for a marked increase in the recommended intake.

With respect to the increased allowance for energy, two major points should be noted. First, it is small compared to the increased allowances for most essential nutrients. The resulting problem is similar to trying to pack a large amount of clothing into very limited suitcase space. The solution, of course, is to pack only those clothing items that are the most useful relative to the space they will occupy. By analogy, the solution in nutrition is to add only those foods which supply the most nutritional value relative to the energy they provide.

FIGURE 17–5. The RDA for the reference woman (R) and for pregnant women (P) age 23 to 50. Changes in allowances cannot be shown graphically for vitamin D or for iron; there is no RDA for vitamin D for the reference woman, and amounts of supplemental iron suggested during pregnancy range from 30 to 60 milligrams daily.

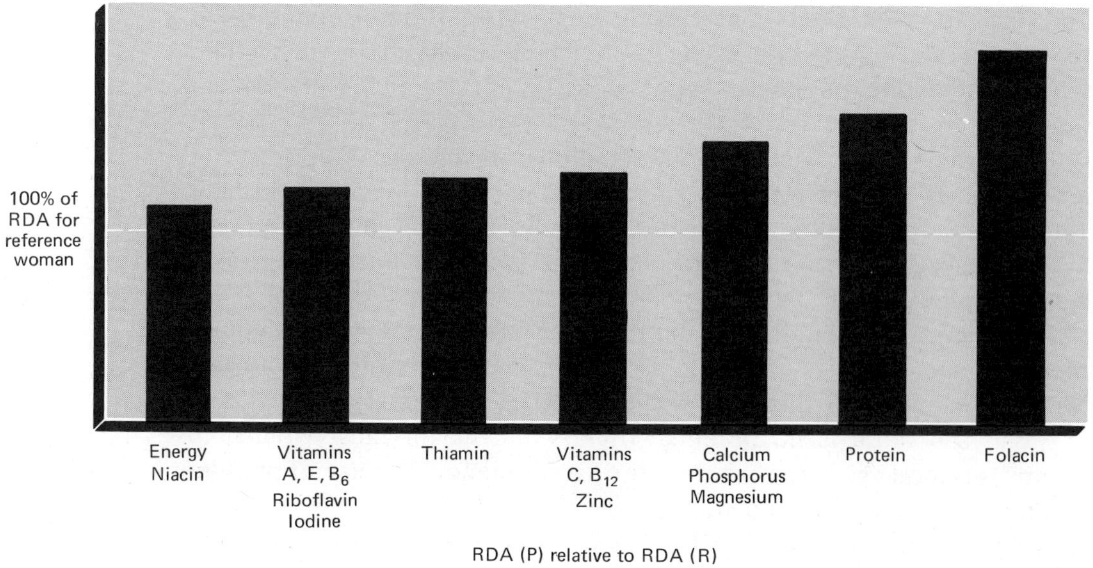

The second point is that the test of energy adequacy is *always* one's body weight. Therefore, if a pregnant woman is gaining weight too rapidly or too slowly, her energy intake is obviously wrong for her, regardless of whether or not she meets the RDA.

From a practical point of view, diet during pregnancy is the same as the diet for the healthy nonpregnant woman, with the following exceptions:

1 Milk should be increased to 4 cups instead of 2. By this change alone, the RDA for calcium, phosphorus, riboflavin, and vitamin D will be met or more than met; 18 of the extra 30 grams of protein will be supplied; and useful amounts of many other nutrients are obtained. If weight gain is a problem, low-fat or skim milk can be used instead of whole milk. All milk should be fortified with vitamin D, and skim milk with vitamin A as well.

2 A small extra amount from the meat group, about the equivalent of 1½ ounces of meat, will supply about 12 grams of protein, plus useful amounts of iron and vitamins. The vitamins vary from one item to another; organ meats such as liver and kidney are very rich in vitamin A and folacin, and nuts and legumes are good sources of folacin, although not of vitamin A.

3 An increase in dark green or deep yellow vegetables and fruits, from one serving every day to 4, 5, or 6 servings weekly, will easily meet the increased RDA for vitamin A activity. In addition, the dark green leafy vegetables ("foliage") are particularly good sources of folacin.

4 Breads and cereals should be of the enriched or whole grain type whenever possible.

Because the usual Basic Four pattern insures that the RDA for ascorbic acid is met for pregnant women as well as for the nonpregnant, no change in good or fair vitamin C sources is indicated. Similarly, the same use of iodized table salt, which is ordinarily a more than adequate iodine source, will also be so during pregnancy.

In summary then, no special foods or unusual diets are really required during pregnancy; doubling the milk intake and slightly increasing the intake of other groups will insure that the RDA are met.

Many obstetricians routinely prescribe multivitamin supplements during pregnancy, sometimes because the woman expects them rather than because she needs them, and this is harmless if a reputable brand is taken. However, it is iron deficiency, rather than any vitamin deficiency, that is most likely to occur in pregnant women if supplements are not taken.

STUDIES OF MALNUTRITION AND MATERNAL HEALTH

In the 1950s, a series of studies, the "Vanderbilt Cooperative Study of Maternal and Infant Nutrition," investigated relationships of maternal nutrition to a number of complications of pregnancy. Over 2000 women were studied by means of dietary, biochemical, and clinical assessments, and eventually over a dozen papers were published on topics such as obstetrical performance and changes in nutritional status and requirements during pregnancy.

These studies are often cited (incorrectly) as having proved that poor nutrition causes major complications of pregnancy. Actually they did no such thing. In fact the authors emphatically stated that complications of pregnancy may cause suboptimal intakes, rather than the other way around; a very ill woman is likely to eat less than normal, whether or not she is pregnant. Obstetricians who care for pregnant women are of course concerned about their nutritional status, but they must necessarily be most concerned with the serious and even life-threatening complications which may occur during pregnancy and delivery.

In particular, *preeclampsic toxemia* (or toxemia of pregnancy) has been studied intensively as a possible form of nutritional disease. Toxemia is characterized by high blood pressure, the excretion of protein (albumin) molecules in the urine, and edema. At one time, it was a major cause of maternal deaths, but modern medical care has greatly improved the situation.

Although postulated causes of toxemia have included protein deficiency, carbohydrate excess, niacin deficiency, and ascorbic acid deficiency, studies have failed to provide evidence that any of these is an actual cause. The strongest correlation between toxemia and nutrition is probably seen in relation to excessively rapid weight gain during pregnancy. Even in this case, much of the weight gained may represent fluid retention rather than fat, so whether excess weight gain is a cause or a result of toxemia is not known.

The main conclusion of studies on nutrition during pregnancy is that the diets of pregnant women can vary widely, in quantity as well as quality, without causing *detectable* effects on the fetus or the woman. There may be more subtle long-term effects (such as effects on the later growth or development of the infant) which are not detected by studies during pregnancy. However, studies of these are confounded by the many environmental factors other than nutrition that can determine postnatal health.

NUTRITIONAL CONCERNS DURING PREGNANCY

The common nutrition-related problems of pregnancy can be considered from two points of view: that of the nutritionist or physician, and that of the pregnant woman. The two points of view do not always coincide.

Weight gain. Current thinking places the ideal weight gain during pregnancy at approximately 20 to 25 pounds. This is far from the

40 pounds or more commonly gained in the days when women believed they should literally "eat for two" during pregnancy. It is also drastically different from the 15 pounds or less to which many obstetricians routinely restricted their patients in the 1960s. Both excess weight gain and too little weight gain are now believed to be incompatible with optimal health of both mother and infant.

The various components of weight gain are shown in Table 17–3. Admittedly, some of the weight gained during pregnancy is fat, which remains after delivery. Most women, however, lose this amount of extra weight without any particular difficulty, especially if they choose to breast-feed their infants.

Calcium and vitamin D intake. The increased activity of the parathyroid glands during pregnancy improves the efficiency of calcium absorption. However, if calcium or vitamin D intake is inadequate, parathyroid hormone's major effect is to remove calcium from the woman's bones. The idea of losing "a tooth for every baby" is incorrect, however; teeth cannot be decalcified, even to meet fetal needs.

The average newborn baby contains about 2 percent as much calcium as the woman does, and a single pregnancy therefore cannot deplete a woman of calcium, even if fetal needs must be met entirely by decalcifying her bones. However, repeated pregnancies, especially if followed by prolonged lactations, can remove significant quantities of calcium from the mother's skeleton. This situation is much more likely to be seen in developing countries than in the United States.

Iron intake. In contrast to calcium, iron is used in very significant amounts in a single pregnancy; typical figures are shown in Table 17–4. Not only is the newborn baby very rich in iron, but the placenta contains considerable iron which must be obtained from the woman. Many animals conserve this iron by eating the placenta after it is delivered—hardly a practical solution to suggest to women.

Some authorities believe that the pregnant woman's hemoglobin level and hematocrit should be maintained at the same levels normal for nonpregnant women. However, total blood volume increases more during pregnancy than does the number of red blood cells (Figure 17–6). If this common phenomenon of *hemodilution,* or "physiologic anemia of pregnancy," is normal, blood values should be expected to decrease somewhat during pregnancy. Certainly anemia should be prevented in pregnant women as in others; but what constitutes anemia during pregnancy is not really agreed upon.

Protein intake. The newborn infant contains approximately 1 pound of protein; another pound is distributed in the placenta, the increased breast tissues, the thickened uterine wall, and elsewhere in the woman's body. Because the protein intake of most American women is high enough to meet the needs of pregnancy even when they are not pregnant, the problem arises only in the case of women whose

TABLE 17–3

Components of weight gain in an average normal pregnancy

	Approximate weight (pounds)
Full-term fetus	7½
Placenta	1½
Amniotic fluid	2
Increase in uterine tissue	2
Increase in breast tissue	2
Increase in blood volume	2
Edema	5
Increase in body fat	up to 6
Total pounds gained	22 to 28

TABLE 17–4

The iron cost of a normal pregnancy

	Average, milligrams	**Range, milligrams**
Iron loss of normal men and non-menstruating women	170	150– 200
Iron in full-term fetus	270	200– 370
Iron in placenta and cord	90	30– 170
Iron in blood lost at delivery	150	90– 310
Cost of pregnancy	680	470–1050
*Plus iron needed for increased total red blood cell mass	450	200– 600

* Iron for the increased red blood cell mass must be provided (from body stores, foods, or supplements) during pregnancy. However, this iron is not considered part of the iron cost of pregnancy because the red cell mass returns to normal after delivery, and iron released from the extra cells is conserved by the woman's body.

From "Iron Deficiency in the United States," Council on Foods and Nutrition, *Journal of the American Medical Association,* 203:407 (1968).

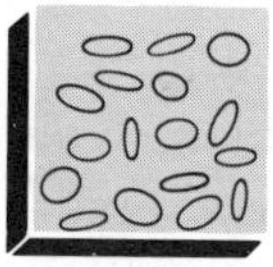

Nonpregnant woman: approximately one-third of blood consists of red blood cells.

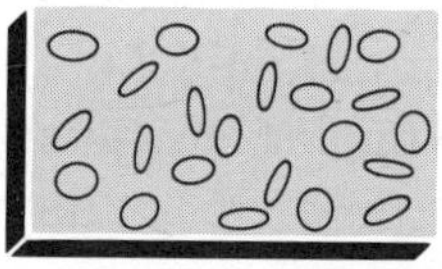

Pregnant woman: blood volume may increase by 50%, while number of red blood cells increases by only 20 or 25%.

FIGURE 17–6. The physiologic hemodilution of pregnancy. Is this anemia or is it a normal change?

usual protein intake is much less than average. It should be emphasized that an increased need for protein is not synonymous with an increased need for meat specifically. Among low-income women, the use of milk and legumes as protein sources should be encouraged.

Pica. Eating nonfoods is called *pica.* The things that may be eaten by pregnant women are truly amazing: chalk, wood, laundry starch, clay. The habit appears to be cultural, "like dipping snuff," as one woman described it, and is particularly common among low-income rural women in the South. Pica can be detrimental by interfering with normal food intake; some women may eat as much as a pound or more of clay or laundry starch daily, crowding out foods. Moreover, some of the items eaten may be toxic, or contain substances that decrease the absorption of certain nutrients. Nevertheless, a blanket condemnation of the habit may be risky; some women believe that they must eat things like clay in order to have a healthy baby, and do not take kindly to the statement that the habit is ignorant or unhealthy.

Cravings. Pregnant women may crave watermelon or fresh strawberries in February, pizza in the middle of the night, or that old classic craving, dill pickles for breakfast. Only a few people seriously believe today that dire consequences will follow if the cravings are not satisfied. Although the cause is definitely not some mysterious "unmet need," there is no harm in a woman's indulging herself in what she particularly wants to eat, so long as the over-all diet is not adversely affected.

Voracious appetite. In some pregnant women, appetite becomes voracity, and weight is consequently gained far too rapidly. The solution proposed by many women to their obstetricians is: Give me drugs to control my appetite, or don't bother me about my weight. Many physicians reply: Control your appetite without drugs, and stop gaining so much weight. This is a perplexing situation; the hazards of drugs must be weighed against the hazards of excess weight, and the possibility of self-control must be measured against the reality of human weakness.

One solution that is definitely *not* advocated is the "feast and famine" technique, in which some pregnant women periodically starve themselves (usually for a few days prior to the next appointment with the obstetrician) to make up for previous excess weight gain. *Ketonemia*—the accumulation of ketone bodies in the blood—is many times greater in pregnant than in nonpregnant women during fasting, and there is some evidence that the resulting high levels of ketone bodies which reach the fetus may be unsafe.

Frequent urination. As the enlarging uterus presses upon the bladder, the bladder responds by the urge to urinate, just as it responds to the pressure of urine from within. Some women seek to avoid this by reducing their fluid intake. This is definitely unwise, because the pregnant woman's kidneys must excrete fetal metabolic wastes as well as her own. The best advice is: Drink plenty of fluids, and don't get too far away from a bathroom so long as this annoying situation lasts.

Constipation. Increased cellulose intake helps to prevent constipation, as does that old standby, prune juice. Laxatives, however, like all drugs, should be taken only on the physician's advice during pregnancy.

Hemorrhoids. Masses of dilated veins in swollen tissue, called *hemorrhoids,* can be very painful. Avoiding constipation can help to prevent them, but surgery or local pain-relieving drugs are sometimes necessary.

"Morning sickness." Nausea, especially in the morning, is very common, occurring in perhaps at least half of pregnant women. The effects on nutritional status depend on *how* nauseated the woman is (some vomit but some just feel sick); *when* vomiting occurs (if it happens when the stomach is almost empty, nutrient losses are minimal); and *how long* it lasts (it generally subsides after the first trimester). A dietary treatment that some women swear by is to eat something dry, such as crisp toast, first thing in the morning. It is sometimes suggested that the woman go to bed with a box of crackers. The punch line, of course, is that "if you'd done that two months ago you wouldn't have this problem now!" *Hyperemesis gravidarum,* or pernicious vomiting, is a very serious but fortunately rare condition of excessive persistent vomiting. Because extreme malnutrition can result, careful medical attention is necessary.

Heartburn. Because of increased intraabdominal pressure caused by the enlarging uterus, the stomach contents are sometimes regurgitated into the esophagus. The resulting burning sensation is caused by hydrochloric acid in the stomach contents, and really has nothing to do with the heart. Eating a large number of small meals helps, because the stomach is not distended by a large amount of food at any one time.

Edema. If edema is severe, the danger of *toxemia* must be considered. However, mild edema, confined mostly to the hands and feet, does not require treatment. Nevertheless, women commonly find the condition annoying and unattractive, and ask the physician for diuretics (drugs which cause the excretion of excess body fluid). Many physicians do not approve of these or other drugs during pregnancy, unless absolutely necessary. A helpful dietary treatment is to decrease the sodium intake, although many physicians believe that this too is unwise. It would seem harmless to decrease the addition of salt to food, and to omit unusually salty foods such as bacon, frankfurters, and cheese. Because iodized salt is a major iodine source, an iodine-containing supplement is recommended if table salt is strictly curtailed.

Leg cramps. Painful spasms of the large muscle in the calf of the leg, usually occurring at night or upon awakening in the morning, are common in the later months of pregnancy. The woman is usually told to avoid lying on her back, and to point "with the heels," rather than "with the toes" when she stretches. Because cramps are related to low calcium and high phosphorus levels in the blood, it may be helpful to take a calcium-containing supplement which does not contain phosphate, such as calcium lactate or calcium citrate. Drinking more milk will not help, because this would raise the already high phosphate level even more than the calcium level of the blood.

Use of alcohol. Most physicians do not disapprove of moderate alcohol use during pregnancy. Excessive use, at the least, interferes with the intake of essential nutrients; at worst, it is possible that it can cause direct injury to the fetus. It is of course not recommended that a woman drink so much alcohol that she falls down a flight of stairs. In one situation, however, excess alcohol is of value: in premature labor, alcohol is used to inhibit secretion of the hormone, *oxytocin.* This can sometimes stop the uterine contractions and allow the pregnancy to continue until the fetus is well-developed enough to survive. However, such treatment is safely done only in a hospital, and is definitely not a "do it yourself" project.

Fainting. Unless it is the result of hunger, as in overly strict dieting, fainting has no relationship to diet during pregnancy.

Skin and hair changes. A so-called "mask of pregnancy" sometimes develops as the skin of the face becomes more deeply pigmented. About half of pregnant women develop red streaks on the abdomen and occasionally on the breasts. These *striae gravidarum,* or "stretch marks," eventually become silvery, but may never completely disappear after delivery. Hair changes include increased growth of body hair, or, occasionally, loss of hair from the head. Contrary to the advertisements for vitamin E, no nutrients are effective in preventing or treating these skin and hair changes, which are apparently caused by hormonal adjustments in the pregnant woman.

LACTATION

During pregnancy, the placenta produces large amounts of *estrogen* and *progesterone,* which stimulate the growth and development of cells of the breasts. Following the delivery of the placenta, estrogen and progesterone levels fall precipitously. It is believed that this permits the anterior pituitary gland to release another hormone, *prolactin,* which stimulates cells of the breast to secrete milk. Large doses of estrogen, which prevent milk production, can be given to women who do not choose to breast feed.

When the baby suckles, yet another hormone, *oxytoxin,* is released from the posterior pituitary gland. This stimulates specialized cells, called *myoepithelial* cells, in the breast to contract, so that milk is ejected from the breast.

Lactation increases nutrient needs differently than does pregnancy, and this difference is reflected in the RDA (Figure 17–7). The RDA during lactation is:

Higher than during pregnancy for energy, vitamin A, niacin, riboflavin, iodine, and zinc.

The same as during pregnancy for vitamins C, D, E, B_6 and B_{12};

thiamin; calcium; phosphorus; and magnesium.
Less than during pregnancy for protein, folacin, and iron.

The reason for the lesser need for folacin is that the postnatal growth supported by milk is largely a matter of increased cell size, which does not require DNA synthesis as does increased cell number. Milk contains so little iron that an increased intake during lactation is not indicated; in fact, extra iron in the mother's diet will not increase the iron concentration of the milk she secretes.

The diet is modified according to the amount of milk produced by the lactating woman and the amount of body fat stored up previously during pregnancy. From a practical point of view, the principal change is an increased need for energy compared to the intake recommended during pregnancy, because the Basic Four modifications recommended for the pregnant woman supply sufficient amounts of most essential nutrients during lactation.

Human milk provides approximately 18 to 22 kilocalories per ounce. However, because energy is used for milk production with only about 80 percent efficiency on the average, approximately 25 kilocalories are required for each ounce of milk produced. This amounts to a total of 750 kilocalories for the total volume, approximately 30 ounces or 850 milliliters, secreted daily by the average lactating woman. Of the 750 kilocalories, it is recommended that 500 come from the diet, with the remaining 250 derived from fat stored during pregnancy.

FIGURE 17–7. The RDA during pregnancy (P) and during lactation (L).

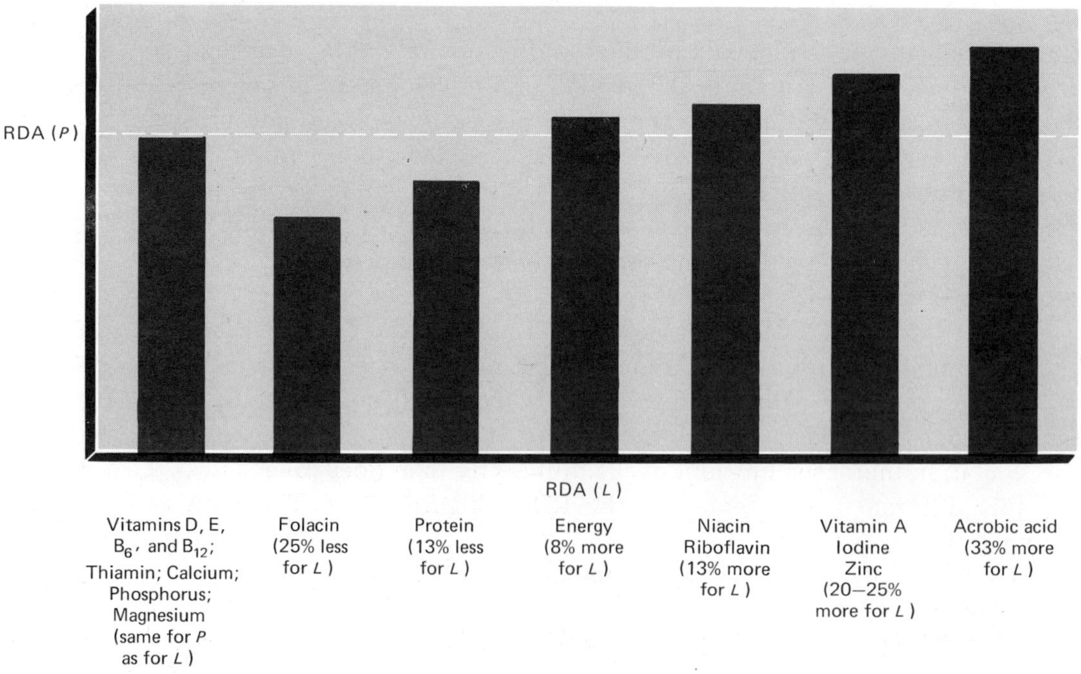

Women who did not accumulate appreciable fat stores must, of course, eat more during lactation in order to avoid becoming underweight.

A good deal of folklore surrounds the subject of lactation. For example, many women believe that certain foods affect the amount or quality of their milk. Some firmly insist that beer, tea, garlic, and yeast are *galactogogues,* which increase the amount of milk produced. Except for the admitted ability of alcohol to encourage the release of milk from the breast by inducing relaxation in the nursing woman, no specific food or nutrient has any effect on milk production. Severe *undernutrition* can decrease the *quantity* of milk produced, but the concentrations of fat, carbohydrate, and protein remain unaffected. However, the concentrations of vitamins may reflect the mother's intake; severe thiamin deficiency in particular may cause a woman to produce milk of such low thiamin content that the baby actually develops beriberi.

Whether specific food components can appear in the milk and "disagree" with the baby is not certain. If a baby appears to be upset by the feeding after the mother eats a certain food, it would appear prudent for the mother to avoid that particular food. However, some women claim that the baby gets diarrhea soon after the mother takes mineral oil, which is obviously impossible.

Whether or not a woman chooses to breast feed, the "baby blues" following childbirth is so common that it should probably be considered a normal human condition. This *postpartum depression* (not *postnatal,* which is a term used to refer to the baby after birth) may be caused by hormone changes, physical fatigue resulting from the care of the new arrival, or emotional reactions to what may at times seem the overwhelming responsibilities of parenthood. The woman should avoid getting so involved with the baby's feedings and other care that she neglects her own needs, such as a good diet, rest, and recreation. Her life as an individual did not begin, nor should it end, with parenthood.

SUGGESTED READINGS

Apgar, V. and J. Beck. *Is My Baby All Right? A Guide to Birth Defects.* New York: Trident, 1972.

Baker, H., O. Frank, A. D. Thomson, A. Langer, E. D. Munves, B. DeAngelis, and H. A. Kaminetzky. "Vitamin Profile of 174 Mothers and Newborns at Parturition." *American Journal of Clinical Nutrition* 28 (1975):59.

Bergner, L. and M. W. Susser. "Low Birth Weight and Prenatal Nutrition: An Interpretative Review." *Pediatrics* 46 (1970):946.

The Boston Children's Medical Center. *Pregnancy, Birth, and the Newborn Baby.* Boston: The Children's Hospital Medical Center, 1971.

Committee on Maternal Nutrition/Food and Nutrition Board, National Research Council–National Academy of Sciences, "Maternal Nutrition and the Course of Pregnancy: Summary Report." Washington, D.C., 1970.

Donaldson, H. H. "Studies on the Growth of the Mammalian Nervous System." *Journal of Nervous and Mental Disorders* 38 (1911):257.

Giroud, A. *The Nutrition of the Embryo.* Springfield, Ill.: Charles C. Thomas, 1970.

Gordon, I. J. *Human Development from Birth to Adolescence,* second edition. New York: Harper & Row, 1969.

Hale, F. "Pigs Born Without Eye Balls." *Journal of Heredity* 24 (1933):105.

Lechtig, A., H. Delgado, R. E. Lasky, R. E. Klein, P. L. Engle, C. Yarbrough, and J. Habicht. "Maternal Nutrition and Fetal Growth in Developing Societies." *American Journal of Diseases of Children* 129 (1975):434.

"Nutrition and Cell Growth." *Dairy Council Digest* 41 (1970):31.

Payne, P. R. and E. F. Wheeler. "Comparative Nutrition in Pregnancy." *Nature* 215 (1967):1134.

Rush, D. "Maternal Nutrition During Pregnancy in Industrialized Societies." *American Journal of Diseases of Children* 129 (1975):430.

Smith, D. W. and E. L. Bierman, eds. *The Biologic Ages of Man.* Philadelphia: Saunders, 1973.

Stiehm, E. R. "Fetal Defense Mechanisms." *American Journal of Diseases of Children* 129 (1975):438.

Trinkaus, J. P. *Cells Into Organs: The Forces that Shape the Embryo.* Englewood Cliffs, N. J.: Prentice-Hall, 1969.

Warkany, J. and H. Kalter. "Congenital Malformations." *New England Journal of Medicine* 265 (1961):1046.

Wilson, J. G. *Environment and Birth Defects.* New York: Academic, 1973.

18

nutrition for infants and young children

A newborn baby may (or may not) be beautiful to its family—but it does not exactly look like the pictures on the baby food packages (Figure 18–1).

The skin is covered with an oily or waxy material called *vernix caseosa.* Because this is believed to serve a protective function, the time-honored tradition of bathing the baby immediately after birth is no longer practiced in many hospitals.

The fingernails and toenails may need to be clipped immediately; babies have a tendency to put their fingers into their eyes, and the long nails can cause serious injury.

Lanugo, fine hair that covered the body in the seventh month of fetal life, may persist until birth, giving a monkey-like appearance which even the new father (and sometimes the mother as well) may remark upon.

The head is disproportionately large, reflecting the amazing growth of the brain before birth. In fact, the newborn's brain weighs 10 percent as much as the whole baby does, in contrast to the adult brain, which accounts for only 2 percent of total body weight.

Although the average baby weighs about 7–7½ pounds at birth, this can vary tremendously. The smallest baby which survived weighed 14 ounces on the third day of life; occasionally a baby is born weighing over 20 pounds. The average length at birth is approximately 20 inches. Thus it can be seen immediately that the average newborn baby has already achieved a length of almost 30 percent of adult height, although weighing less than 5 percent as much as the average adult weighs. This seemingly strange situation is to be expected, for as a rough biological rule, weight increases as the *cube* of the increase in length. So, because the length approximately triples from birth to adulthood, the weight increases by a factor of *about* 3^3, or 27. Naturally this varies greatly, depending on factors such as sex, genetic background, and postnatal environmental factors. Therefore, there is no point in trying to predict a person's adult size from the birth weight or length.

At birth, the baby must make a number of crucial adjustments to the new environment of extrauterine life. The most immediate adjustment required is the onset of breathing. Changes in the circulatory system shunt blood to the lungs instead of to the placenta, where gas exchange took place before birth. After breathing is established satisfactorily, as it is in the vast majority of babies, three other basic needs must be met:

1 **The need to meet energy and nutrient needs.** Several inborn reflexes are present to insure this. The *rooting* reflex causes the baby to turn the head toward a nipple (or any other object for that matter) which touches the cheek. The *suckling* and *swallowing* reflexes automatically

allow the baby to obtain food from a nipple. By contrast, the *extrusion reflex* stimulates the baby to spit out anything which is placed on the front of the tongue rather than on the back, where milk from a nipple is delivered.

2 **The need to eliminate waste.** No longer can the baby empty metabolic wastes via the placenta into the mother's bloodstream, to be excreted by her kidneys. The baby's own kidneys must perform this function. Intestinal excretion also must begin, although this may not occur for several days after birth. *Meconium,* the first intestinal excretion, is a sterile, dark greenish or blackish material which accumulated in the digestive tract before birth. Thereafter, intestinal wastes consist of materials similar to those in the feces of other human beings and vary depending upon the baby's diet.

3 **The need for protection.** From a purely physical point of view, the newborn needs protection from danger and from cold; the infant has little ability to regulate body temperature, being unable even to shiver to produce extra body heat. Although it is assumed that the baby needs to be held and comforted for emotional security as well, how much this matters to the newly born is not really known.

From the point of view of nutrition, two outstanding characteristics of the newborn must be considered: the body composition and the lack of maturity.

THE BODY COMPOSITION OF THE NEWBORN BABY

The body composition of a newborn baby is very different from that of an older infant or an adult (Table 18–1).

The water content is high—some 75 percent of body weight—which allows the baby to survive for several days without fluid. This must have been an important survival mechanism in earlier times, when the only fluid available was that from the mother's breasts, ordinarily secreted only after several days following delivery. New parents sometimes become alarmed at the weight lost by their baby during the first few days, but most of this weight loss represents merely fluid. The parents can be reassured that the loss is normal and harmless, and that even giving the baby large amounts of fluid will not prevent it.

Compared to the chubby older baby, the newborn is thin; only about 12 percent of the body weight is fat. However, compared to many other mammalian species, such as the rat, cat, or dog, the human newborn is remarkably fat.

The *total* protein concentration at birth is similar to that at other ages, although numerous *specific* proteins are present in very low concentrations, which rise as the baby matures.

The iron concentration is approximately twice as high in a newborn baby as in an adult, partly because of the high hematocrit and hemoglobin concentration in the blood, and partly because of large stores of iron in the newborn's liver.

FIGURE 18–1
A healthy newborn baby.

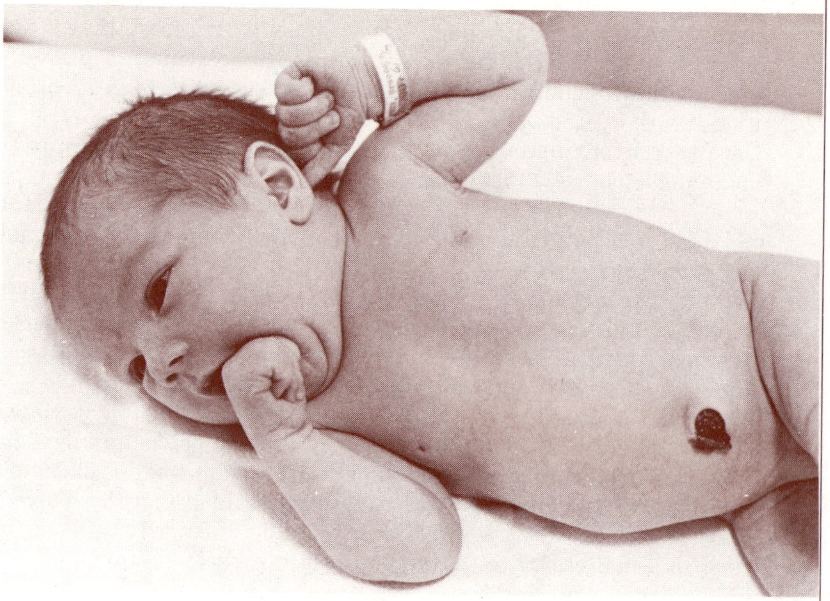

TABLE 18–1
Comparison of body composition of normal infants and adults

	Approximate percent of			
	Water	**Fat**	**Protein**	**Other***
Newborn	75	11	11	2.5
One-year-old	59	24	15	2.5
Adult	60	14 (male) 20 (female)	16	5

* Includes minerals, carbohydrates, vitamins, and other body components. Marked age-related differences in this category include the following:

Iron Water-soluble vitamins in general	Significantly higher concentrations at birth than at later ages
Calcium Fat-soluble vitamins in general	Significantly lower concentrations at birth than at later ages

Data on percent of body components for newborn and one-year-old obtained from S. J. Fomon, *Infant Nutrition,* 2nd Ed., Philadelphia: Saunders Company, 1974.

Calcium and phosphorus are present in relatively low concentrations in the newborn, because the bones are poorly mineralized before birth. This may be a means of facilitating birth; poorly mineralized bones are flexible and therefore tend to bend readily during the process of birth.

Water-soluble vitamins, actively transported across the placenta before birth, are ordinarily present in concentrations greater than those in maternal blood. Therefore, even if the mother is mildly or moderately deficient, the baby is likely to have obtained, at her expense, the water-soluble vitamins needed. Fat-soluble vitamins, although less readily transported from maternal to fetal blood, are generally present in at least adequate amounts in the normal newborn baby.

Vitamin K is the one vitamin very commonly present in less than adequate amounts in the newborn. Because it is fat-soluble, vitamin K does not cross the placenta as readily as do water-soluble vitamins; and because there are no bacteria in the intestine until some time after birth, vitamin K is not supplied through bacterial synthesis either. Uncontrolled bleeding, called "hemorrhagic disease of the newborn," can result from vitamin K deficiency, and this vitamin is therefore routinely given by injection to newborn babies. This is especially important for breast-fed babies, because human milk contains only one-fourth the concentration of vitamin K that cow's milk does.

IMMATURITY OF THE NEWBORN BABY

Immaturity refers to a lack of development, which normally will be corrected with the simple passage of time. Compared to other species which bear one offspring at a time, such as cattle or horses, the human newborn is very poorly developed. This is true by any standard—the ability to forage for food, neuromuscular coordination, the ability to communicate, or any of a number of other parameters. This immaturity has one great advantage to our species, however. A longer gestation, which would allow the fetus more time to mature, could also result in a head size disproportionate to the relatively narrow pelvis of a human female. Because of its large brain (and hence its large head) perhaps the human infant must be born "early" (compared to other mammals) in order to be born at all!

Some specific examples of immaturity that have important nutritional implications are the following:

The digestive system

The digestive tract of the newborn produces quite different kinds and amounts of digestive fluids than it will later. The flow of saliva is scanty, which is no real disadvantage so long as the diet is liquid. "Drooling" usually starts at about the age of three months, when saliva flow increases, but the baby is still too immature to swallow the excess flow. Perhaps this indicates that three months, rather than a much earlier age, is physiologically right for adding solid foods to the diet.

"Spitting up" of small amounts, common during the first few

months, usually subsides as the digestive system matures. Vomiting, however, especially if it is forcible and in large amounts, may be a sign of illness and should be reported to the doctor.

Infantile colic is the name given to excessive crying in the early months. Because the crying appears to be associated with intense pain, the condition can be extremely unsettling to the parents. Unfortunately the causes are not understood, and no reliable treatment is available. Some believe that food allergy is the culprit and that changing the formula will help; others believe that tension in the parents causes colic in the infant; and others insist that it is the colic that causes the parents' tension! Fortunately, in the vast majority of babies, the excessive crying subsides after the age of three months, regardless of what treatment is tried. Curiously, most babies eat well and grow well despite apparent frequent pain. The parents' feelings of helplessness and anger probably need relief more often than the baby's colic.

Kidney function

The young infant's kidneys have little ability to produce concentrated urine. This means that, in order to excrete a given *solute load* (urea, uric acid, creatinine, excess minerals, and other components of urine), the baby must excrete a relatively large volume of water. Ordinarily, this is no problem because the baby is on a fluid diet. It becomes a problem, however, in the following situations.

If the formula is prepared incorrectly, the resulting concentrations of solutes, such as urea or minerals, may be too high for the immature kidneys to cope with. In one hospital, several babies died after they were given formulas in which salt had been used by mistake in place of sugar. *Protein dehydration* results when very excessive protein levels are fed, because of the large amounts of urea which result. Excessive amounts of water can also be lost by extrarenal routes (routes other than the urine), as when sweating is profuse or when the baby has diarrhea. Finally, the *total* fluid intake can be too low, as may happen if a baby becomes ill and refuses the breast or bottle.

Because dehydration of a serious degree can develop much more rapidly in infants than in children or adults, prompt medical treatment is necessary whenever it occurs.

Immature levels of specific proteins

The following examples of immaturity of enzyme systems and other specific proteins are of particular importance to nutrition.

The baby apparently lacks an adequate level of one or more enzymes involved in the synthesis of *histidine;* this amino acid, nonessential for adults, is therefore essential for infants.

Newborn babies are commonly unable to catabolize two amino acids, *phenylalanine* and *tyrosine,* normally. Abnormally high levels, especially of tyrosine, therefore accumulate in the blood. The condition, known as *transient neonatal tyrosinemia*, is innocuous, and should not be confused with serious genetic diseases in which abnormal blood levels of amino acids are also found. Not all physicians agree that the condition should be treated at all, because the simple passage of time will correct it. However, it can be treated if desired. Ascorbic acid, which is the cofactor for several of the enzymes involved in phenylalanine and tyrosine metabolism, stimulates cells to produce mature levels of the enzymes more rapidly than they would otherwise. The condition will therefore disappear more quickly if ascorbic acid intake is increased, and if protein intake is *moderately* reduced in order to avoid excess phenylalanine and tyrosine.

The liver of the newborn contains low levels of enzymes known as *drug metabolizing enzymes*, which convert foreign compounds to other substances. Because the products are *generally* (although not always) less toxic than the original compounds, the enzymes are also sometimes called *detoxifying enzymes*. Their relative lack of these enzymes causes babies to be highly sensitive to doses of foreign compounds harmless to an adult. For this reason, addition of preservatives and other additives to baby foods is strictly controlled by the Food and Drug Administration. Even so, foreign compounds may be ingested by a baby, as when a drug taken by a lactating mother appears in the milk. If this happens, it may be better to discontinue breast feeding rather than risk harmful effects in the baby.

The baby is born with a supply of antibodies, derived before birth from the mother's blood, which confer a certain degree of immunity to diseases. After birth, the antibody levels decline, reaching a low point at about the age of one month. Levels then rise again as the baby gains the ability to produce its own antibodies, in response to experience with microorganisms. The nutritional implication of the changing antibody levels is that some degree of sanitation is necessary, but exactly how much care is needed in this regard is a matter of controversy. In past decades, almost everything the baby touched was routinely washed with disinfectant, or boiled. Today it is generally assumed that a healthy full-term baby can withstand the onslaught of a reasonable number of microorganisms, and a more relaxed attitude toward sterilization is the result.

The hemoglobin present in the red blood cells before birth is different in structure from the hemoglobin produced later, and this difference causes fetal hemoglobin to bind oxygen more tenaciously than does adult hemoglobin. The fetus can thus compete effectively for oxygen, because oxygen in the pregnant woman's blood is attracted to fetal hemoglobin in preference to the mother's adult hemoglobin. Starting shortly before birth and for some months afterwards, the baby gradually destroys its fetal red blood cells and produces new cells of the adult type. The iron released from hemoglobin is conserved and reused for production of new hemoglobin molecules. This recycling of iron, plus the iron stores present at birth, allow the baby to remain in good health on a low-iron diet (milk) until the age of 3–4 months.

Jaundice—yellowing of the skin because of accumulation of the pigment *bilirubin*—is very common in new born babies. It is caused by a combination of two factors. One is the very rapid production of bilirubin, a product of hemoglobin breakdown. The other is the newborn's lack of the enzyme which catalyzes the conversion of bilirubin to a compound which the kidneys can excrete. Although there is no dietary treatment of the jaundice, exposure to blue light can speed up the decomposition of bilirubin. It is important to note that the yellowing of the skin caused by excess carotene intake is *not* jaundice; *hypercarotenemia* and jaundice are caused by accumulation of two completely different yellow pigments, and excess carotene accumulation can be entirely prevented by avoiding excess carotene intake.

INFANT FEEDING

Socially and psychologically, food is of enormous importance to the infant. Psychologists refer to infancy as the *oral stage* of psychosexual development because the infant derives gratification primarily through stimulation of the mouth parts during feeding. Highly specialized diets —at first liquid and later soft—are needed during early infancy, but the food intake usually changes so rapidly that by the age of one year many infants are eating diets similar to those of adults.

Lifelong eating patterns may be largely established during infancy; the term *nutritional imprinting* is used to describe the tendency of the young to accept certain kinds and amounts of foods as "normal." However, it is not known whether food habits established this early in life actually resist later modification. A few generations ago, infants were commonly fed exclusively on milk throughout the first year of life; although for other reasons this diet is not adequate, rejection of most foods as a result of lack of early experience with them remains unproved.

From the point of view of physical health, there seems to be little doubt that the decreased infant mortality seen in developed countries during the twentieth century has been largely the result of advances in knowledge of infant feeding. Problems of two aspects of feeding—nutrition and sanitation—caused many infant deaths until well after 1900. Infants who could not be breast fed, and therefore had to be given cow's milk, faced one of two problems. If the cow's milk was *not* boiled, the baby could be exposed to a dangerously large number of infectious microorganisms, as well as the relatively indigestible protein of unboiled milk. If the milk *was* boiled, the small amount of vitamin C present was destroyed, with scurvy commonly resulting. Either way, cow's milk was an unsuitable food for infants until the basic problems of sanitation and nutrition had been solved.

Whether malnutrition during infancy causes permanent damage to various organs is unknown. The final level of growth of each organ is affected maximally by the conditions which existed during the period of maximum growth rate, and this critical period for the brain is during late fetal life and infancy. Therefore, it is reasoned, brain growth and hence mental ability may be permanently impaired by severe early undernutrition. It is probably safe to say that *if* postnatal malnutrition causes permanent mental retardation at any stage, it is more likely to do so during infancy than during later stages. This is as far as we can go at present, because it is possible that if malnutrition is severe enough to cause actual brain damage, it is also so severe as to be fatal.

Despite the vast amount of knowledge about infant feeding that has been accumulated during the twentieth century, certain problems of infant feeding persist. These problems remain, not because of a lack of available information, but because this knowledge is not always put into practice.

IS BREAST BEST?

Intuitively, most people would agree that human milk is an ideal food for humans during the first few months. However, there is no consensus on the best diet for a young baby, and a number of generally accepted beliefs regarding breast feeding are questionable or erroneous. Those conclusions based on facts should be distinguished from those based on emotional fervor.

LaLeche League, an organization consisting mostly of lay people rather than of professional nutritionists, is the largest organized group of proponents of breast-feeding in the United States. Although few would disapprove of their motive to encourage breast feeding, a number of objections can be made to the information they provide. The following are examples of the kinds of questionable claims made by LaLeche League.

Colostrum—the liquid produced by the breasts for a few days before true milk secretion begins—is said to be extremely important as a source of antibodies; a few extremists even believe that an infant who receives colostrum has no need for inoculations to prevent diseases. Although colostrum is an important postnatal source of antibodies for some species, such as the pig, human infants are born with a supply of maternal antibodies obtained *prenatally* from the mother's blood. Pediatricians and nutritionists generally agree that in humans colostrum is of little value in providing protection against diseases.

A common claim is that breast feeding provides psychological benefits, both to the mother and to the baby, that cannot be obtained in any other way. Studies are cited to "prove" that infants must be breast-fed in order to develop emotionally in a normal manner. However, many other studies could be cited to show that emotional development is as normal in formula-fed babies as in those who are breast-fed. (Remember, Jack the Ripper and Adolph Hitler were undoubtedly breast-fed.)

Another advantage cited is that breast milk is always at the right temperature, which spares parents the work of warming the bottle. However, babies readily accept unwarmed formula, straight from the refrigerator, with no apparent ill effects. Mothers, more often than babies, may reject the idea of cold formulas, perhaps because of the emotional connotations of cold feedings.

Economy is often stressed as an advantage of breast feeding. Certainly, equipment for preparing formulas must be purchased, whereas the equipment for breast feeding is provided free by nature. However, the milk, which is the principal expense over the long run, is certainly not free, whether it is produced by cows or by humans. In fact, cows convert inexpensive feed to milk so efficiently that a cow's milk formula prepared at home may actually cost slightly less than the extra food needed to support lactation in a woman.

Definitely incorrect is the claim that breast milk alone is sufficient for an infant for at least the first six months, or even throughout the entire first year. In particular, human milk is lacking in vitamin D and in iron, and these nutrients should be supplied from other sources, at least after the first three months.

Finally, it should be emphasized that breast feeding does not provide for a natural spacing of births, as is commonly claimed. Women are *generally* unable to conceive for some three or four months after giving birth, and breast feeding usually prolongs this period of natural sterility for a month or so more. But many women have discovered, to their dismay, that breast feeding is an extremely unreliable form of contraception. Those who do not wish to have babies very close together would be well advised to choose a more effective method of preventing conception.

But breast feeding does have a few proven advantages. Allergies to human milk are extremely rare, which would be something to consider in families troubled by allergies. Breast feeding is definitely superior to formula feeding in situations where there is a lack of knowledge, motivation, or equipment needed to prepare and store a formula properly, as may be the case among people in lower socioeconomic groups. The advantages become progressively less among well-informed, conscientious people, who are able to breast-feed or formula-feed their babies with equally satisfactory results.

Breast feeding is contraindicated if the mother has active tuberculosis; cannot produce a sufficient quantity of milk; chooses to return to work or to social activities which keep her absent from the home for considerable periods of time; is taking drugs (including many oral contraceptives) which are excreted in the milk; or finds that breast feeding is a disadvantage physically, socially, or psychologically. No woman need feel guilty, inadequate, or unfeminine if she decides that, for her, breast is *not* best.

PREPARING AN INFANT'S FORMULA

Because there are so many possible ways to prepare a baby formula from cow's milk, no one "right way" can be recommended. The principles are:

1 Add water to dilute the milk.
2 Add carbohydrate (syrup or sugar).
3 Heat to destroy bacteria and to make the protein more digestible.

The reasons for these steps can be seen in Table 18–2. Further details of formula preparation depend upon the condition of the baby and the preferences of the mother and the pediatrician. A few important points are the following:

Evaporated milk is most commonly used for an infant's formula, but some pediatricians recommend pasteurized whole milk. Sweetened condensed milk is *not* suitable because its sugar content is too high. *Raw* or *certified* milk, which has not been pasteurized, is not considered safe for an infant or anyone else unless it is heated to kill bacteria.

The formula can be sterilized in either of two ways. In the *aseptic* method, a sterile formula is prepared and poured into previously sterilized bottles, after which sterile nipples are put on. In the *terminal-heating* method, an unsterilized formula is put into clean but unsterilized bottles, the nipples are put on, and the filled bottles are then sterilized by boiling in a kettle of water. Many brands of presterilized disposable plastic bottle liners cannot be boiled, and the aseptic method must be used with this type of bottle.

Prepared canned formulas, which need only be mixed with water, are somewhat more expensive than those made "from scratch." However, they are very convenient, and their use minimizes the possibility of errors in measurement.

Whether breast- or formula-fed, the newborn will at first need to be fed at intervals of three or four hours, day and night. Even if the parents do not set up a schedule, the baby will usually establish a feeding pattern, for example 7–11–3 o'clock, or 6–10–2 o'clock. By the age of four to six weeks, most babies can sleep through the 2 or 3 A.M. feeding, and by three months, most can skip the late evening (10 or 11 P.M.) feeding as well. The total amounts of milk and solids are then of course redistributed among the four remaining feedings.

The formula-fed baby should be held during feeding, just as the breast-fed baby is. Propping up the bottle is not recommended, espe-

TABLE 18–2

Composition of 100 milliliters of milk*

	Human milk	Cow's milk
Energy (Calories)	71.0	69.0
Fat (grams)	3.8	3.7
Lactose (grams)	7.0	4.8
Protein (grams)	1.2	3.3
Minerals (total milligrams)	200.0	700.0
Calcium (milligrams)	33.0	125.0
Phosphorus (milligrams)	15.0	96.0
Iron (milligrams)	0.1	0.1
Vitamins		
A (IU)	176.0	113.0
Carotene (IU)	45.0	63.0
D (IU)	0.4	2.4
E (milligrams)	0.56	0.06
K (Dam–Glavind units)	26.0	100.0
Ascorbic acid (milligrams)	4.3	1.6
Folacin (micrograms)	0.18	0.23
Niacin (milligrams)	0.17	0.09
Pantothenic acid (milligrams)	0.20	0.35
Pyridoxine (milligrams)	0.01	0.05
Riboflavin (milligrams)	0.04	0.16
Thiamin (milligrams)	0.016	0.042
Vitamin B_{12} (micrograms)	trace	0.56
Bacteria	Normally absent	Often present

Note: Compared to human milk, cow's milk has *higher* concentrations of minerals and protein, and a *lower* concentration of carbohydrate (lactose). Therefore cow's milk must be diluted and sugar must be added to make its composition suitable for feeding human infants.

* Slightly adapted from "The Composition of Milks," Food and Nutrition Board: Pub. No. 254, National Academy of Sciences—National Research Council, Washington, D.C., 1953.

TABLE 18–3

Three options suitable for babies up to three months old

Option 1	Option 2	Option 3
a. Vitamin D-fortified evaporated milk formula prepared at home b. Vitamin C source: regular orange juice, any "baby food juice" (because all are vitamin C-fortified), or vitamin C in drops c. Fluoride (drops) if this is lacking in the water used for formula preparation d. Cooled boiled water (offered as dictated by baby's acceptance)	a. Commercial infant formula containing all necessary nutrients (as well as some which may not be necessary) b. Water to dilute formula, according to directions c. Cooled boiled water (offered as dictated by baby's acceptance)	a. Breast feeding b. Vitamin D source (drops) c. Fluoride (drops) even if water supply contains adequate fluoride, as this mineral is not excreted in significant amounts in milk d. Cooled boiled water (offered as dictated by baby's acceptance)

cially for very young babies, because the baby is too likely to choke if the milk flows too fast.

OUTLINE OF DIET DURING THE FIRST YEAR

Except for babies with special nutritional needs, any one of the three options shown in Table 18–3 will be suitable for the first two or three months.

People are sometimes surprised to learn that solid foods such as cereals and strained fruits are not really necessary during the first two or three months. Although it is customary in developed countries to begin feeding solids to babies only a few weeks old or even younger, there is no evidence that this is necessary for the baby. The greatest benefits probably accrue to the mother, who can impress her friends with the news that her 3-week-old is already eating as many different things as the 4-month-old up the street is. Parents may mistakenly believe that early acceptance of a wide variety of foods is a very important developmental step, and heaven forbid that the baby should be unable to compete successfully.

By the age of three months, however, solid foods should be part of the diet, because most babies of this age have used up the store of iron which they had at birth. Even if the formula is fortified with iron, solid foods are still recommended in order to accustom the baby to foods other than liquids. The foods that are offered at first are actually only semisolid, in order to give the baby an opportunity to adjust to this strange new texture. The amount of liquid is then gradually reduced, until a truly solid type of diet is being fed.

As was true in the case of the earlier diet, more than one option is possible:

Option 1	**Option 2**
Commercially prepared baby foods	Home-prepared foods made by straining, blending, or mashing some of the family's food

Chopping, blending, and mashing small amounts of foods can be time-consuming and messy compared to opening and possibly warming a jar of already prepared food. Therefore, although it is entirely possible to feed a baby well without the use of convenience foods bought specially for the baby, the overwhelming majority of parents in developed countries use at least some commercial baby foods. Commercial baby foods available on the retail market are the following:

Precooked cereals. The traditional "first solid" given to babies, these are bland, easily digested, and ready to serve after simply adding liquid. Because iron, thiamin, riboflavin, and niacin have been added in very useful amounts, baby cereal is a "best buy" in terms of nutritional value relative to cost. Rice cereal is commonly given before the other grains are, not because it is more nutritious but because allergies to rice are rare compared to allergies to other cereals.

Cereal and fruit combinations. These are packed in jars, and save the trouble of mixing the cereal with liquid; however, the cereal may not be enriched, as are the dry cereals. Therefore, whether their greater convenience is worth a possible loss of nutritional advantage is questionable.

Strained meat. Although definitely more convenient to buy than to attempt to prepare at home, strained meat is probably not really necessary in a baby's diet. Milk can provide adequate protein, and baby cereals provide far more iron and vitamins than equal amounts of meats contain.

Egg yolk. Half a century ago, egg yolk was a more important iron source in infant diets than it is today, because it was much easier to strain at home than meats were. Today, with commercially prepared strained meats and iron-fortified baby cereals available, feeding egg yolk is more a tradition than a nutritional necessity. Egg *whites* are generally not recommended until after the first year, both because allergies to the white are much more common than allergies to the yolk, and because the iron of an egg is almost entirely in the yolk.

Strained fruits. These vary greatly in nutritional value. Some, such as applesauce, are good sources of bulk or cellulose, which is important in preventing constipation. In fact, many mothers vary the fruit intake almost entirely on the basis of the baby's bowel movements. Some, notably apricots, are significant vitamin A sources. Others are good sources of vitamin C, but not, oddly enough, because the fruits contain high levels of vitamin C at harvest. Rather, the vitamin is added as a preservative to prevent darkening of the food when the jar is opened and the contents exposed to air. Vitamin C is always used for this purpose in strained bananas; for other fruits, the label must be read in order to find out whether vitamin C has been added.

Strained vegetables. Like fruits, these contain cellulose, which can help to prevent constitpation. In addition, vegetables are usually more nutritious than fruits, particularly the green and yellow vegetables, which are excellent sources of vitamin A value. However, fruits are generally fed more often than vegetables, because babies like the sweet flavor of fruits. And parents tend to offer those foods that the baby accepts more willingly, rather than those that are of greatest nutritional value. Getting the baby to like vegetables is commonly the new parent's first experience with the little darling's amazing strength in resisting the parent's offerings.

Vegetables and meat combinations. These "combinations" are actually vegetables with a trivial amount of meat added for flavor. They should be used as alternates to plain vegetables, never as alternates to meat. "High meat dinners," however, consist of a mixture of approximately one-third meat and two-thirds other ingredients, such as vegetables and starchy fillers. They are better protein sources, and of course are more expensive, than either plain vegetables or vegetables and meat combinations.

Desserts. These are so low in nutritional value, relative to both cost and sugar content, that both parents and babies would probably be better off without them. However, babies like them and parents enjoy giving their babies what they like, so perhaps it is more realistic to recommend that their use be confined to an *occasional* dessert served *after*, rather than in place of, a meal consisting of more nutritious foods.

"Junior" baby foods. These are identical to the strained products, except for the texture, which is coarser. They should be introduced when the baby is about seven or eight months old; otherwise, an occasional baby may become so accustomed to the smooth texture of strained foods that later it may be difficult for him or her to learn to tolerate lumps in food without gagging—a very unpleasant situation for everybody else at the table, as well as for the child. As was true during the earlier months, home-prepared junior foods can be used instead of commercially prepared foods, merely by chopping or mashing some of the family's food, just until it is slightly lumpy.

During the first year, it is considered desirable to introduce a reasonable variety of flavors so that the baby can become accustomed to many different flavors. However, the *nutrient* needs can be supplied by a diet based upon nothing more than milk or formula, baby cereal, and a source of vitamin C, if this is not already in the milk or formula. People who cannot afford liberal amounts of more expensive foods should be reassured that the baby can be adequately nourished without them.

Three meals a day

By the age of about 6–8 months, most babies eat less at one of the usual four daily meals than at the others, and this is a signal for the change to a three-meals-daily pattern, with one or two *planned* snacks to satisfy the baby's continued enthusiasm for eating (Figure 18–2). The meal pattern might look something like this:

Breakfast: cereal, milk, juice
Midmorning: juice, crackers
Lunch: vegetable, meat or egg, milk
Midafternoon: milk or juice, crackers or toast
Dinner: cereal, fruit, milk

There is nothing magical about such a pattern; it is only a suggestion, and if meat for breakfast and cereal for lunch fits in better, this is fine.

Weaning: when and how?

Although babies will generally accept sips of liquids from a cup or glass by the age of 5–6 months, most are unwilling to give up the breast or bottle completely before the age of a year or so. Even then, many babies cling tenaciously to the old familiar way of sucking milk rather than

FIGURE 18–2

In a healthy baby, eagerness for food is usually very obvious. (Photo courtesy Gerber Products Company, Fremont, Michigan.)

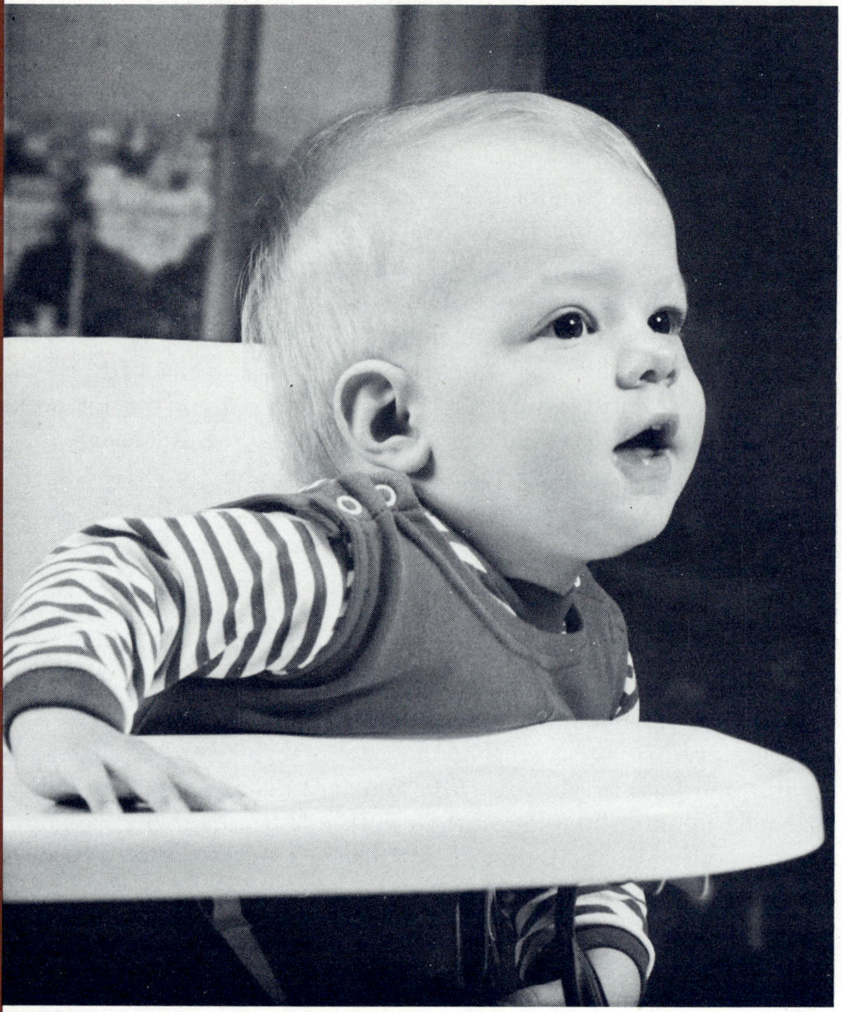

sipping it. Ideally, weaning from the breast or bottle should be accomplished gradually, one feeding at a time, between about 9 and 12 months. However, if a baby appears to be frantically unhappy about being weaned, this should be discussed with the physician. The "right" age for weaning varies from one baby to another, and only the baby knows how much the breast or bottle means in the way of emotional security.

SOME COMMON ERRORS IN FEEDING BABIES

Overfeeding, usually by overenthusiastic feeding of solid foods to young infants, is probably the most common mistake parents make in feeding babies. People do this for a variety of reasons: They believe that a fat baby is a healthy one; they hate to waste the rest of that jar of baby food; they think the baby will not have to be fed so often if each feeding is as large as possible. The common result is obesity, which is no more a sign of health in babies than in anyone else.

Excessive salting of baby food is common. There is no evidence that a high salt intake is of any value to babies, and some evidence that it may predispose to hypertension later in life. Parents should recognize that babies readily accept unsalted or very slightly salted foods, even though adults find them too bland.

Careless handling of baby foods can result in infectious diseases. A portion of food should be transferred from the jar to a clean dish, and the remainder of the jar should be refrigerated immediately; feeding directly from the jar should be done only if the baby can finish the whole jar at one feeding. Otherwise, organisms from the air and from the baby's mouth can get into the food, where they multiply rapidly. Also, the starch-digesting enzyme in the baby's saliva gets into the food and liquifies it, resulting in a watery puddle too unappetizing to feed to anyone.

Failure to provide adequate water occurs if parents assume that the formula or breast milk alone provides enough water. The baby should be offered plain water several times daily, especially in hot weather, when sweating may be profuse, or during illness, when water may be lost because of diarrhea or vomiting.

Let's face it: *occasional* mistakes in caring for infants are very likely, because parents are human. However, errors can be kept to a minimum if people are reasonably well-informed on the care and feeding of babies, and if a physician is consulted regarding any question about the baby's health.

PRESCHOOL CHILDREN: TODDLERS, DAWDLERS, TALKERS, AND WALKERS

Preschool children—those between the ages of one and five years—are much more complex than infants, socially and psychologically as well as physically. Discussion of this age group must therefore necessarily be limited to those characteristics most relevant to nutrition.

Putting the brakes on: growth and appetite

Preschool children grow at a slow rate compared to infants (Figure 18–3). During the first year, weight increased by about 14 pounds, and length by about 10 inches. If this growth rate were to continue, the average child would weigh almost 80 pounds and be nearly 6 feet tall by the fifth birthday. Obviously, marked deceleration of growth must occur during the preschool years.

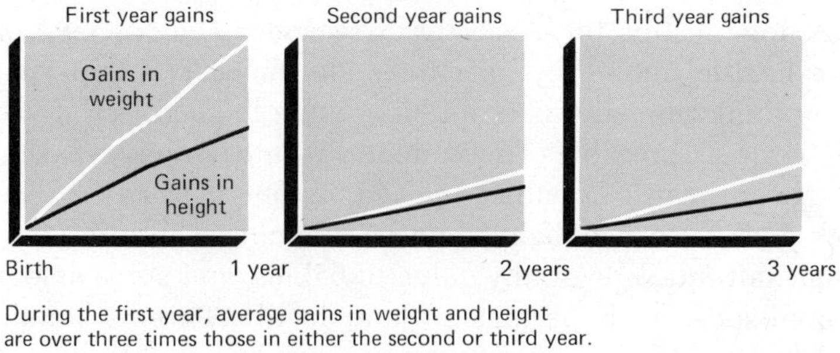

FIGURE 18–3. The reason for decreased appetite after infancy: the slow growth of young children compared to infants. (Photo courtesy Gerber Products Company, Fremont, Michigan.)

Along with the decreased growth rate there is a decreased need for food, and the child responds by eating less. Because it is normal, the decreased appetite is called *physiologic anorexia,* to distinguish it from the loss of appetite caused by physical illness or emotional stress. The problem that sometimes results is not (at least at first) in the child. Rather, the parents may become concerned because they mistakenly believe that children should eat as ravenously as they did when they were infants. "Doctor, this child doesn't eat enough to keep a bird alive," is one of the commonest complaints physicians hear from the mothers of preschool children, especially when the child is between one and a half and three years old. Actually, if a child has a normal amount of body fat, the individual energy need is being met, whether or not the mother thinks so.

Streamlining for action

Compared to the chubby baby, the child has a lean, streamlined appearance, with a smaller percent of body fat. This is to be expected; a streamlined design is ideal for a body that moves, and moving is one thing that most preschool children seem determined to do. Child psychologists refer to a basic developmental task of the one- to two-year-old as "the active motor exploration of the environment." Parents sometimes put it a bit more succinctly: "That kid gets into everything."

Increased physical activity of course requires increased energy. However, this is more than offset by the lower energy need resulting from decreased growth rate. The *net* effect, then, is that the preschool child needs an estimated 100 kilocalories for each kilogram of body weight. Although this is far above the estimated 35–40 kilocalories per kilogram of body weight recommended for adults, it is less than the corresponding values during infancy (Figure 18–4).

Special needs and limitations of young children

No special foods are actually needed for the preschool child, although some parents continue to feed chopped baby foods or special "toddler"

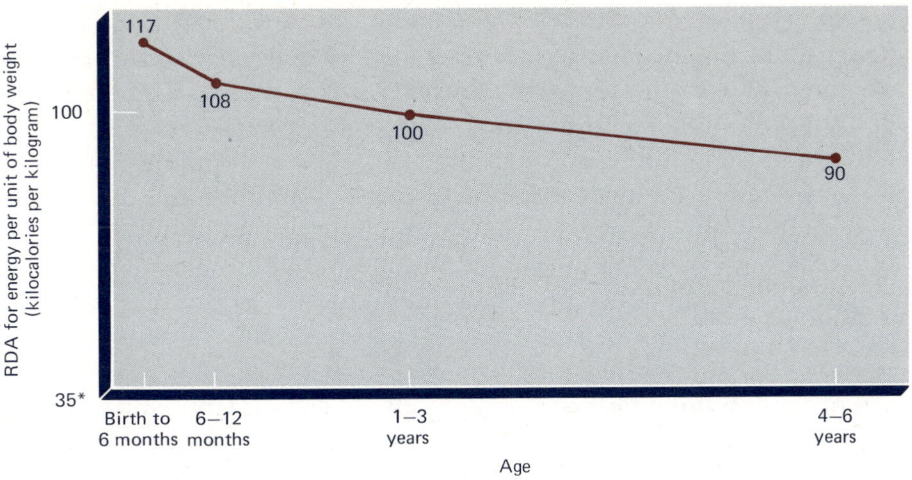

*Approximate RDA for energy (kilocalories per kilogram of body weight) for an average adult female. The approximate RDA for adult males is 40.

FIGURE 18–4. The RDA reflects decreased needs for energy after the rapid growth period of infancy.

meals until the age of two years or more. However, the most nutritious baby food, baby cereal, is unfortunately often discontinued long before the baby is a year old; the usual family cereals that replace it are often highly sugared, and are less valuable sources of nutrients—especially of iron. By extending the period during which baby cereals are fed for at least another year or two, parents would considerably increase the iron intake of most preschool children.

Some of the common eating problems of young children have nothing to do with food itself but with the equipment necessary for eating. The chair may be too low, or the glass may be so big that a small hand can hardly lift it without risking a spill. Even in ideal surroundings, spills and messiness are inevitable during the self-feeding learning process. Remember, there is no such thing as a "spoon-feeding reflex," or an innate ability to eat neatly at the table. Children usually want to have a try at feeding themselves with a spoon at least by about the age of fifteen months, and there is no point in postponing it until they learn to be neater. Learning requires practice, and a messy dining room table and floor may therefore be part of quite a few meals until the technique is more or less mastered.

Social aspects of food for preschool children

During the preschool years, the child must learn to adapt and conform to others in many ways. Experts in child development speak of the basic developmental task of establishing "self-identity versus social conformity" between the ages of two and three years. (Parents may say that the child is at "that awful no-no stage.") Many necessary social adaptations have to do with aspects of life other than nutrition: cooperative play with other children, control of bowel and bladder function, gaining independence, accepting the fact that he or she is not, after all, the center of the universe. However, other social adjustments are quite directly related to nutrition. The child is expected to eat meals with the family; although two or three snacks may be allowed, no more will feeding be "on demand"; and family expectations and opinions as to what is eaten, how much is eaten, and how fast it is eaten now come into play far more than during infancy. The child observes and learns, mostly by imitation, and develops food habits and patterns that may last for the rest of his or her life.

One very important part of socialization that takes place by the age of two or three years is sex-role identification. How much this affects food intake is unknown, but even at this age, boys generally eat more than girls, possibly as a result of the parents' subtle encouragement of greater physical activity in boys. Certainly as boys and girls get older the activity difference, and hence the energy requirement, becomes more marked. Whether this is an inborn sex difference is very difficult to determine. Boys are expected to be more active, aggressive, and rowdy than girls are, and sex-role stereotyping can exert strong influences even in the very young.

NUTRITIONAL STATUS OF PRESCHOOL CHILDREN

In developed countries such as the United States, both the infant and the preschool child are in a favored position nutritionally. The only common nutrition-related problems seen in preschool children are the following:

Iron deficiency anemia. This is almost always the result of excess milk drinking, which crowds out iron-containing foods, and is most commonly seen in the child who has not been weaned from the bottle by the age of one year. (The American child who is still being breastfed after the age of one year is a rarity indeed.) A very large number of people simply are unaware that a child can drink too much milk, or that late weaning encourages excess milk drinking; some even believe that a child needs a quart of milk daily for good health. Actually this is far too much; one pint daily is plenty for preschool children.

Overweight. Overweight children may be overeating spontaneously because of boredom or of an overly strong emotional association of food with love. Other children may overeat because of outside pressures—the "eat, eat, my child" urging of the oversolicitous mother, who thinks that a child should eat constantly to be healthy, or perhaps to prove that the child appreciates Mother's efforts.

Some overweight children, however, really eat no more than other children; their problem is primarily underactivity. The child's need to be distracted and to find amusement and novelty no longer requires physical movement, as it did in previous times. Television, in particular, can bombard a child with constantly changing stimuli without any effort on the child's part. If this is the situation, parents can and should provide more motivation for physical activity, starting perhaps by pressing the "off" button on the television set.

Underweight. Underweight of a severe degree in an otherwise healthy child is uncommon in the United States. Of first importance is a thorough physical examination to rule out underlying physical diseases such as allergies, chronic infections, or previously undetected disorders of the heart or other organs. If there is no demonstrable physical defect, underfeeding as part of a pattern of neglect may be suspected. In other children, spontaneous undereating or hyperactivity may be responsible. Prompt medical attention is indicated in order to determine the underlying causes.

Temporary infectious diseases. These rarely interfere seriously with food intake. Parents can be reassured that a healthy child will not become severely malnourished as the result of a few days of decreased appetite during a cold or a childhood disease.

Teething. Although tooth eruption does not cause rashes, diarrhea, or similar problems for which it is commonly blamed, teething can cause discomfort and decrease appetite in some children. Because all 20 deciduous ("baby") teeth erupt between the ages of six months and two years in the average child, the occasional child who experiences discomfort with the initial eruption of each tooth is obviously going to be uncomfortable much of the time. Fortunately, most children suffer few or no ill effects from teething.

Pica. This is most common between the ages of one and three years, when the child is mobile enough to get into things but too lacking in judgment to avoid eating them. The preschooler may happily ingest dirt, leftover pet food, household cleaning supplies, marbles, pennies, paint, and a host of other things that are nonnutritious and unsanitary at best, and potentially lethal at worst. The parents should, however, walk a thin line between the penalty for their carelessness and the danger of overconcern, because a completely safeguarded environment can be an obstacle to normal learning. Sound judgment and parental supervision without overprotection is the goal they should seek.

Food jags. Many preschool children go on jags, refusing all except one or a few foods. However, whether this is really a problem depends upon which foods are the chosen few. For example, a child may decide to eat nothing except peanut butter sandwiches, orange juice, and milk. Granted, the diet may not meet the standards of the RDA (or of the exasperated parents). Still, it isn't actually bad, at least for a few days or weeks. If a jag continues for longer than this, a physician should be consulted in order to determine whether the unorthodox food intake is a sign of some underlying emotional problem, such as a desire for more attention.

RECOMMENDED NUTRIENT AND ENERGY INTAKES FOR YOUNG CHILDREN

Are the RDA for preschool children realistic? Consider the two-year-old as an example. Although he or she weighs only about one-fifth as much as an adult, it is reasonable that the RDA is set somewhat higher than one-fifth of the RDA for adults, because the child is still growing. However, for most nutrients the RDA is from 50 to 100 percent of adult levels (Figure 18–5). Some of these allowances are easily met; for example, just one pint of milk daily virtually assures meeting the RDA for calcium, phosphorus, protein, and riboflavin.

However, other nutrients, particularly iron and vitamin A, are likely to be present in less than recommended amounts in the diets of preschool children. A diet furnishing only 1300 kilocalories will not supply 15 milligrams of iron unless highly fortified foods are used, or liver (hardly a favorite food of most children) is eaten often. As for vitamin A activity, the principal common food sources are the dark green and deep yellow fruits and vegetables–a list of which almost looks like a list of foods most frequently disliked by young children.

Surveys therefore commonly show that the diets of many preschool children do not meet the RDA, and that iron and vitamin A intakes are

FIGURE 18–5. The RDA for young children (taking the midpoint of the values for children one- to three -years-old) compared to the RDA for adult males.

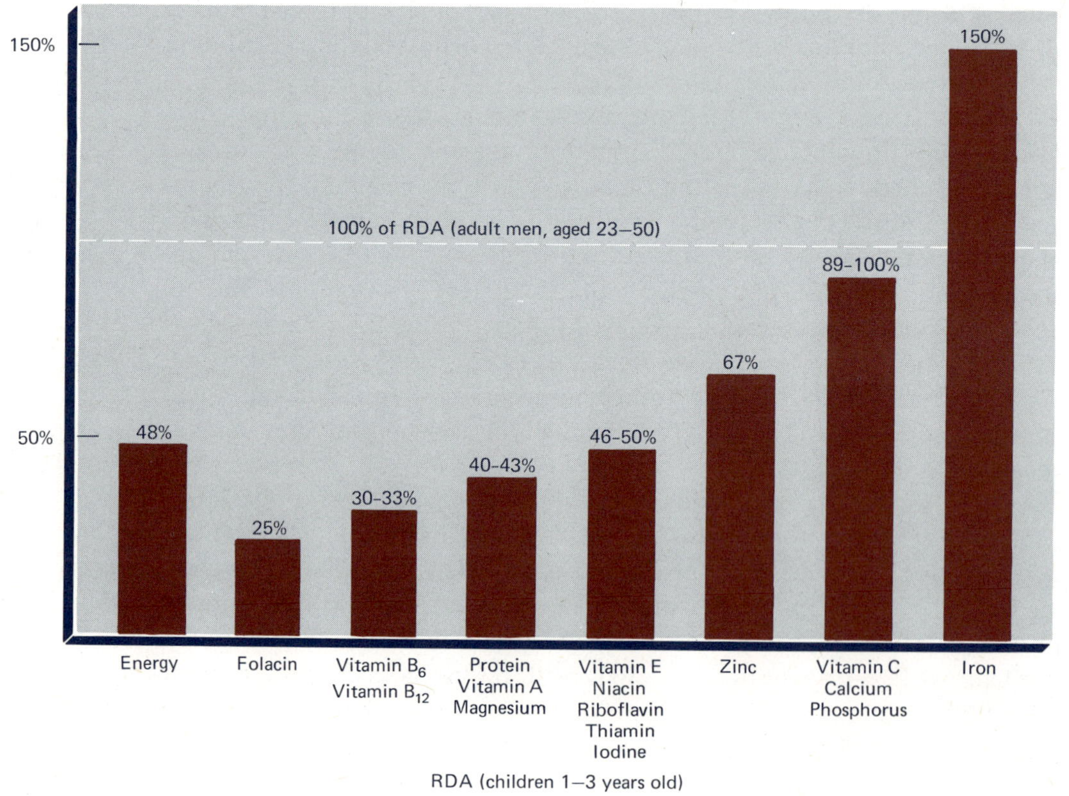

most frequently short of the allowance. This information may be published in the popular media, with frequent (and incorrect) conclusions that malnutrition appears to be very common in young children in the United States. Such statements can cause a good deal of unwarranted concern on the part of the mothers of young children, particularly in those parents who are most receptive to information on nutrition and whose children are therefore most likely to be well nourished. The result is usually an increase in the number of supplements given to children whose diets are already adequate, whereas many children whose diets actually need improvement are likely to be unaffected.

DEVICES TO HELP A CHILD TO EAT WELL

The most common problem related to feeding preschool children in the United States is not that of obtaining or preparing a suitable diet, but in getting the child to eat it. It can be exasperating to the parents to see a child push food around the plate, eat two or three bites, and then announce, "I'm full." The following suggestions may help:

Keep the portions small. A young child can feel overwhelmed by a plate overflowing with food. A general rule of thumb is to give 1 tablespoonful of meat, fruit, or vegetables for each year of age; for example, a three-year-old can be expected to eat three tablespoons of peas, rather than the $\frac{1}{2}$ cup serving suitable for older children or adults. A child with a very small appetite may respond better to even smaller servings.

Let them help themselves. Like anyone else, children like to feel that they have some freedom of choice as to what and how much is put on the plate or poured into the glass. This does not, of course, mean that the parents must remain silent in the face of an entire meal of bread and catsup (Figure 18–6).

If manners must be corrected, do it tactfully. Children are not bothered by their own dirty hands or by the fact that they chew with their mouths open, and it is puzzling to them that others find such things objectionable. Gentle reminders repeated often may be necessary.

Allow eating with fingers as much as possible. Fingers *were* made before forks, and children develop good hand-to-mouth dexterity long before they can aim a fork or spoon at their mouths accurately.

Recognize the limited chewing ability of young children. Meat, in particular, may be very difficult for a child to chew even if it is tender by an adult's standards. It may be necessary for the parents to cut meat into very small bits. Otherwise, the child confronted with large pieces of meat may simply give up on it, or may try to bolt it whole.

Respect a child's need for moderate temperatures in foods. Very hot and very cold foods can actually be painful to a child's sensitive

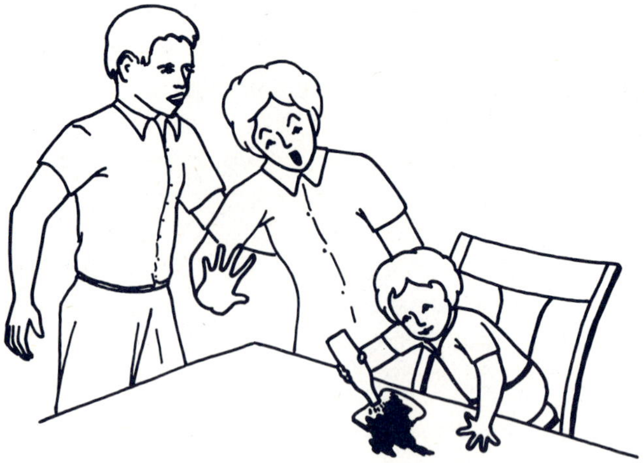

FIGURE 18–6. In feeding, as in every other aspect of raising children, permissiveness may get out of hand!

mouth, and although lukewarm mashed potatoes and runny ice cream may not appeal to adults, they are often preferred by children.

Capitalize on a child's delight in color. Bright colors, not only in the food but in dishes, glasses, and napkins, catch a child's eyes and direct attention toward the meal.

Don't force a child to eat. If a child categorically refuses to eat a disliked food, to try a new one, or to eat more of a given food, forcing him or her to eat it proves only that a parent is bigger and stronger than a child. It is very unlikely that anyone will learn to like a food as the result of force-feeding or coercion.

Allow enough time. If the rest of the family "eats and runs," the preschooler may be only halfway through when everybody else is finished. Urging him or her to "hurry up so I can get the dishes done" can create frustration in the child who cannot keep up with the rest. Conversely, the family that lingers at the dinner table should not expect a young child to remain patiently for polite conversation after eating.

Avoid moral judgments on eating. The child who is praised for being a "good eater" or criticized for being "picky" can come to believe that eating is done to please or displease others. Children, like all other people, should eat for their own benefit.

ARE THERE ANY FOODS NOT RECOMMENDED FOR CHILDREN?

As a general rule, young children's diets are built around the same Basic Four Plan suitable for all other healthy people beyond the age of infancy, with only the serving sizes being different. However, a few foods are generally not recommended for infants and young children for reasons indicated as follows:

Nuts, popcorn, and raw raisins are easy to choke on and may be inhaled into the lungs. Foods such as cooked raisins and peanut butter are of course perfectly all right.

Fruits with pits, such as prunes, olives, and cherries, should be pitted for children, and bones should be removed from fish; otherwise children often swallow or choke on the pits and bones.

Whole small vegetables and fruits, such as corn, peas, and berries, may pass unchanged through a child's digestive tract, so they should be mashed slightly for young children.

Caffeine-containing drinks, such as coffee, tea, and many soft drinks, are not recommended because of their stimulant effect. However, many parents give in occasionally and allow their children to have these desirable "grown up" drinks in small amounts, and this is probably harmless if the amounts are truly small.

Candy, cookies, jelly, jam, syrup, and other concentrated sweets should be kept at a minimum. Forbidding them entirely is impractical, for sooner or later all but the most protected child learns that these delights exist, and occasional indulgence is a legitimate pleasure of childhood. However, sweets should not be used as rewards for being "good," or withheld as punishment for being "bad." And it goes without saying that sweets should not be given just before a meal or in place of a meal.

Raw carrots are so often one of the few sources of vitamin A activity liked by young children that it seems a shame to say that they are not recommended for this age. However, the possibility of choking on the small flinty pieces is so great that many pediatricians recommend that raw carrots not be given to children less than five years old.

Other than the above, the foods suitable for the rest of the family are generally suitable for the preschool child as well. As a result, how the rest of the family eats will greatly influence the biological, social, and psychological roles food plays in the child's life—not only now, but perhaps far into the future as well.

SUGGESTED READINGS

Ascoli, W., M. A. Guzmán, N. S. Scrimshaw, and J. E. Gordon. "Nutrition and Infection Field Study in Guatemalan Villages, 1959–1964." *Archives of Environmental Health* 15 (1967):439.

Bryan, M. S. and M. E. Lowenberg. "The Father's Influence on Young Children's Food Preferences." *Journal of the American Dietetic Association* 34 (1958):30.

FAO/WHO/UNICEF Protein Advisory Group. "Lives in Peril: Protein and the Child." Food and Agriculture Organization, Rome, 1970.

Fomon, S. J. Infant Nutrition, second edition. Philadelphia: Saunders, 1975.

Foman, S. J. and T. A. Anderson, eds. *Practices of Low-Income Families in Feeding Infants and Small Children.* Rockville, Md., U.S. Department of Health, Education, and Welfare, 1972.

Gersh, M. J. *How to Raise Children at Home in Your Spare Time.* New York: Stein and Day, 1966.

Gordon, J. E. "Weanling Diarrhea; A Synergism of Nutrition and Infection." *Nutrition Reviews* 22 (1964): 161.

Puffer, R. R. and C. V. Serrano. *Patterns of Mortality in Childhood* (excerpts). Washington, D.C.: Pan American Health Organization, 1973.

Smith, C. A. Overuse of Milk in the Diets of Infants and Children. *Journal of the American Medical Association* 172 (1960):567.

Solomon, J. B. *Foetal and Neonatal Immunology.* London, North-Holland Publishing Co., 1971.

Sutherland, J. M., H. I. Glueck, and G. Gleser. "Hemorrhagic Disease of the Newborn: Breast Feeding as a Necessary Factor in the Pathogenesis." *American Journal of Diseases of Children* 113 (1967):524.

Tanner, J. M., G. R. Taylor, and the editors of Time-Life Books. *Growth.* New York: Time-Life, 1965.

Wallace, W. M. "Why and How Are Children Fat?" *Pediatrics* 34 (1964):303.

Winick, M. and A. Noble. Cellular Response in Rats During Malnutrition at Various Ages. *Journal of Nutrition* 89 (1966):300.

19

nutrition after early childhood

When children leave the apron strings to start their formal education, they enter the period that corresponds roughly to what is called the *latent* stage of human development. The term *latent* suggests that for most children this is a relatively quiescent interlude, with the frustrations and tantrums of early childhood left behind and the emotional storms of adolescence lying far in the future. Between about the ages of five and fifteen years, children live in what has been called the "golden age of immunity," during which they enjoy the years of the lowest mortality rates for almost every infectious disease. This high degree of resistance may be partially masked, however, by the increased exposure to infection from others at school.

Several influences other than the family become important in affecting the eating behavior of school-aged children. These are:

1 Teachers
2 Organized school feeding programs that may be available
3 Peer groups

THE TEACHER AS A NUTRITION EDUCATOR

To a large extent, the effectiveness of school teachers as nutrition educators depends upon the same qualities which determine success in teaching any other subject. Does the teacher select subject matter appropriate to the abilities of the various children in the class? Are facts presented through methods which arouse interest and discussion rather than being simply recited (Figure 19–1)? Elementary-school children, for example, are usually very interested in a simple animal-feeding experiment which shows that a well fed animal grows faster, acts more lively, and looks healthier than an animal fed on cookies and soda pop. What they learn by actually doing the feeding and observing the results can be much more meaningful than what they merely hear or read about food, growth, and health.

In addition to general teaching ability, the effective teacher of nutrition needs a basic knowledge of the facts of nutrition. In some states, a course in nutrition is part of the curriculum for students who plan to teach in public schools. However, many states do not have this requirement, and as a result teachers may be ill prepared to teach the subject with confidence.

A genuine interest in nutrition is another valuable attribute, for if the teacher lacks the conviction that food is important to health, no amount of factual material will convince the children. Equally important is the personal example the teacher sets. For example, an obese teacher is not likely to be effective in convincing children that good nutrition can improve people's health and appearance. The teacher who eats in the school lunchroom, or who is otherwise visible to the children while eating, should be willing to practice what is preached by eating the foods recommended to the children during class.

However, because eating is a personal matter, tact is also important in teaching nutrition. Rigid condemnation of certain foods can seem, to a child, to represent a threat. Children, particularly those from low-income families, may quite correctly see food that they enjoy (regardless of nutrient content) as one of the few good things in their lives. The teacher should therefore always be mindful of the social and psychological values of foods, as well as their biological function, that of supplying nutrients. Good eating practices can be encouraged and reinforced without placing undue emphasis on "bad" practices which may be representative of many of the students' family eating patterns.

One problem with regard to teaching nutrition is that the limited school day is already crowded with competing subjects. Thus, although nutritionists are understandably enthusiastic about having their subject occupy a prominent place in the school curriculum, teachers and administrators do not always place an equally high priority on this goal. Yet public schools have managed to fit into the curriculum other subjects, such as sex education and information on drug abuse, in response to pressure from groups that are convinced of the value of these subjects. Nutrition would certainly seem to be equally important.

If nutrition is to be taught in the public schools, which concepts are the most important ones to be communicated? There is a good deal of honest difference of opinion on this subject, and what one nutritionist considers important may be expendable in the eyes of another. To serve as a guideline for educators, the Interagency Committee on Nutrition Education has approved four basic concepts of human nutrition for use in educational programs. These concepts, shown in Table 19–1, can be taught to people of all ages, and of all social and economic levels. This is accomplished by using different terminology, facts, and examples appropriate to the abilities and interests of various groups. Admittedly these four concepts cannot encompass all that is known about the subject, but they do include a great deal of the basic information needed to make informed choices about food and nutrition.

THE SCHOOL LUNCH AND OTHER ORGANIZED PROGRAMS

The *primary* purpose of school feeding programs is of course to provide food. This is most important for those children with the poorest home diets; the *National Nutrition Survey* showed that school lunches made a significant contribution to the total energy and nutrient intake of children from low-income families. Food does not only improve nutritional

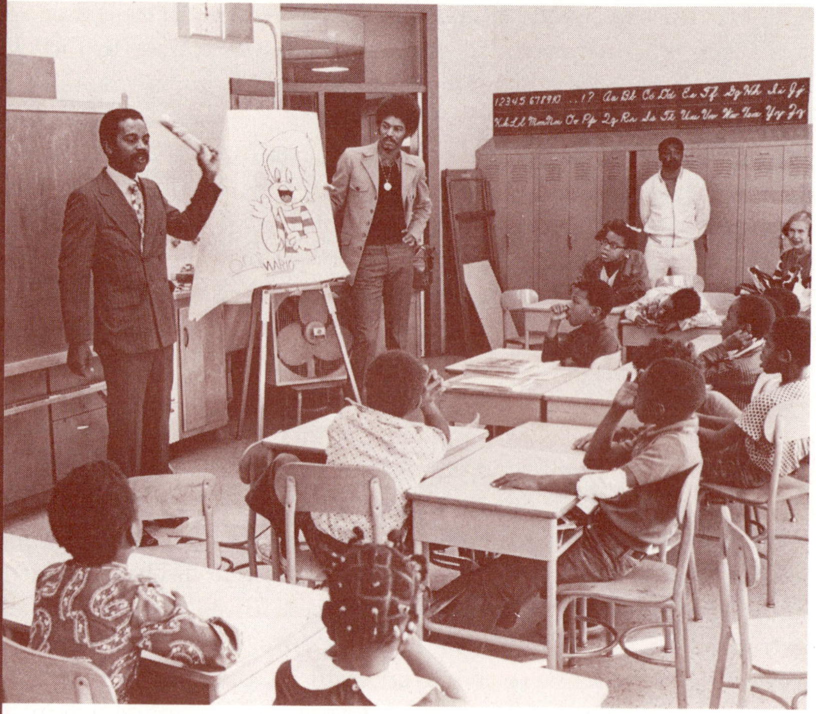

FIGURE 19–1

The writer and the artist of a comic strip talk about nutrition to fourth graders. A cartoon character whose bad eating habits get him into trouble makes nutrition a lively subject for these children. (USDA photo.)

TABLE 19–1

Basic concepts for use in nutrition education

1. Nutrition is the food you eat and how the body uses it.
This concept emphasizes that nutrition is not just food, but also the dynamic biological processes of digestion, absorption, metabolism, and excretion by which food is transformed into life. It emphasizes the broad dimensions of nutrition, and avoids the implication that nutrition is "eating what you ought to whether you like it or not."

2. Food is made up of different nutrients needed for growth and health.
This concept points out that essential nutrients can and should be obtained from a variety of ordinary foods, so that no supplements or special "health foods" are ordinarily needed. Food guides such as the Basic Four Food Group Plan are based on this idea.

3. All persons, throughout life, need the same nutrients, but in varying amounts.
This concept is a generalization of the RDA, which recommends varying amounts of nutrients for people of different age, sex, and size. It emphasizes that no nutrient need is peculiar to one particular group of people, and that products sold on the basis of the "special needs" of any group, such as the elderly, are therefore unnecessary.

4. The way food is handled influences its nutrient content, safety, appearance, and taste.
This concept emphasizes the importance of retaining and preserving the characteristics of foods, while recognizing the necessity of sometimes compromising one value in favor of another. Thus, for example, people can accept the fact that pasteurization of milk results in an insignificant loss of ascrobic acid, offset by a great gain in protection against infectious disease.

status; it allays hunger as well. This is important because, although the *structure* of the brain is essentially completed long before school age, the *functioning* continues to be influenced by the environment. An otherwise well nourished but hungry child may be unable to concentrate on school work; perhaps this is related to a low blood glucose concentration caused by lack of recent food intake, or perhaps it is the result of the sheer physical discomfort of hunger, which children feel keenly. At any rate, food may allow a child to settle down and learn, undistracted by hunger.

It should be recognized, however, that the most well-balanced and most abundant school lunch cannot entirely compensate for a very poor diet at home. Lunch is, after all, intended to be only one-third of the day's meals. Considering vacations and holidays when children are not in school, this amounts to only about one-fourth of the meals during an average school week, and one-sixth of the total meals on a year-round basis. Therefore, the school lunch in itself could not eradicate hunger and malnutrition in children, even if every child could participate in the program.

Aside from providing food, a second value of the school lunch is to serve as an integral part of the total education program of the school. Children can be introduced to new foods and can see examples of balanced meals, which may not be available in the home (Figure 19–2).

Laws first affect the food offered when children begin to participate in a school feeding program. The National School Lunch Act places responsibility for setting the nutrient requirements for school lunches with the United States Department of Agriculture, and the meals served must follow the general pattern specified by federal and state regulations. The *Type A lunch,* as it is called, is based on nutritional needs, not on the type of financing involved. The general menu is shown in Table 19–2.

The amounts served are based on the nutritional needs of ten- to twelve-year-old children, although portions may be adjusted upward or downward for younger or older children. To qualify for federal funds, the Type A program *must* operate on a nonprofit basis, and meals *must* be available free or at reduced prices to children from low-income families.

Nutritionists overwhelmingly approve of the basic meal pattern, which provides approximately one-third of the RDA for nutrients for ten- to twelve-year-olds. A greater difference of opinion revolves around the specific foods offered in the school lunch. Some nutritionists adamantly insist that school children should learn flexible food habits, and should overcome their dislikes of certain nutritious foods. However, whether a child learns new food habits at school depends upon many factors. The home, not the school, is the most powerful educational institution, and most children enter school with well-established food

FIGURE 19–2
The school lunch program can be a valuable educational experience as well as a feeding project.

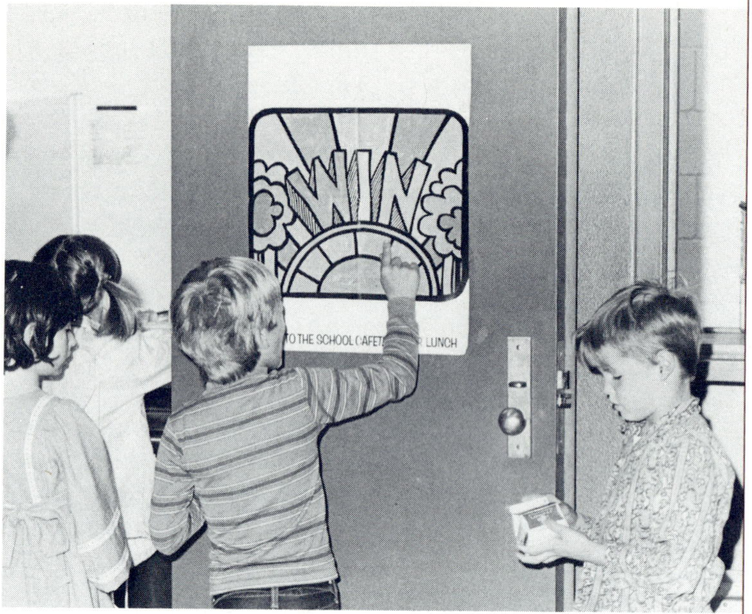

TABLE 19–2
Basic pattern of the Type A school lunch

1. One slice (1 ounce) bread: whole grain or enriched
*2. Two ounces of cooked meat, cheese, fish, or poultry, or
   1 egg, or
   $\frac{1}{2}$ cup cooked dry beans or peas, or
   $\frac{1}{4}$ cup peanut butter, or
   equivalent combination of the above
3. One-half pint milk: whole, 2 percent, skim, chocolate, or buttermilk
4. Three-fourths cup (total) of two or more vegetables or fruits
5. One teaspoon butter or vitamin A-fortified margarine

* **Note:** The alternates within the meat group are not all nutritionally equivalent; 1 egg and $\frac{1}{2}$ cup of cooked dry legumes are each equivalent to 1 ounce, not 2 ounces, of cooked meat. However, the amounts listed above are those specified by federal law at present.

habits and definite likes and dislikes. How these are handled varies from school to school. In some school lunch programs, children are required to eat everything offered, regardless of whether they like it. In other schools, children are urged to try at least one bite of every food. In others, the children are given only those foods that most of them like anyway; hamburgers, hot dogs, pizza, and sloppy joes may be served day after day. Opponents of such a program point out that the children are not learning to expand their food habits. But admittedly, no food is nutritious unless it is eaten, and a child will therefore benefit from a well-balanced school lunch only if it is acceptable to that child.

THE PEER GROUP (THE OTHER KIDS)

Upon starting school, a child is suddenly exposed to a large number of other children, all of whom have their own ideas and habits. Parents of kindergarten children are sometimes horrified to hear certain words from the lips of their presumably innocent children. Nevertheless, for good or for ill, the beginning of the school years marks the start of an ever increasing influence of what "the other kids" say and do. This influence, detectable even in the early elementary grades, rises most rapidly at about the beginning of adolescence, until for many teen-agers the peer group is the all-important influence on thought and behavior.

Just as language, clothing style, hair length, bedtime, and study habits are influenced by the peer group, so are food habits. A child who hears friends talking about "yukky" green vegetables may decide that broccoli is indeed "yukky," even though the child may have previously liked it. Fortunately, for young children most meals are still largely family affairs and the rejection may therefore be only verbal rather than a real influence on behavior. However, as children get older, and especially as they eat away from home with their friends more frequently, it becomes more and more likely that peer group pressure will determine actual choices. The very existence of choices may be determined by where they choose to eat. And the choices made—milk or cola, for example—may be determined by what the others choose rather than by nutritional value, or even by the preferences of the child. Certainly nutrient content often ceases to be a significant influence on food habits after food becomes an important part of a young person's social life.

GROWTH AND APPETITE IN ELEMENTARY-SCHOOL CHILDREN

Physical growth during the elementary-school years is fairly slow and steady, with occasional spurts of growth. Although biological sex differences in growth and behavior are not marked enough to justify setting separate allowances for boys and girls below age eleven, social factors can greatly influence the energy needs. A 10-year-old boy who plays baseball and climbs trees is proclaimed to be a "real boy"; a girl who does the same things at this age may often hear the exasperated question, "Are you going to be a tomboy all your life?"

In general, elementary-school children have good appetites, and seldom does a parent complain that the child eats too little at this age. In fact, parents may feel that they spent most of their time urging a child to eat more during the five years or so after infancy, only to spend the next five years or so urging the child to eat less. However, *what* the child eats may also become an issue as the child asserts greater independence: "No, you can't have a can of pop instead of milk with your dinner." "Get out of those cookies; you know what the dentist said." "If you're too hungry to wait for lunch, have a slice of bread—not candy." The child's usual response to this is, "I'm not *that* hungry."

After age seven, children can be expected to eat the adult-size servings of food recommended in the Basic Four Plan. This is worth mentioning because mothers sometimes continue to serve very small portions of foods (especially vegetables, which are generally not the child's favorites) long after this is appropriate. Perhaps out of habit, the mother may feel that the child's capacity is still very limited. In this case, it might be well to notice how the capacity usually increases when dessert is served.

The most common exception to the rule of good appetite is a lack of interest in breakfast. Sometimes this is related to a situation in the home. If bedtime rules are not enforced, the child may oversleep and be too tired and rushed to think about food in the morning. Late evening snacking, or a late dinner hour, may not allow time for a child to become hungry by morning. The mother, perhaps occupied with the care of a younger child or some other responsibility, may mistakenly assume that school-aged children are old enough to see to their own needs at breakfast time. Although many people assume that children often miss breakfast because of a working mother who leaves for work before her children are fed, studies show that whether or not the mother is employed outside of the home has little effect on whether children eat breakfast before school.

Feelings toward school can also determine whether a child is willing, or even able, to eat breakfast. In extreme cases, an actual school phobia can develop; the child may be afraid of the teacher, or unable to feel at ease among other children, or fearful of venturing away from the security of home and mother. Emotional support, not forced breakfast-feeding, is needed by these children. However, the problem still remains: how can children function effectively in school if they eat nothing until lunchtime? The answer is that they probably cannot. Sometimes it helps to give the child a sandwich to eat in school during the morning (assuming, of course, that the teacher is informed of the reason for this). Above all, the causes for the child's inability to eat breakfast should be determined so that the underlying problems can be corrected.

Orthodontics, or tooth-straightening, is a common procedure which interferes with the intake of certain foods. Happily, however, this can actually improve the diets of some children, because foods which should be avoided by a child with braces include chewy and hard candies. The child is warned about breaking a brace by biting into a hard food such as a raw carrot or an apple, but this is no problem if the foods are cut into pieces.

The "fat spurt"

In many children between the ages of 8 and 10 years, body weight increases more rapidly than height does, so that the proportion of body fat increases. This phenomenon, known as the "fat spurt" and commonly called "puppy fat" or "baby fat," is often laughed off by parents, but may be a source of great distress to the child. It may be helpful to keep the following points in mind:

The fat spurt is normal, and is probably a storing of excess energy to serve as a buffer during the rapid growth of adolescence which is soon to follow. Both boys and girls experience the fat spurt, although it may be more marked as well as more psychologically distressing in girls.

Although "baby fat" occasionally continues to the point of obesity, this is not the usual course. Therefore, attempts to reduce a child's weight should be made only if a physician agrees that the weight is excessive enough to constitute a real physical, emotional, or social problem for the child. Certainly a child of any age can be offered low-calorie alternatives, such as skim milk in place of whole milk and fruit instead of sweets for dessert (Figure 19–3). However, *vigorous* attempts to reduce the weight of a child too often fail. The result is a child who, because of the failure, feels even less adequate than before, and who in most cases is as fat as ever. For these reasons, the recommended course of action is to try to prevent more weight gain while allowing the child to "grow into" the height more appropriate to the weight.

Diet surveys in school children

School-aged children are generally a pleasure to have as subjects in a diet survey. They are usually cooperative, honest about the information they give, and curious about the study. And, of course, they are easily accessible, because practically all children of school age attend school in developed countries.

Repeated diet surveys show that nutrient intakes of most children of elementary-school age are above recommended allowances, with two common exceptions. These are vitamin A and ascorbic acid, which indicates that vegetables and fruits could be emphasized more than they are in the diets of this age group.

As children approach adolescence, however, the quality of the diet usually declines from its previously high value. Especially among the girls, this is largely related to the beginning of conscious attempts to lose weight, beginning as early as age ten in some areas. Fortunately, few children of this age can restrict their food intake rigidly for long periods of time, and "dieting" therefore tends to be a short-lived activity which seldom creates real nutritional problems before adolescence.

FIGURE 19–3
Children can learn to enjoy nutritious sweets such as fruits in place of at least some of the low-nutrient sugary foods they so often eat.

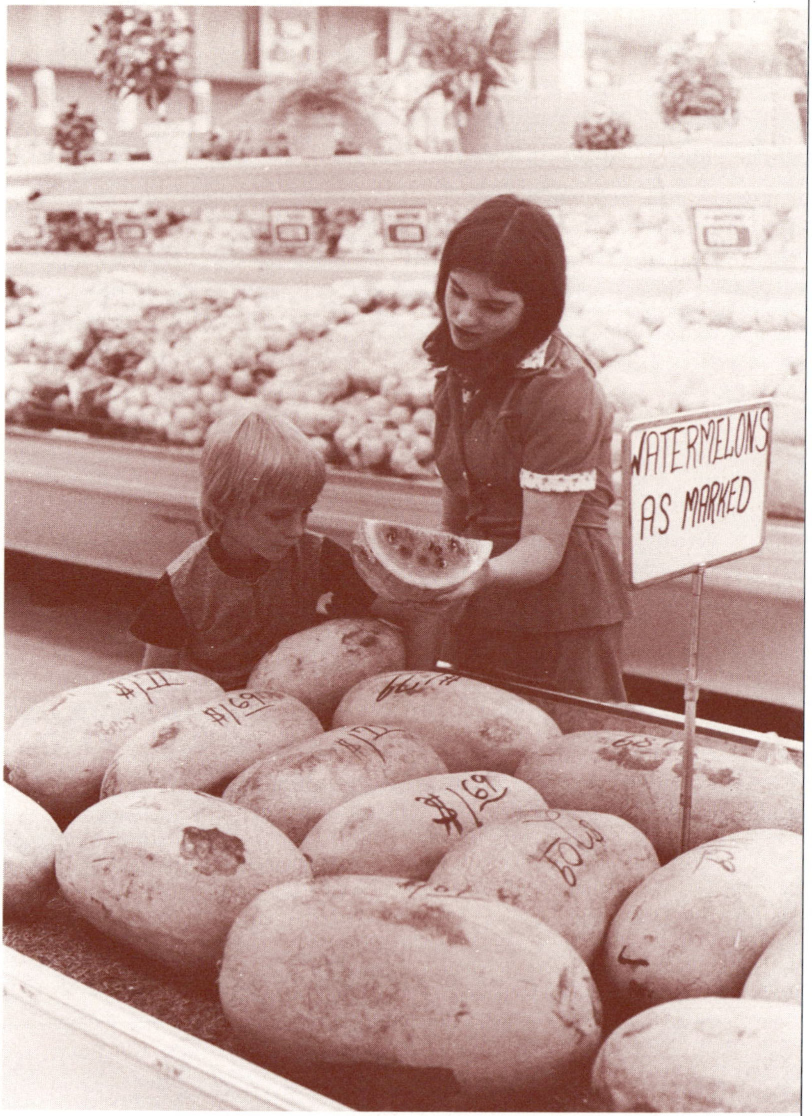

PUBERTY AND ADOLESCENCE

Puberty and *adolescence* should not be used as synonyms, as they so often are. Puberty is the stage of maturation at which reproductive capacity is attained. In girls, the usual criterion of puberty is the *menarche,* or onset of the menses. In boys, there is no adequate single criterion; sperm cell production, the growth of body hair, and the urinary excretion of male sex hormones have all been used. Certainly chronological age is completely useless as a point of reference after childhood, for one fourteen-year-old may be a biologically immature child, and another may already be a parent.

Severe undernutrition can delay the onset of puberty, but many factors other than nutrition can also affect this; genetic variation, for example, appears to be important. There is also a marked sex difference; females begin to mature earlier and complete their growth and maturation sooner than males. Contrary to popular opinion, climate is *not* an important factor. Although puberty generally occurs earlier in children living in temperate zones than in those in the tropics, this difference appears to be the result of the better total environment in developed countries compared to developing countries, most of which are tropical or subtropical.

The tendency of children to grow faster and to mature earlier today than in the past, known as the "secular trend in growth and development," is not completely understood. Improved nutrition and control of infectious diseases which previously impaired growth and development are believed to be important. However, another factor may be the greater likelihood that people of the present time will marry someone distantly related, rather than someone in the same small area as in previous eras. This greater mixing of genetic stocks may produce larger and faster-growing children, a phenomenon similar to the *hybrid vigor* seen when distantly related plants or animals are bred. Other hypotheses have little support; for example, it is probably safe to discount the suggestion that children mature earlier today because of excessive exposure to the sexually stimulating ideas of our permissive modern society.

In girls, moderate overweight is associated with earlier than average puberty. However, this does not necessarily mean that excess energy intake *causes* earlier maturity; so many factors are involved in both overweight and the age of puberty that the only definite statement that can be made is that the two are often correlated.

Adolescence, in contrast to puberty, is not a single age or stage but a range of years during which an individual develops from a child to an adult. In addition to the enormous amount of physical growth and development that occurs during these years, adolescents experience psychological and social changes without which they would never reach the real end-point of adolescence: the ability to leave the families in which they grew up and to function as adult members of their society.

The *adolescent growth spurt,* which refers primarily to the physical growth that occurs during adolescence, has the following characteristics:

1. **It is rapid.** Despite the advertisements that refer to the "Wonder Years Age One Through Twelve," the real "wonder years" of growth are during infancy and during adolescence (Figure 19–4).

2. **It is very different in boys than in girls.** Girls begin their adolescent growth spurt so much earlier than boys that the average girl is taller and heavier than the average boy between the ages of 11 and 13 years and heavier, although not taller, between the ages of 13 and 14 years—the only times during the human life cycle that females on the average are larger than males. The peak of most rapid growth also

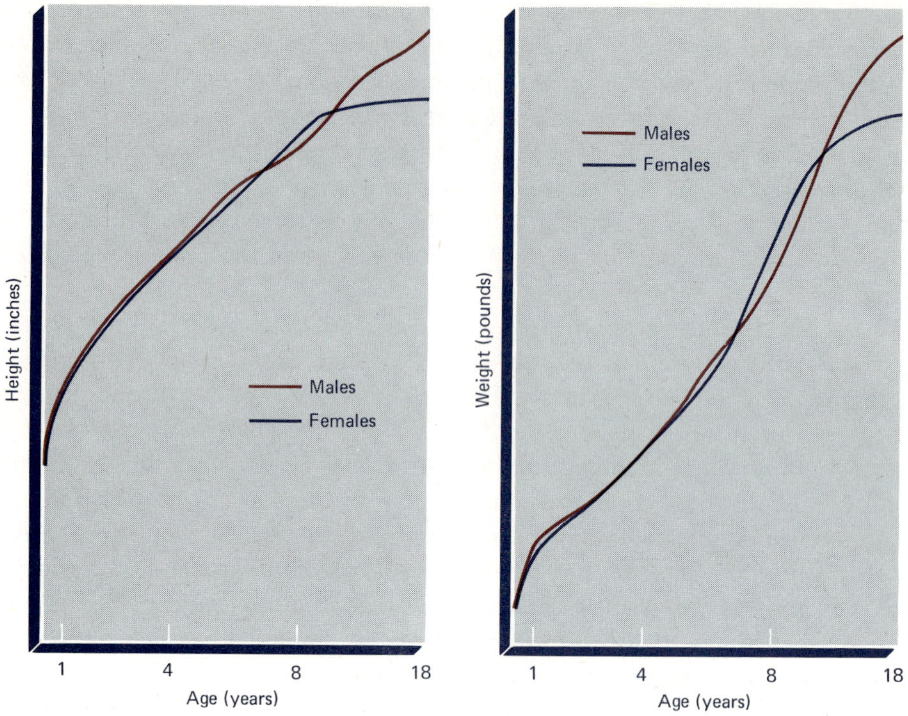

FIGURE 19–4. The real "wonder years" of growth: infancy and adolescence. These curves, which represent the growth of boys and girls at the 50th percentile, could be very different for normal individuals above or below the 50th percentile.

occurs earlier in girls; growth is most rapid at age twelve to thirteen in girls, but at age thirteen to fourteen in boys. However, when the boy's growth spurt does occur, it is much more intense than that of the girls; the increase in lean body mass occurring during the adolescent growth is actually twice as great in boys as in girls.

3. **It is relatively brief in a given individual.** The RDA is set high all through adolescence in order to cover the needs of early and late maturers as well as the average adolescent. However, the peak of growth, during which the young person seems to "shoot up" overnight, lasts for only a fraction of the total years of adolescence.

4. **It is final.** Physical growth ends at maturity, and this can be disturbing to adolescents, who must come to grips with the realities of their own growth and development. The short boy realizes that his earlier dreams of growing tall will never be fulfilled; the stocky girl must accept the fact that she is not destined to become willowy and long-legged.

5. **It is related to changes in sex hormones.** Increased *growth* in both sexes is caused by increased secretion of *androgens,* by the testes and the adrenal cortex in males and by the adrenal cortex alone in

females. Sexual *development*, however, depends upon male sex hormones in boys and female sex hormones in girls. Many of the sex differences in various body parts are of course established long before adolescence; the most obvious example is in the genitals, which develop differently in males and in females early in fetal life. Other less well-known examples could be given; for example, the length of the index finger relative to the length of the ring finger is apt to be greater in females than in males. Many differences, however, arise as the direct result of changes in the secretion of sex hormones during adolescence. Males develop larger muscles, females more fat; the shoulders broaden in the male, the pelvis widens in the female; the concentration of hemoglobin in the blood increases so much more in males than in females that separate standards must be used for blood tests thereafter. These changes result from male sex hormones in boys and from female sex hormones in girls, in contrast to the height increase during adolescence, which is caused primarily by male sex hormones in both sexes.

The principal effects of hormone changes on nutrient requirements of adolescents are the following:

Both boys and girls need more energy as well as more essential nutrients to support physical growth. The growth rate and hence the needs of boys are greater than those of girls, a difference which is reflected in the RDA (Figure 19–5).

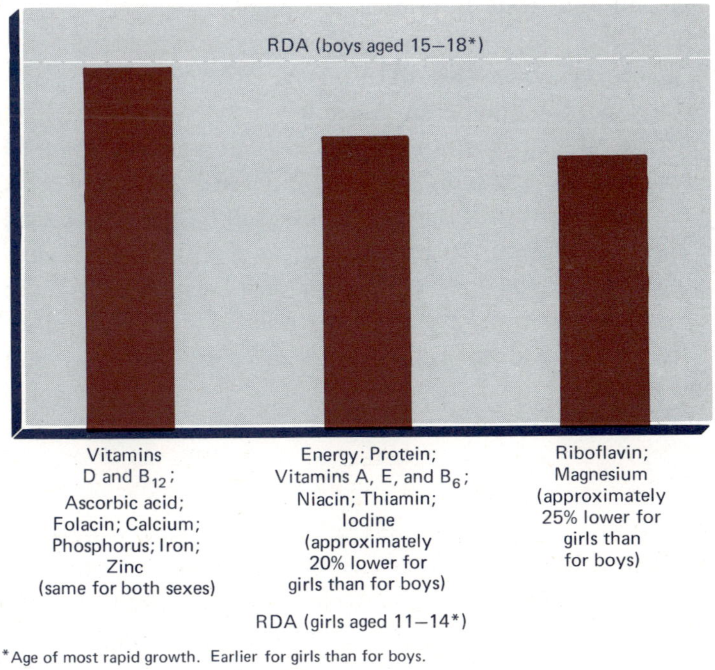

FIGURE 19–5. The RDA for adolescents reflect the greater food needs of boys compared to girls.

FIGURE 19–6
Freedom of choice, as in this cafeteria-style school lunch, can make the program acceptable to adolescents. (USDA photo.)

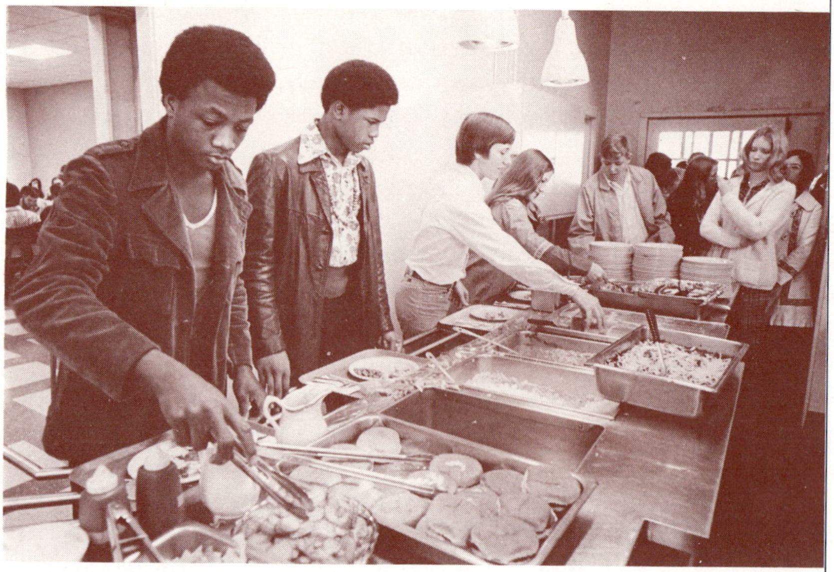

A specific increased iron requirement is brought about by the onset of the menses, resulting from hormone changes which cause the female reproductive system to mature. However, the greater growth rate and hemoglobin synthesis in adolescent boys compared to girls offsets the greater need of girls for iron to replace that lost in the menses. Hence the RDA for iron is set at 18 milligrams for both sexes between the ages of eleven and eighteen years.

The effects of sex hormones on physical activity, and hence on energy needs, are not known. Teen-age boys are generally more active than girls, a behavioral difference which some believe is caused by the higher levels of androgens in males. However, others believe that this difference has nothing to do with biology, but is, instead, a culmination of years of social conditioning, during which children are led to believe that boys are "naturally" active and aggressive and girls are "naturally" passive and gentle.

DIETS OF ADOLESCENTS

According to almost all diet studies of adolescents, the nutrients most often below the RDA are iron (in girls' diets), and calcium, vitamin A, and ascorbic acid (in both boys' and girls' diets). The diets of girls are almost always poorer (by the standards of the RDA) than those of boys.

Skipping breakfast is an established habit for many adolescent girls, for reasons the same as those of younger children, plus two more: determined attempts to reduce weight, and the desire to spend morning time on sleeping, grooming, and makeup rather than on eating.

Snacking on nonnutritious foods is very common; in some adolescents, more than half of the day's intake may consist of high-energy, low-nutrient foods such as soft drinks, potato chips, and candy bars. Eating may be very irregular, hurried, away from the family table, and governed by the timing of social events, club meetings, and similar activities—almost everything but nutritional needs.

Adolescents often complain about the school lunch program, and some of their discontent is justified; the lunchroom may be crowded and noisy, the lunch period too short, and the food not selected or prepared to their liking. However, at least some of the complaints may represent nothing more than the objections voiced to any other type of institutional feeding program: griping about food is a socially acceptable way of relieving tensions. A school lunch program that offers a choice of well-liked, nutritious foods can be very well accepted by adolescents (Figure 19–6).

For girls, two particular foods—milk and eggs—become much less acceptable than they previously were. It has been suggested that this is caused by emotional factors: eggs represent fertility, milk represents maternity, and so forth. Perhaps so. Then again, perhaps it is simply because eggs are generally served at breakfast (which girls often skip) and milk is incorrectly considered fattening as well as "childish." Because of an unrealistic standard of slenderness held by many teen-age girls, many girls who are not actually overweight nevertheless believe that they need to lose weight.

Do these findings indicate that malnutrition is rife among adolescents? Some nutritionists believe so. However, against this opinion is the fact that the great majority of teen-agers are healthy, have a degree of vitality envied by their elders, and show few signs of malnutrition other than overweight or underweight. It seems more fruitful to determine which nutritional problems actually exist rather than to assume that malnutrition is the inevitable result of snacking, hurried eating, bizarre meals at midnight, and the like.

NUTRITION-RELATED PROBLEMS OF ADOLESCENTS

Because the diets of teen-agers are so often assumed inadequate, a faulty diet is sometimes blamed for many or even most of the ills of adolescence.

The frequent colds and other infections, some believe, may be the result of certain vitamin deficiencies. However, it must be recognized that adolescents are exposed to infections much more than younger children because of their greater independence, and that nonnutritional factors, such as adequate rest, are also important in resistance to infections.

Acne, or common pimples, caused by male sex hormones acting

on sebaceous glands in the skin, is a very distressing problem to a large number of adolescents. Nutrition comes into the picture because restriction of certain foods is often part of the treatment—although dermatologists do not at all agree on the value of these restrictions. Most believe that rest, cleanliness, and emotions are far more important than diet. Particular foods, and perhaps poor diet in general, may aggravate the condition in certain individuals; however, people vary so much in this regard that a physician's advice is always indicated.

Tooth decay, very common in adolescents, is at least somewhat related to diet, because frequent snacking on high-carbohydrate foods can increase the rate of decay. This is a local effect, in which sugars support abundant growth of microorganisms which produce tooth-eroding acids in the mouth. However, most of the dietary factors that affect dental health, such as the intake of calcium and fluoride, operate almost entirely during the time when the teeth are developing, long before adolescence. Therefore, although it is certainly desirable for teen-agers to get adequate amounts of all essential nutrients, these cannot increase resistance to dental decay after the teeth have already formed.

Although some have suggested that the high accident rate of teen-age boys may be the result of night blindness caused by vitamin A deficiency, there is really little evidence for this. A combination of youthful exuberance and inexperience would seem to be at least an equally likely explanation.

Pregnancy is far more likely to be difficult in teen-age girls than in adult women, especially if the girl is less than seventeen years old. However, many factors other than nutrition affect the outcome of pregnancy. The reproductive system of a young girl is not fully mature; also, a disproportionate number of pregnancies in very young girls occur under generally unfavorable circumstances: low socioeconomic status, failure or inability to obtain adequate medical care, unmarried status, psychological problems, and perhaps rejection by the family, the school, and society in general. Therefore, although pregnant teen-agers certainly need nutritional guidance, this is not their only, and perhaps not even their major, need.

The problem of nutrition during pregnancy in teen-agers is often assumed to be acute because the average age of first-time mothers in the United States is less than twenty. However, this is somewhat misleading, because the great majority of these young mothers are seventeen, eighteen, or nineteen years old—not the rapidly growing younger girl who is far more likely to have a difficult pregnancy.

Of the health problems common during adolescence, three are definitely related to nutrition in that dietary changes can correct the condition. These are obesity, underweight, and iron deficiency anemia.

Obesity in adolescents

Although obesity is more common in girls than in boys, a considerable number of teen-agers of both sexes are afflicted. Concern about obesity in adolescents is partly based on its effects on physical health; obesity is associated with decreased life expectancy and with increased probability of many causes of death. There are two notable exceptions: tuberculosis and suicide are actually *less* common in obese people than in those of normal weight. No explanation is yet available to account for these statistics.

To the obese adolescent, physical damage that may occur years hence is not of primary importance; instead, the social and psychological aspects are most distressing. A small proportion of obese teen-agers manage to compensate for their appearance through their accomplishments or their personalities, but a much larger number find themselves socially disadvantaged at an age when acceptance is all-important.

Psychological tests, such as word-association tests and sentence-completion tests, show that obese adolescent girls respond differently from girls of normal weight. Obsessive concern about weight is indicated by their tendency to respond to test items with answers related to topics such as food, calories, fat, and overweight. For example, the word *outdoors* might suggest only picnics and barbeques to an obese girl, whereas to a nonobese girl, the word might suggest sports or sunbathing. Obese girls therefore appear to be extremely preoccupied with their body image, even though they may pretend to be unconcerned about it.

Another outstanding characteristic of obese girls is passivity. For example, the sentence, "When school gets too hard for me, ———" may be completed with the words "I cry" or "I feel bad," rather than with active responses such as "I try harder" or "I find someone to study with." Life seems, then, to be something that *happens* to many obese girls, rather than something they actively live.

Obesity should not, however, be assumed to *cause* emotional problems in adolescents. It is equally possible that the emotional problems preceded the obesity and, in fact, contributed to obesity, rather than the other way around (Figure 19–7).

As with people of any age, an important part of treating adolescent obesity is determining the causes of the positive energy balance which led to the condition. Does the girl eat voraciously? If so, is this caused by temporary emotional tensions, or is it a continuation of long-standing habits? Is she aware of the energy value of her own diet? Teen-agers frequently know very little about calories, although they may talk about them a great deal; a girl may shun a slice of bread because it is "fattening," but eat a second helping of meat, which furnishes far more energy than the bread. Education regarding the energy values of common food portions is obviously imperative in such cases.

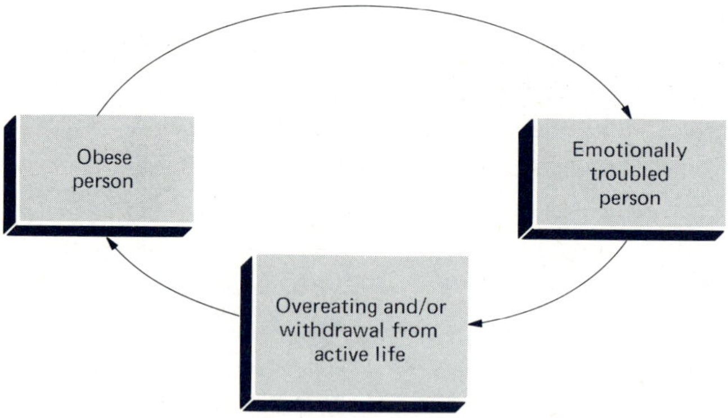

FIGURE 19–7. Which comes first: obesity or the commonly associated emotional problems?

In a surprising number of obese adolescent girls, however, the intake is no greater than that of normal girls, and positive energy balance is the result of abnormally low energy output rather than unusually high intake. In a minority, the low output is related to hypothyroidism, a not uncommon condition in adolescent girls; treatment with thyroid hormone is successful for these. In the majority, however, low energy output is caused by lack of physical activity. Inactivity and obesity of course reinforce each other: the obese girl, embarrassed by her appearance, often shrinks from participation in physical exercise. This in turn makes positive energy balance even more likely, and leads to even greater obesity. Thus, whether inactivity was the original cause or is the result of overweight, the two act together, each contributing to the other.

Underweight in adolescents

In boys, temporary underweight can result despite an enormous food intake if the demands for growth and the level of physical activity are simultaneously high. Urging a boy to force himself to eat more is not likely to help, and of course one would not want to slow down the boy's growth, even if this were possible. The most effective approach is to attempt to persuade the boy to cut down on at least some of his activities. This is not easy, because social pressures and masculine pride may demand that boys participate in sports, work at part-time jobs, and stay out as late as possible almost every night. Parents can at least take comfort in the fact that moderate underweight during adolescence is usually self-limited, often ending when the adolescent growth spurt ends. In fact, the adult male who continues to eat like a teen-ager will almost certainly change from a thin adolescent to an overweight man.

In adolescent girls, underweight is not commonly related to excessive physical activity or extremely rapid growth. Far more often, it is the result of strict dieting, motivated by the girl's conscious desire for extreme slenderness. Girls often try to emulate models and popular entertainers, who may be thin to the point of emaciation. In some girls, deliberate extreme weight loss definitely appears to be related to emotional problems: fear of "getting fat like my mother," anxiety about the "sexiness" associated with fat deposition on the breasts and hips, or a desire to relieve deep-seated guilt feelings through self-denial of the pleasure of eating. Also, some girls are unaware that fat deposition on the breasts, hips, thighs, and abdomen is normal and healthy in adolescent females. Sex education, as well as nutrition education, is needed by these young women.

Anorexia nervosa, a psychoneurosis occurring mostly in young females, is the extreme example of aversion to food and consequent underweight (Figure 19–8). Fortunately rare, this affliction can lead to severe malnutrition unless the girl is given prompt medical treatment. Of primary importance is hospitalization so that the patient can be fed, by tube if necessary; in addition, psychotherapy to uncover the reasons for the compulsive refusal of food may be necessary to prevent the patient from again starving herself as soon as she leaves the hospital.

A teen-aged girl who announces that she is "going on a diet to lose a few pounds" should be watched rather closely. Unless she knows more about nutrition than most girls do, she may omit many essential nutrients along with the energy. If she continues dieting beyond the point of attaining normal weight, she can become unattractively and unhealthily thin rather than normally slender. And in extreme cases, self-starvation may continue to a dangerous, and occasionally fatal, conclusion.

Iron deficiency anemia

Although failure to meet the RDA for iron is much more common in adolescent girls than is actual iron deficiency anemia, anemia is nevertheless more common in American girls than deficiency of any other specific nutrient. The advertising for iron-containing supplements stresses the fact that the need for iron increases in females after puberty. Nutritionists agree that it would be far better for people, including adolescent and adult females, to obtain the iron they need through food rather than from pills. Adolescent girls should be given the information they need on the iron content of foods. For those who then choose not to eat a diet which meets their need for iron, a supplement containing perhaps 50 to 100 percent of the RDA for iron would seem to be a reasonable alternative.

Nutrition and the teen-age athlete

Adolescent boys sometimes go on unusual diets, but for entirely different reasons than those of girls. The most peculiar diets common to teen-age boys are those that are supposed to increase their muscle development and improve their performance in sports.

FIGURE 19–8

Anorexia nervosa: a pathetic victim of self-imposed starvation in the midst of plenty. (Photo by Dr. W. Stewart Agras, courtesy of Newsweek.)

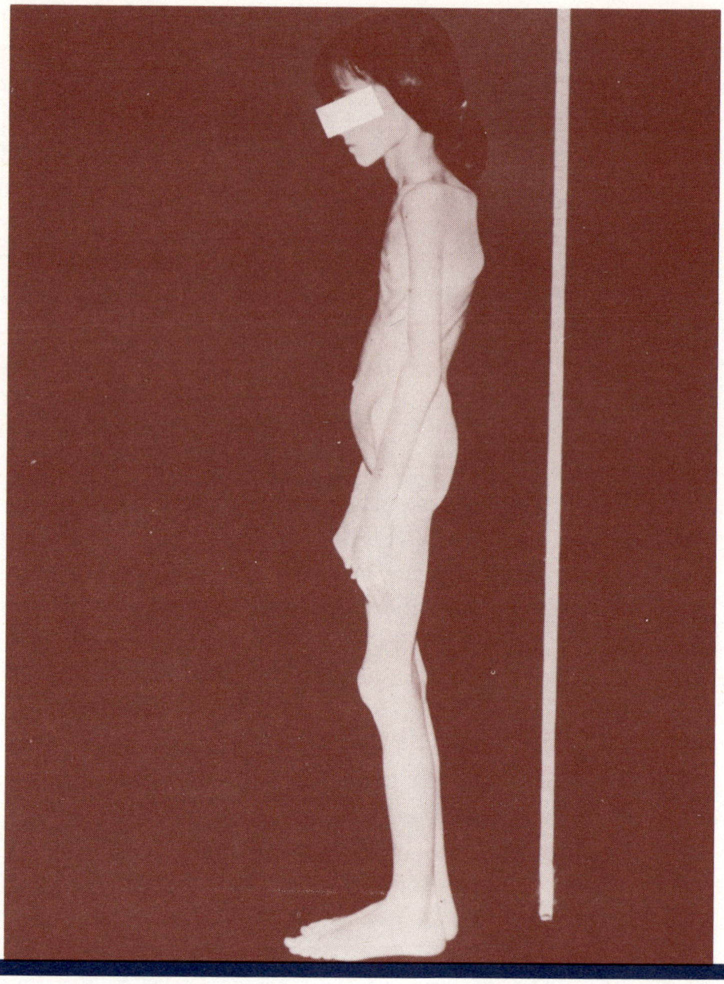

Although athletic coaches and physical education teachers should be sources of reliable nutrition information, not all of them are knowledgeable about the subject. Physical activity actually increases dietary needs in only three respects: increased energy is needed to support the work of muscle contraction, and additional water and salt are necessary if large amounts of these are lost through sweating. Yet coaches often recommend practices that are of no value, and even potentially harmful. Athletes may be told that they must have an enormous protein intake "to replace the protein torn down in muscles during exercise." Milk is sometimes banned because it is supposed to cause "cottonmouth," a dry feeling in the mouth. Some coaches tell their young charges to avoid spinach because the oxalic acid in it "robs the body of calcium." Special "sports drinks," which are actually only an expensive form of water, sugar, and salts, may be recommended. Wrestlers are commonly subjected to excessively strict weight-reduction programs in order to compete in a given weight class. Supplements containing protein, vitamins, and minerals are all too often recommended in enormous amounts. All of these practices are deplorable, in light of the potential help that coaches and physical education teachers can give to adolescents.

Helping adolescents improve their diets

Anyone interested in improving a teen-ager's diet might start by trying to answer the following questions.

1 *Do you honestly see nutrition as an issue, or merely an excuse for an intergeneration argument?* If parents resent the adolescent's obvious preference for eating with friends rather than with the family, they should state this frankly—not hide behind the "we're-only-thinking-of-your-health" routine.

2 *Are you sure that the teen-ager's diet really needs improvement?* Snacking per se is not bad; missing a meal *occasionally* does not necessarily lead to nutritional disaster; and the nutrients in a cold left-over cheeseburger that an adolescent may enjoy are no less valuable just because an adult finds cold cheeseburgers nauseating.

3 *Have you set good examples?* Actions speak louder than words, and adults who go on crash diets, drink to excess, and have doughnuts and coffee for breakfast can hardly expect their advice on nutrition to be taken seriously.

4 *Can you express your honest opinions about nutrition without talking down to the teen-ager?* Adolescents are more willing to accept guidance on any subject if they feel they are being treated as responsible young adults, not as children whose opinions and ideas are beneath consideration.

5 *Are your claims for nutrition realistic?* Adolescents are generally far too sophisticated to believe that good nutrition alone will bring them glossy hair, clear skin, and popularity. In fact, some of the most attractive and popular boys and girls have diets that some nutritionists might call atrocious—and adolescents know it.

6 *Would you really want a teen-ager to be completely lacking in rebellion, with regard to diet or any other subject?* A certain amount of resistance to adult values is normal and desirable; without it, adolescents might never achieve the ultimate goal of responsible independence.

7 *Do you remember the many concerns of adolescence—grades, sex, clothes, being accepted, growing up—that made nutrition seem a rather minor problem by comparison when you were that age?* Many adults tend to forget that teen-agers have many problems which, although perhaps trivial by adult standards, are of paramount importance during the final years preceding adulthood. You can most profitably discuss health as a value and nutrition as one factor in health if you consider the adolescent's many other values as well.

ADULTHOOD AND AGING: WHEN DO THEY BEGIN?

Adulthood is commonly viewed as a somewhat uniform plateau, enviably free from both the earlier stresses of growth and the later problems of old age. In reality, however, young and middle-aged adults have their share of necessary adjustments.

In their twenties, young people are expected to "settle down," choose a career, have children, and in general make most of the major decisions that will largely determine the rest of their lives.

In their thirties, people are subjected to cultural forces which spur men on to greater economic success and encourage most women to concentrate largely on the continued rearing of children—whether or not the individual really enjoys these roles.

In the forties and fifties, numerous potentially stressful changes occur for both men and women. At about the time grown children leave home, grandparents reach the age at which they may need financial and personal assistance. The man may have to give up long-cherished illusions (he is not going to become president of the company after all). Many women must consider the possibility of a completely new career, unless they are content to be professional grandmothers and mothers-in-law for the remainder of their lives.

Sometime during the forties or early fifties, the ovaries cease to function and women lose the capacity to reproduce. This period, known as the *menopause* or *climacterium,* can be accompanied by profound psychological changes, perhaps particularly severe in the woman whose very identity has been limited almost entirely to motherhood. The relative contributions of hormone changes and psychological factors remain an enigma.

Many men in their forties or fifties also experience an identity crisis analogous to the female menopause. However, in normal males the condition is not related to hormonal changes or loss of reproductive capacity, but to psychological stresses associated with the loss of youth, which men can regret as acutely as women can.

Nobody would claim that proper nutrition or any other single factor can solve all of the problems of adults. Nevertheless, maintenance of health can contribute to productivity and personal satisfaction at any age, and nutrition is one of the preventive means of maintaining health. *In fact, the one most common preventable factor in illness and death in adults is obesity, which is entirely preventable by a maintenance diet that matches the energy intake to that appropriate for the level of physical activity.*

What is aging, and at what point does it begin? This is a subject of lively controversy (Figure 19–9). Some see aging as degenerative changes resulting in a progressive loss or decline of functions, first appearing several decades after maturity is attained. Others think that aging begins at the time the individual reaches physical maturity. Still others view aging as synonymous with development, and believe that the changes seen in very early development, even before birth, are consequences of the aging process, just as the changes in later life are.

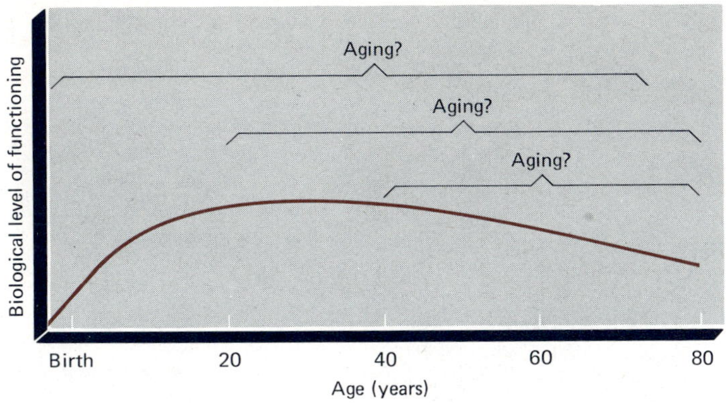

FIGURE 19–9. Aging: when does it begin?

Certainly it is difficult to decide when a person should be called aging, old, aged, or elderly. Age sixty-five and over is often used synonymously with "the elderly" because social security benefits begin and retirement is often mandatory at this age. Biologically, the definition is meaningless; in many nursing homes, some of the employees are chronologically older than some of the elderly patients they care for.

The causes of aging are of great interest in the field of *geriatrics,* the branch of medicine concerned with treating the problems of the aging, and in the science of *gerontology,* the scientific study of the aging process. The "wearing out" theory holds that aging is caused by the sheer wear and tear of functioning, which causes cells, like machines, to break down eventually. The "rusting out" school of thought claims that lack of use, rather than overuse, causes the body to deteriorate. However, despite the fact that many biological and psychological changes occurring with age have been described, the causes of these changes are largely unknown.

The same factors which affect growth and development help to determine the rate of aging and the length of the life span, or longevity. Genes are important, as shown by the fact that the life span of a human or other animal is related to the life span of the parents. Individuals with the rare genetic disease, *progeria,* may start to show signs of advanced aging at the age of one year, and may die at age ten to fifteen of heart disease similar to that seen in very old people.

Hormones were once believed to be a veritable fountain of youth, and quack treatments utilizing ill-defined "glandular extracts" still abound. These treatments are entirely different from reputable therapies, such as treatment of postmenopausal women with estrogens, the purpose of which is not to rejuvenate, but to alleviate certain symptoms of estrogen deficiency such as loss of minerals from the bones.

Of the environmental factors which may affect the aging process,

FIGURE 19–10
Elderly people may need special help in order to have an adequate diet. (USDA photo.)

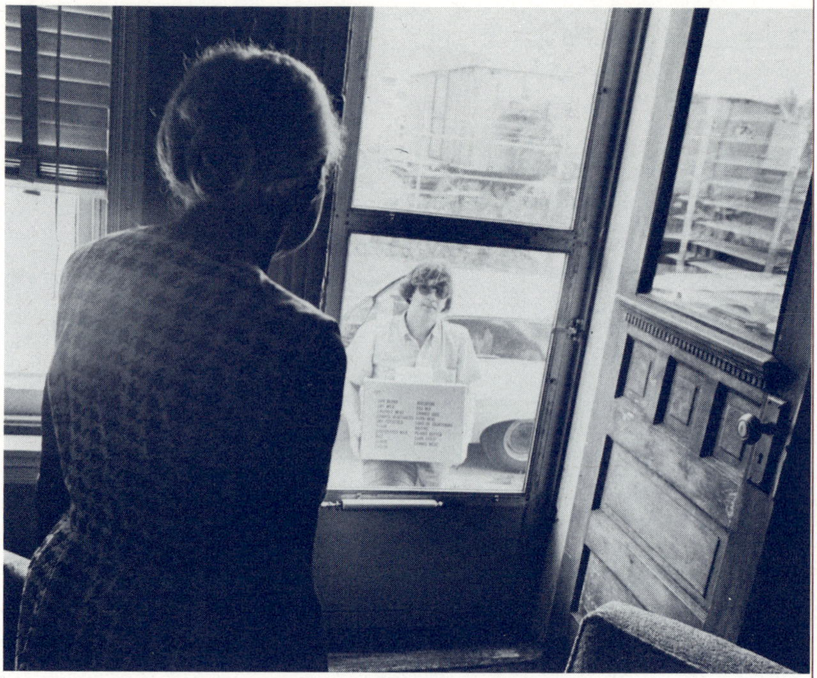

nutrition is one that has been studied very intensively. Perhaps the most well-documented finding is that restriction of energy intake substantially increases the life span of rats. The restricted rats maintain a youthful appearance at an age when unrestricted rats appear senile, and show a decreased incidence of degenerative changes in organs such as the heart and kidneys.

However, the degree of restriction used in many of these experiments was so severe that it inhibited growth, and in some cases even prevented maturation. How can we apply the results of such studies to humans? Certainly we would not want to underfeed infants and children severely enough to impair their growth and development. The studies may, however, have implications for our practice of *overfeeding* infants and children, and for the common belief that maximum growth during early life is necessarily optimal for health in later life.

Almost certainly to be discounted are stories of people who live to be 120 or 150 years old by virtue of their diets. Such people are generally claimed to have been found in some area remote from civilization, where their simple way of life and diet have remained unchanged for centuries. In all cases, the claims for remarkable longevity are based on unverified statements by the people themselves, or on pure conjecture by the writer who claims to have discovered them. Because birth records never seem to be available for these individuals, accepting the claims regarding their astonishing life spans is a matter of faith rather than of acceptance of documented evidence.

Many studies have shown that physical well-being and lowered mortality rates are related to adequate nutrient intakes. The problem in interpreting these findings is that diet may have been affected by the state of health, rather than the reverse. Certainly at present, too little is known about the relationships of diet to aging to make many definite recommendations regarding the optimal nutrient intakes for a healthy old age or a long life span. For example, the life expectancy of women in the United States now surpasses that of men by seven years, although diet surveys consistently show that women's diets fail to provide recommended intakes more often than men's diets do!

However, we know much more about the effects of aging on nutrition than on the effects of nutrition on aging. Nutritional changes seen in aging persons fall into two major groups: those primarily related to social and psychological factors, and those with underlying biological causes.

Social-psychological changes with aging

Golden agers? Sunset years? For many, these glowing terms are appropriate. But many other elderly Americans can say, with justification, that they are treated as an ignored minority group rather than as individuals deserving full acceptance in society. They are old in a youth-fixated society, and unemployed or unemployable in a work-oriented culture which defines people's roles in terms of gainful work. They are perhaps living in poverty at a time when there is no certainty of assistance from neighbors or grown children, and they are often lonely among people who fail to comprehend that social isolation is devastating to people of any age.

Some elderly people maintain to the end of life a large share of the things they cherish. Others lose these one after another: the home now too large to care for; the husband or wife; friends their own age; sight, hearing, and other biological functions; the previously adequate income. Small wonder, then, that many elderly people have nutritional problems as well. Food and drink may be used as the only available source of pleasure, with obesity as the result. Or the individual may become so disinterested in life in general, including food, that serious undernutrition develops. Indeed, a disproportionate number of elderly people live in such extreme poverty that they cannot even purchase food enough to meet their needs, unless special efforts are made to help them (Figure 19–10). Old people are sometimes found dead of starvation in their own homes, right here in the United States.

Physical changes with aging

Just as the various systems of the body develop at different rates early in life, so their decline is far from uniform. A seventy-year-old may

TABLE 19–3

Age-related biological changes important in nutrition

Change	Comments
Atrophy of salivary glands	May cause difficulty in swallowing, especially of dry foods.
Loss of taste buds	May make eating less pleasurable. Many elderly people use increased amounts of seasonings because food is tasteless otherwise.
Loss of teeth	Although not inevitable, very common with aging. Diet need not suffer if properly fitted dentures are worn. However, if the necessary dental treatment cannot or will not be obtained, the diet may be limited to soft foods that do not require chewing. Such diets are commonly inadequate unless the person knows more about nutrition than most people do.
Decreased secretion of stomach acid	Common but far from universal in old age. Certain minerals are absorbed less efficiently when stomach acid secretion declines.
Decreased secretion of intrinsic factor	Magnitude of decrease too small to significantly impair vitamin B_{12} absorption in most elderly people.
Decline in basal metabolic rate	It is common for elderly to feel cold at temperatures comfortable to younger people. In the Bible we read in I Kings 1:1 that "King David was old and stricken in years and he gat no heat." (The treatment recommended was that King David lie with a young virgin. Elderly men today may have to content themselves with electric heating pads.)
Decreased size and activity of thyroid gland	Probably a response to decreased need for thyroxine to regulate metabolism of lean body mass (see below).
Increased proportion of fat to lean	Universal in aging people as dying cells are progressively replaced with fat cells rather than with the type of cell that died.
Decrease in height	The only time in the life cycle that this normally occurs. Decrease is slight in healthy elderly people, reflecting loss of material between vertebrae. However, height may decrease by several inches in those with serious bone disease.
Decreased physical activity	Impaired coordination, decreased speed and strength of neuromuscular reactions. However, the basis may also be social and psychological: lack of opportunities for previously enjoyed group activities; limited funds for activities such as golfing and bowling; loss of companions with whom activities were formerly shared.
Decreased brain volume	Not necessarily accompanied by decreased intellect. Apparent lack of mental activity in many elderly people may reflect a lack of social stimulation rather than actual intellectual decline. Remember, the words *senator* and *senior* are derived from the same Latin word as *senility* (senex = an elder).
Increased incidence of many chronic diseases	Decreased ability to obtain, prepare, and eat an adequate diet, as in crippling diseases such as arthritis. Diseases can impair the digestion, absorption, and metabolism of nutrients. Drugs necessary to treat the disease may have further adverse effects on nutrient utilization.

have well over half of the kidney function that was present at twenty, but only one-third of the taste buds. Thus, although all of the systems of the body decline with aging, this functional loss varies from one cell type to another in a given individual, as well as varying from one individual to another. Some of the age-related changes relevant to nutrition are shown in Table 19–3 and Figure 19–11.

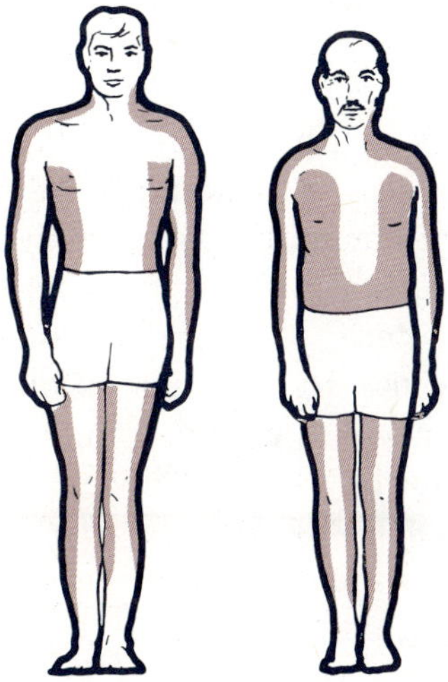

FIGURE 19–11. "I haven't gained an ounce since I was twenty." True perhaps for total weight; but the percentage of fat (shaded areas above) in the body unavoidably increases after maturity. (From R. M. Deutsch, The Family Guide to Better Food and Better Health. Des Moines: Meredith, 1971.)

Nutrient needs of the elderly

A large number of nutrient supplements are sold for the purpose of meeting the supposed "increased needs" of elderly people. Are these nostrums useful? In order to answer this question, the Recommended Dietary Allowances for older people can be compared to those for people twenty-two to fifty years old (Figure 19–12).

In most cases the recommendations are the same; a few allowances are actually decreased for the older population. A lower energy intake is recommended because of the decrease in basal metabolism and in physical activity. Niacin, thiamin and riboflavin are recommended in correspondingly decreased amounts because the need for these vitamins is closely related to the metabolism of energy nutrients. Because thyroid gland function decreases, the allowance for iodine is less for the older person. Iron is recommended in smaller amounts for women over fifty because iron is no longer lost in the menses. An individual woman may of course experience the menopause much earlier or somewhat later than age fifty, and this will determine her need for iron at any particular age.

Vitamin B_{12} absorption decreases in many elderly people, but the magnitude of this decrease is too small to justify an increase in the

RDA for this vitamin. The one outstanding conclusion that can be drawn from the data in Figure 19–12 is that in no case is an allowance *increased* for the elderly population. The healthy older person has the same nutritional needs as the young adult has, except for *decreased* requirements for energy and for a few essential nutrients. "High-potency" supplements and health foods sold to cover the purported "increased needs" of the elderly are therefore an unnecessary expense, useless in improving the nutrition of the aged.

One vitamin deserves special mention because it is so commonly advertised as being specifically useful in flagging the failing sexual powers of elderly men. This is vitamin E. Advertisements sometimes show a silver-haired gentleman playing with a young child (presumably his), while his wife (invariably much younger) stands by with a satisfied smile on her face. Because sexual potency is mostly controlled from the neck up, some elderly men may well feel more potent after taking vitamin E; but they could get the same effect from a sugar tablet.

What about the elderly person who actually does have unusual nutrient needs because of a physical disease? Certainly nutrition is an important part of the treatment. However, this should always be part of an individualized program of treatment by a physician, rather than indiscriminate self-medication.

FIGURE 19–12. The altered nutritional needs of the elderly, as reflected in the RDA, are in the direction of decreases rather than increases.

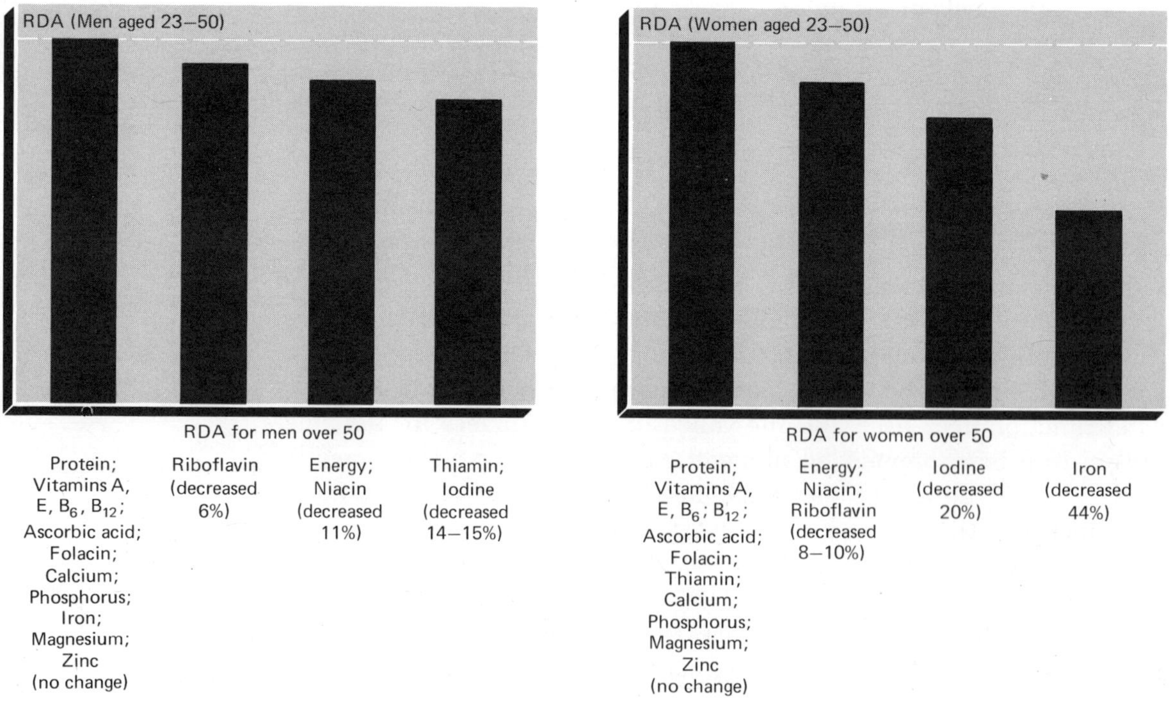

Some practical proposals for improving nutrition in the elderly

Free or low-cost medical and dental care should become an accepted right of every human being. Because medical and dental disorders so often underlie the nutritional problems of older people, the elderly would particularly benefit from changes in the health care delivery system.

Every elderly individual should have an income sufficient to cover the costs of adequate food, housing, clothing, recreation, and other needs, regardless of previous employment or changes in the cost of living.

For the benefit of those elderly people who are no longer able to live independently, supervision of nursing homes and similar institutions should be strengthened to insure that all aspects of living, including diet, are adequate.

Nutrition education programs for the elderly should consider the fact that group-decision techniques may be more effective than the lecture method suitable for teaching younger adults. One *can* "teach an old dog new tricks" if one of the right approaches is used (Figure 19–13).

Elderly people should be provided with services to help them to shop for food and to cook meals if it is impossible for them to cope with these problems without assistance. Group meals, offered at schools or other community centers, can provide much-needed social interaction as well as physical nourishment. Home-delivered meals, such as those available through the Meals on Wheels program, should be provided for those who can neither prepare their own meals nor go to a group-meal center (Figure 19–14).

Society has long ignored the plight of the elderly. Perhaps this is understandable; certainly it is more pleasant to concentrate on early development (the end-point of which is maturity) than on the process of growing old (the end-point of which is death). Would it not be prudent, however, for those who are young today to work toward all of the social and economic changes needed to insure improved nutrition and a generally better life for the elderly of the future as well as for those who are old today?

SUGGESTED READINGS

Bettelheim, B. *Food to Nurture the Mind.* Washington, D.C.: The Children's Foundation, 1970.

Bruch, H. "Perils of Behavior Modification in Treatment of Anorexia Nervosa." *Journal of the American Medical Association* 230 (1974):1419.

Bullen, B. A., L. F. Monello, H. Cohen, and J. Meyer. "Attitudes Towards Physical Activity, Food, and Family in Obese and Nonobese Adolescent Girls." *American Journal of Clinical Nutrition* 12 (1963):1.

Butler, R. N. "Why Are Older Consumers So Susceptible?" *Geriatrics* 23 (1968):83.

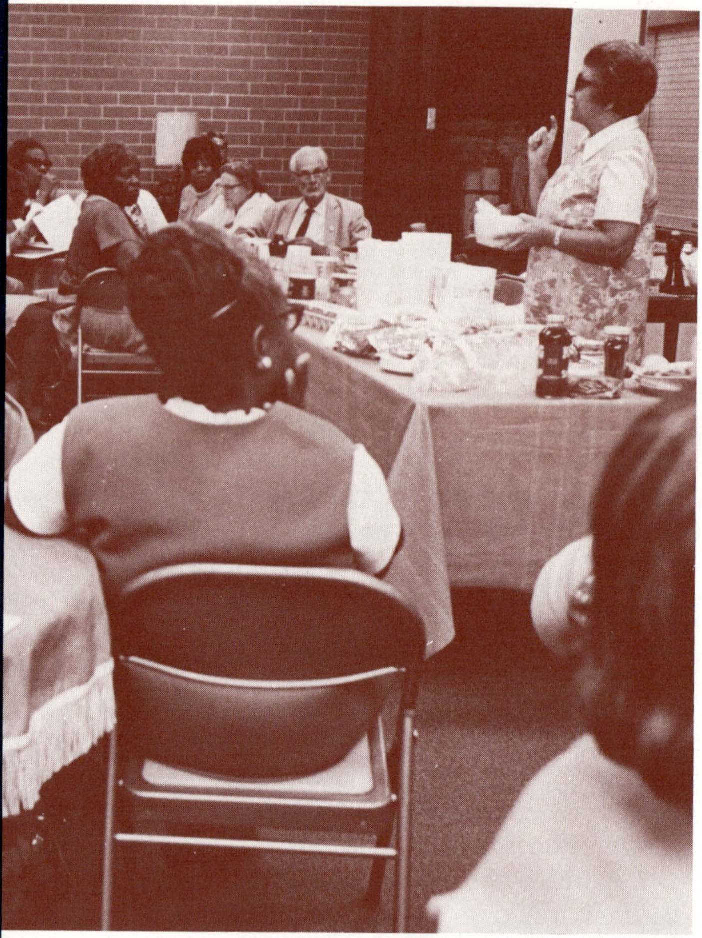

FIGURE 19–13
If the methods of teaching are suitable, we are never too old for education—including nutrition education. (USDA photo.)

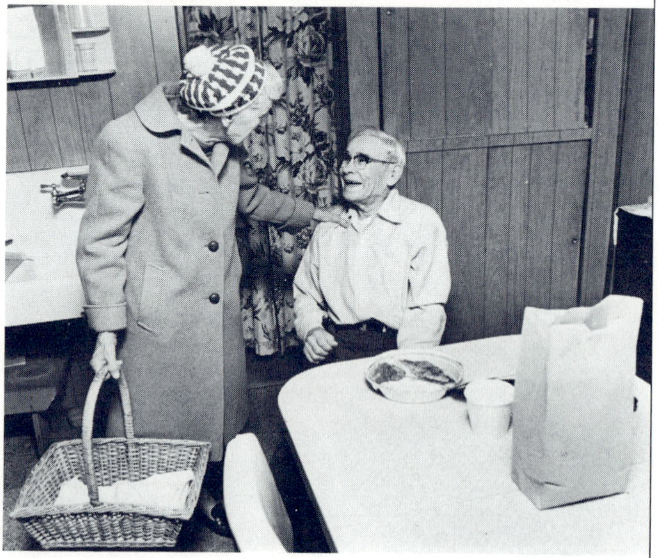

FIGURE 19–14
Home-delivered meals provide much-needed social interaction as well as good nutrition for elderly people who otherwise cannot or will not obtain an adequate diet. (USDA photo.)

Carrier, R. "Learning Nutrition by Doing." *Nutrition News* 34 (1971):13.

Deutsch, R. M. *The Family Guide to Better Food and Better Health.* Des Moines: Meredith, 1971.

Dwyer, J. and J. Mayer. "Psychological Effects of Variations in Physical Appearance During Adolescence." *Adolescence* 3 (1968):353.

Goldstein, S. "The Biology of Aging." *New England Journal of Medicine* 285 (1971):1120.

Gussow, J. "Counternutritional Messages of TV Ads Aimed at Children." *Journal of Nutrition Education* 4 (1972):48.

Heald, F. P., ed. *Adolescent Nutrition and Growth.* New York: Meredith, 1969.

Hill, M. M. *Food Choices: The Teen-Age Girl.* New York: The Nutrition Foundation, 1966.

"Home and Garden Bulletin No. 17: Food Guide for Older Folks." Washington, D.C., USDA, 1971.

"Home and Garden Bulletin No. 194: A Guide to Budgeting for the Retired Couple." Washington, D.C., USDA, 1971.

Josselyn, I. M. *Adolescence.* New York, Harper & Row, 1971.

Klinger, J. L., F. H. Frieden, and R. A. Sullivan. *Mealtime Manual for the Aged and Handicapped.* New York, Simon and Schuster, 1970.

Kohn, R. R. *Principles of Mammalian Aging.* Englewood Cliffs, N. J.: Prentice-Hall, 1971.

Leverton, R. M. Basic Nutrition Concepts for Use in Nutrition Education. *Journal of Home Economics* 59 (1967):346.

Leverton, R. M. The Paradox of Teen-Age Nutrition. *Journal of the American Dietetic Association* 53 (1968):13.

Mann, G. V. "Relationship of Age to Nutrient Requirements." *American Journal of Clinical Nutrition* 26 (1973):1097.

McCay, C. M., M. F. Crowell, and L. A. Maynard. "The Effect of Retarded Growth upon the Length of Life Span and upon the Ultimate Body Size." *Journal of Nutrition* 10 (1935):63.

Root, A. W. "Endocrinology of Puberty: Normal Sexual Maturation." *Journal of Pediatrics* 83 (1973):1.

Schlenker, E. D., J. S. Feuring, L. H. Stone, M. A. Ohlson, and O. Michelsen. "Nutrition and Health of Older People." *American Journal of Clinical Nutrition* 26 (1973):1111.

Shock, N. W. "Physiologic Aspects of Aging." *Journal of the American Dietetic Association* 56 (1970):491.

Tanner, J. M. "Earlier Maturation in Man." *Scientific American* 218 (1968):21.

20

personal choices in nutrition

Consider the poor koala, that Teddy Bear-like inhabitant of Australia. Perched on a branch, it munches away on the only food it can accept and utilize—the leaves of certain *Eucalyptus* trees. The price of this lack of nutritional diversity is a precarious existence, for if the *Eucalyptus* trees ever disappear, so surely will the koala.

Other animals are much less narrowly specialized than the koala in their ranges of food options. Of all species, however, humans have the greatest dietary diversification because of two outstanding characteristics:

First, humans have developed biologically in such a way that they are innately able to accept and to utilize as food a very wide variety of organisms, both plants and animals.

Second, we have developed a technology that makes even more dietary variability possible. We are not limited to what is available in a given ecological niche; we can travel to, and obtain food from, virtually every location on land, in the waters, or in the air. Also through technology we can process food: cooking, canning, freezing, drying, and, in many cases, manufacturing the already wide range of raw foods that humans can use (Figure 20–1).

As a result, people are confronted with many choices regarding food. As consumers, we understandably want to know: Which choices will bring about the greatest benefit to me or to others who are affected by what I choose?

Although people commonly assume that their own cultural practices are automatically best, it must be admitted at the outset that there is no one "right way" that is best for everybody. For example, in most Western nations it is almost a matter of faith that meat is part of a good diet, and vegetarianism is therefore viewed as a peculiar cult or fad which must somehow be inferior to the "normal" diet. Yet the fact remains that many people who have chosen not to eat meat are in excellent nutritional status on well-selected vegetarian diets. There is no evidence that they are any more healthy than meat-eaters, but neither is there any evidence that they are any less healthy. Thus, whether vegetarianism is a fad, a cult, or a good diet depends upon one's definitions of these terms. Vegetarianism, like any other diet that satisfies an individual's biological, psychological, and social needs, can be the "right diet" for one person, even though it may be entirely wrong for another.

On the other hand, although no one choice is right for everyone, some choices are definitely *not* sound. This is not a moral judgment, but a statement of fact: some personal decisions in nutrition are incompatible with meeting people's needs. The human ability to think and learn, which enables people to choose rationally, was gained only at the cost of giving up what other animals have retained to a much greater degree: the ability to make appropriate choices, in eating as well as in other forms of behavior, by instinct alone.

NATURE VERSUS NURTURE IN NUTRITION

With the rise of modern psychology came a wave of interest in allowing people to follow their natural basic drives, unsuppressed by society. Accordingly, many people believe that completely free choices, based on instinctive desires, must somehow automatically be best. The belief is that already well-nourished people would involuntarily select foods that would maintain the present state, and those who are malnourished would, through some mysterious "wisdom of the body," gravitate naturally toward those foods which contain precisely what is needed.

These beliefs are based upon two main fallacies. The first is that animals and "primitive people," knowing nothing of the science of nutrition, invariably select adequate diets by following their natural instincts. The second is that this ability has actually been demonstrated in children, presumed free of the supposedly damaging pressures and inhibitions of society.

The role of instinct in meeting energy needs

With regard to energy needs, humans, like other animals, apparently have at least some ability to match intake to needs without a great deal of conscious thought. Appetite increases as energy requirements rise: during rapid growth, pregnancy, and lactation; when people are very active physically; and in larger people compared to smaller ones. These differences all indicate the existence of some innate kind of regulation which allows energy intake to vary as needs change. That this control is imperfect is shown by the large number of people who maintain their ideal weight only by consciously struggling to control their food intake, their level of exercise, or both. Nevertheless, the fact that we do not all have to fight the "Battle of the Bulge" continuously indicates that nature provides some automatic control of energy intake.

The role of instinct in meeting nutrient needs

When it comes to demonstrating an instinctive ability to meet specific *nutrient* needs, we are on much shakier grounds than in the case of meeting energy requirements. For example, what about the "binges" that people sometimes experience, during which they crave specific foods—pickles, strawberries, potato chips, ice cream? Do these consuming desires represent an instinctive drive to obtain something desperately needed by the body, or are they purely psychological? To answer this question, it is helpful to consider the results of controlled

FIGURE 20–1

Many new orange products retain the nutritive benefits of fresh oranges. These are Milk-Orange Drink (MOD) in pitcher, Orange-Ho in bowl, reconstituted instant orange juice powder in glass, and orange juice powder and tablets in small dish. (Photo courtesy USDA)

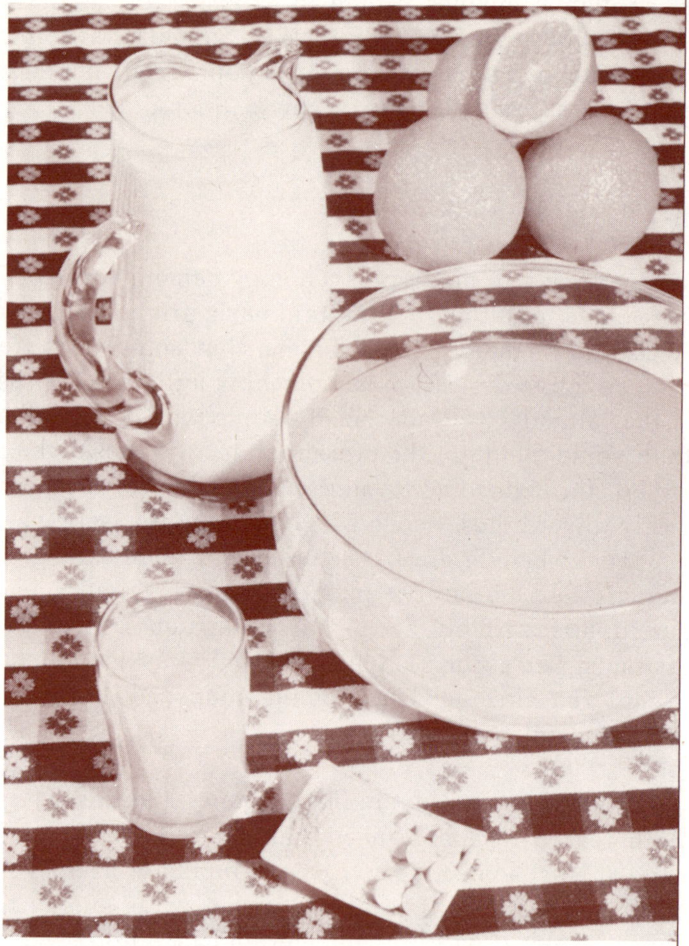

experiments with animals; in this way we can avoid the complex emotional connotations which people attach to foods.

The simplest situation in which animals can be studied with respect to instinctive drives for nutrients is one in which a single nutrient is lacking, such as that shown in Figure 20–1. If an animal's adrenal glands are removed, sodium deficiency develops quite rapidly. This is because one of the hormones secreted by the adrenal glands is aldosterone, which conserves sodium in the body by preventing excessive excretion of the mineral in the urine. Lack of aldosterone leads to a lack of sodium in the body, severe enough to be fatal within days. This can be prevented, however, if the intake of sodium is great enough to replace the amount lost in the urine.

Rats that have been made sodium deficient (as shown in Figure 20–2) respond in two very different ways, depending upon their previous diets: those that are nutritionally naïve—not previously accustomed to any particular taste, such as sweetness—generally select salt solution in preference to plain water if they are offered a choice of the two. However, rats that have previously learned to like the taste of sugar characteristically choose what they *like* (sugar solution) instead of what they *need* (salt solution), even though death inevitably results from the choice.

What conclusions can be drawn from such studies? First, an animal suffering from severe deficiency of a specific nutrient tends to increase its intake of that nutrient. This may represent an instinctive drive to obtain what is needed; on the other hand, it may represent the ability

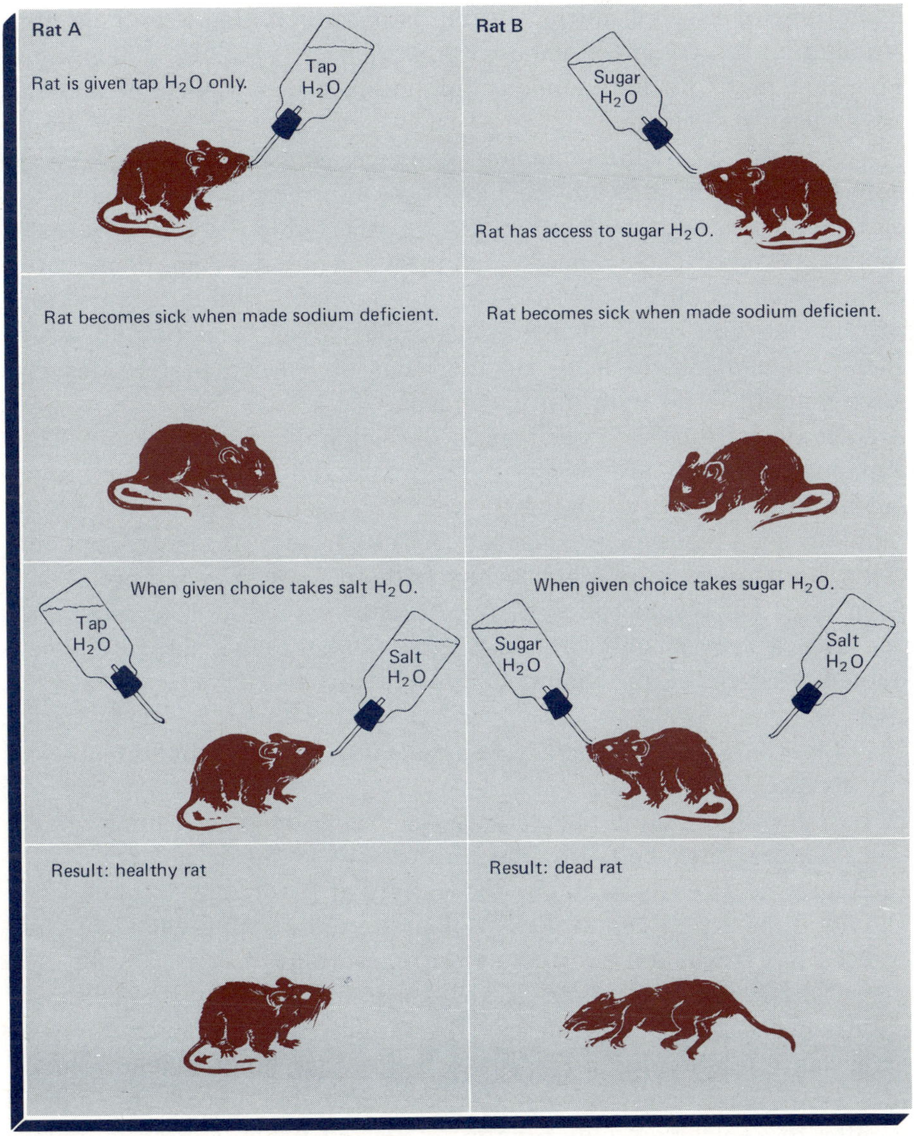

FIGURE 20–2. The wisdom of the body?

of rats to learn to associate the taste of salt with a prompt feeling of improved well-being as the necessary sodium is absorbed into the body.

However, rats that have learned to like a certain taste (in this case, sweetness) show very little "wisdom of the body." Indeed, the stupidity of the body under certain conditions is strikingly shown by the rat's lust to obtain what it likes in preference to what it needs, even though it is dying as a result of its choice.

As the result of many experiments of this kind, it must be concluded that appetite is *not* a reliable guide to obtaining the specific nutrients needed, even for rats. Nevertheless, a good many people persist in believing that the *human* appetite is controlled by the presence or absence of essential nutrients in the body. According to this idea, a shortage of a given nutrient in the body affects the taste buds, thus stimulating the person to choose foods rich in that particular nurient. Precisely how the individual could possibly detect the nutrient has never been explained.

Consider, now, the abundant evidence against this belief. For example, people in parts of the Far East often continue to choose unenriched white rice rather than brown rice, which is much richer in thiamin, even after advanced thiamin deficiency develops. Their preference is based on factors such as appetite, habit, and the status value of refined grain, rather than on nutritional value. Does this not prove that food choices are made on the basis of learned preferences that have nothing to do with nutrient needs?

No, insist those who believe in the value of natural instinct. They explain that people are born with an innate ability to meet their nutrient needs, but that this naturally healthy appetite is perverted by the prejudices and biases of society. Therefore, they reason, if appetite could be allowed to operate freely, without interference from others, good nutrition would follow naturally and inevitably. These opinions are based on a misinterpretation of a much-quoted, and often misquoted, series of studies done over 40 years ago.

The Clara Davis studies: Self-selection of diets by infants and children

During the 1930s, many people held very rigid ideas on feeding infants and children; they believed that the number of meals, the amount of food allowed at each meal, and the variety of foods offered to children should all be strictly controlled. When, how much, and what the *child* wanted to eat was not considered very important.

Clara Davis, a physician who was interested in the nutrition of children, decided to test the hypothesis that children could safely be given more freedom with respect to their eating habits. Over a period of several years, she observed 15 children for periods ranging from 6 months to $4\frac{1}{2}$ years. At the time of admission to the study, the babies were from seven to ten months old, and had only recently been weaned;

having had no experience with any food other than milk, there was no possibility that their appetites had been "perverted," by society or in any other way.

Until the babies were old enough to feed themselves, a nursemaid was available to help, but she was not allowed to talk or to offer any food other than what the baby reached for or touched. After the babies became able to feed themselves, they received no assistance except for waitress service to assure that a baby's selection would never be limited by unavailability of any choice. In short, no control was exerted over either the amounts or the kinds of foods selected from what was offered.

Most of the children ate large amounts of meats and fruits. Vegetables were much less popular than fruits, and green leafy vegetables in particular were generally rejected (any parent could have predicted this finding). Each child developed an individual eating pattern, which might fluctuate enormously from meal to meal or from day to day; a given child might make an entire meal of ten eggs, or of lamb only. Yet over a period of time, all of the children at least tried practically all of the foods offered, and most ended up eating a variety of foods which apparently provided adequate amounts of essential nutrients. At any rate, none of the children developed an actual deficiency disease, and none were remarkably overweight or underweight. Consequently, it is often stated that this study proved that children can remain vigorous and healthy if they are allowed free choice in their eating.

However, a glance at the list of foods offered shows that choice was actually far from free:

The only beverage was milk, either plain or soured—no cola drinks, uncola drinks, or sweet, artificially flavored "juice substitutes."
The meats were served steamed or raw, with no salt or other seasonings; eggs were hardboiled or raw, and unseasoned.
Fruits were unsweetened, and vegetables unflavored with salt or butter; the only variation was raw versus cooked.
The only grain products available were Ry-Krisp, raw whole grain cereals, or cooked porridge, none of which were served with cream, milk, or sugar. There were no snap, crackle, pop cereals; no presweetened or shot-from-guns products.

Each of these foods contains useful amounts of a number of essential nutrients, and none of them was pleasing enough that a child would be likely to select it exclusively, at the expense of other foods. The key to the success of this study now becomes obvious: it was inherent in the list of foods offered to the children. All that the study actually showed is that children select an adequate diet *if nothing except nutritious foods are available.* It offers no evidence whatever that children choose a nutritious diet if they are allowed completely free choice of all the foods available in the average home. A child free to choose between milk and soft drinks, or between carrots and candy, may very well choose the soft drinks and the candy, but this certainly does not indicate superior nutritional value for the choices. When food selection is really free, children, like people of any other age, may well select the foods they *like* in preference to those which contain the nutrients they *need.*

CHOICES OTHER THAN "WHAT" AND "HOW MUCH"

A food grouping plan such as the Basic Four, although a useful guide, cannot answer many of the questions that arise in translating a general guide into actual human eating patterns; personal choices other than kinds and amounts must be made. People must consider factors such as life style, time, money, and effort, and not all of these are equally important to each of us. A discussion of such factors can point out certain facts and fallacies; but it is then up to each individual to decide whether or not to incorporate this information into her or his personal living pattern.

How many meals or snacks daily?

Each culture considers its own behavior patterns the norm, an attitude which includes the number of meals and the times for eating them that are considered "proper." Nevertheless, as we see in our own society, many people develop eating patterns that may vary greatly from those characteristic of the majority.

Some people eat whenever they are hungry, even if this means six or more meals daily. Naturally those who eat six times daily must avoid eating as much at each meal as they would on a three-meals-daily pattern. However, there is no valid objection to frequent eating unless *total* food intake is excessive.

The opposite pattern, that of eating only once or twice a day, is generally decried by nutritionists. They point out that skipping one or more meals daily can decrease efficiency, and cause indiscriminate snacking, overeating at the next meal, omission of foods which are generally unavailable in the rest of the day's meals, and other possibly dire nutritional consequences.

In view of these objections, it seems almost heretical to give even tentative approval to a pattern of less than three meals per day. However, there are at least two reasons for doing so. The first is that some people do manage to function quite effectively on only two meals per day; for example, controlled tests show that although skipping breakfast impairs the efficiency of some people, it has no apparent adverse effects on others. Confirmed breakfast-skippers may have adjusted to this pattern so well that they function quite efficiently under conditions which would impair the performance of others.

It is also questionable whether skipping a meal necessarily leads to nutrient shortages. Certainly it is not a good idea to skip a meal if this invariably drives you to snack on candy bars, soft drinks, or sweet rolls in order to relieve hunger. However, some people snack on foods such as sandwiches, fruits, and milk after skipping a meal, or do not snack at all, and there is no logical reason to object to these practices.

Many people who skip meals, especially breakfast, do so in an attempt to lose weight. A frequently voiced objection to this practice is that it is futile, because skipping breakfast causes overeating later in the day. Statements such as this should be eschewed if one is to avoid creating a credibility gap, because, quite simply, many people know from experience that skipping breakfast does *not* necessarily cause later overeating. Studies of school-aged boys have shown that the intake at lunch and dinner increases if they skip breakfast. However, the only conclusion that can be drawn from this is that boys who are not attempting to lose weight tend to make up for skipped meals; it is hardly valid to conclude that the same is true for people who are consciously trying to lose weight. Although those who are convinced that meal-skipping is unwise are understandably eager to cite evidence to support their view, this does not justify making statements that are questionable or actually inaccurate.

A generation or so ago, nutritionists commonly warned that skipping breakfast could decrease appetite for the next meal. The motive was good; nutritionists were concerned that breakfast-skipping dieters might then skip lunch and perhaps dinner as well. However, if any statement could be guaranteed to cause dieters to skip breakfast, it is the warning that skipping one meal may cause loss of hunger for other meals! At any rate, it is not true that most people are less hungry after skipping a meal. The idea that your stomach "shrinks" as a result of going hungry is pure myth.

Omitting meals to the extent of eating only *one* meal daily is less defensible than milder degrees of meal-skipping. Eating only one meal daily is not uncommon in areas of some developing countries, because a meal may involve lighting a fire and searching for more fuel—conditions under which it becomes very difficult to eat often. People may consequently see a single meal daily as the only practical solution. In developed countries, although very few people find it necessary to eat only once a day, some do this by choice. However, this "meal" may actually consist of several hours of intermittent eating, usually in the evening. It is certainly possible to get enough energy in this manner; in fact, some of the people with this kind of eating pattern are very obese. It is also possible, with careful planning, to get sufficient amounts of essential nutrients in a "meal" lasting from 6 P.M. to perhaps midnight. Nevertheless, nutritionists offer two valid objections to this practice. One is that almost everybody will feel better and function more efficiently if at least something is eaten other than what is crammed into an interval of a few hours. The other is that cells utilize nutrients more effectively if they are supplied in small, frequent batches rather than in one lump. It is true that some animals habitually gorge themselves only once a day, or even less frequently, with no apparent ill effects. And it is a fact that a python can go without food for weeks after swallowing a pig, but this does not prove that the same habit would also be a desirable eating pattern for humans.

One very common misconception regarding meal timing is that food eaten late in the day is more likely to be converted to body fat than the same food eaten earlier. Food eaten at night will of course "go to fat" if it is in addition to, rather than in place of, food eaten earlier. However, a given *total* energy intake has the same effect on body weight whether eating is followed by exercise or by sleep—just as you will get the same mileage from a given amount of gasoline whether the gas tank is filled just before starting a trip or the night before.

The value of variety—how important is it?

Nutritionists quite logically stress the importance of variety in foods, because increased variety gives greater assurance that the diet will supply adequate amounts of all essential nutrients.

However, people sometimes place undue stress on the need for variety for psychological reasons. Although animals generally are stimulated by change, and response is deadened by monotonous repetition, it does not necessarily follow that we *all* need frequent changes in diet —such as new foods, new methods of preparing familiar foods, and different table settings. The fact is that some people genuinely prefer having the same foods, prepared and served in the same way, day after day. Children and elderly people, in particular, may find comfort and security in food which deviates little from time to time. After all, people do many things besides eating, and those who experience sufficient variety in their work and play may have little need to seek novelty per se in foods. At any rate, nobody should be criticized for getting into a nutritional rut merely because of the *assumption* that variety is everybody's emotional need; one person's rut is another person's comfortable routine, and this should be respected. (If you are intimidated by people whose diets are so varied as to include foods such as snails in wine, you might find comfort in one person's definition of a gourmet: "A hog in a tuxedo.")

Meals as family occasions—do they bring us together?

In many families, at least one daily meal is a pleasant family occasion, an opportunity for conversation and interactions between the family members. For these people, mealtime is a social occasion which may be the most rewarding occasion of the day.

However, social changes have reduced the number of meals the family has together. Children often eat at school instead of coming home for lunch; adults of both sexes generally eat lunch at or near their work, and work is no longer as home-centered as it was in former times.

Does this mean that the family structure is inevitably being weakened? Such a gloomy prediction hardly seems justified. Most families can manage to eat together at least occasionally if they really want to, and even if meals are never used as family occasions, there are many activities other than eating which people can do together as a social unit. In fact, one family member may best be fed *away* from the rest of the family. This is the infant or young child who has not yet learned even the rudiments of social graces. If other family members (older siblings even more often than parents) object to such sights as finger painting with creamed spinach, it may be best to feed children separately until they are old enough to eat in a manner that does not interfere with *other* people's enjoyment of eating. (Some parents say that this ability is achieved at about age two—some say age five—a few would say age eighteen or so!)

SURVIVAL IN THE SUPERMARKET

The average American adult or adolescent consumes about *one ton* of food each year, practically all of which is purchased rather than produced by the family. Food is, then, a major expense, accounting for about one-sixth of the average family's income, and of course a much larger proportion for low-income families.

The following suggestions are of proven value in minimizing the shock at the check-out counter:

1. Make out a shopping list, and follow it. Impulse buying, especially of expensive unneeded snacks, can send the cost soaring.

2. Avoid taking children along if at all possible, unless you have somehow managed to train them not to beg for, or even look longingly at, items such as the cereal with the free toy inside the box and the candy displayed near the check-out line.

3. Never go shopping when you are hungry. Most people buy more when they shop on an empty stomach, because everything looks so good that it is difficult to make the most economical choices.

4. Don't be too easily impressed with the "large economy size." The large size may not be any more economical (8 ounces of cereal for 62 cents and 12 ounces for 93 cents are the same in cost per serving), or the difference may be trivial (for example, a 1 pound package of something for 49 cents versus the 2 pound package for 95 cents). Even if the price per unit of weight is less for the larger package, it may not be an economy, for if storage space is too limited or the package very large the food may spoil before it is all used.

5. Compromise between the desire to use new foods and the established likes of the family. A new food may become a family favorite after it is introduced several times; on the other hand, it will just be

FIGURE 20–3

Read and understand food labels if you want to be informed about the package contents. (Photo courtesy General Mills.)

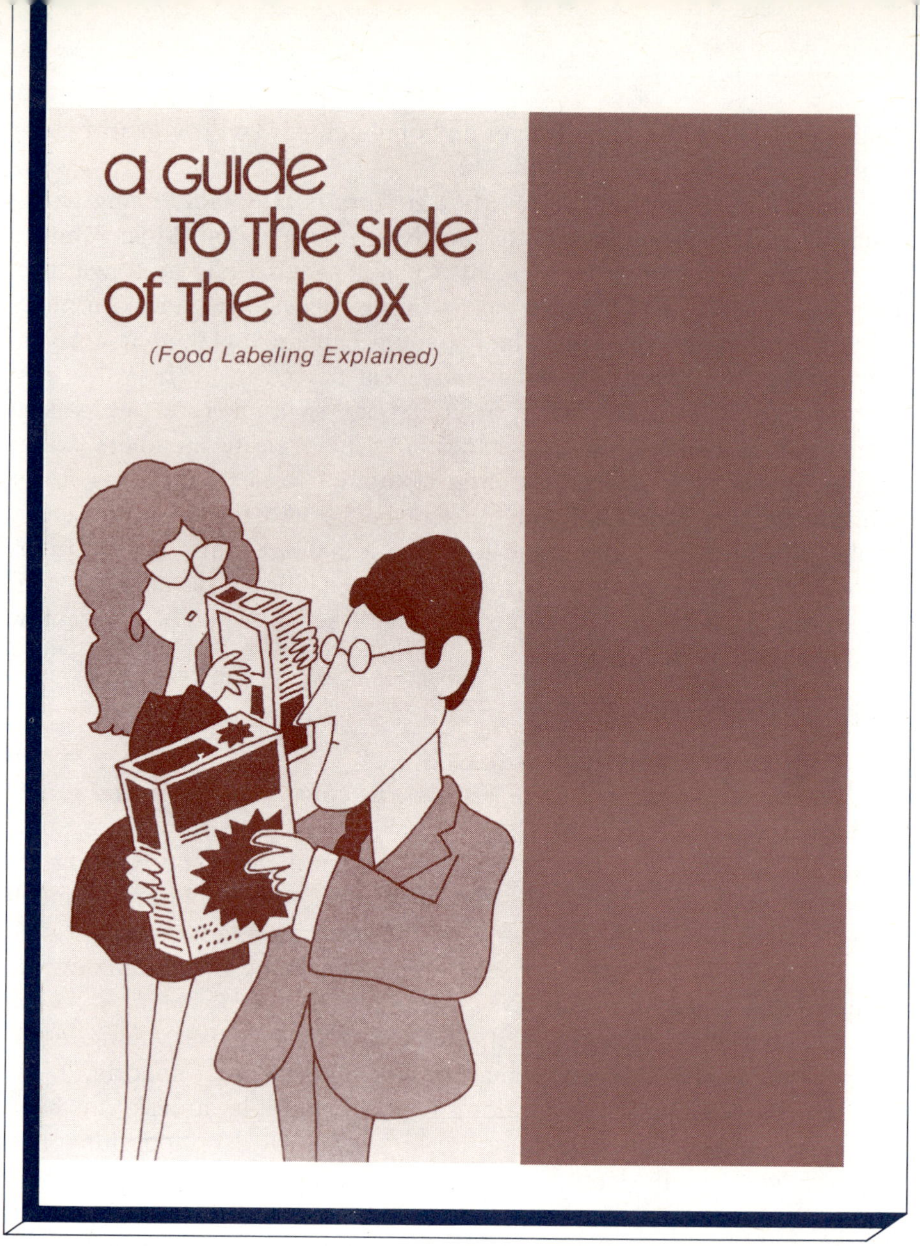

thrown out time after time if the family refuses to accept it. It seems the better part of wisdom to know when to give up trying to get people to change their opinion of a food.

6. Check the newspaper for advertisements on sales, but remember that it is no economy to spend a dollar on gasoline driving from store to store in order to save pennies on food, and that the time and energy spent in store-hopping may be more valuable than the money saved.

7. Ask yourself how "special" those advertised specials really are. That "specially reduced price" may be no lower than the regular price, and unless you know the regular prices of items, you cannot know whether the "special" price is lower. Foods are often advertised in

order to promote a new or slow-moving product, not to inform the public of genuine price reductions.

8. Learn to read labels on foods as carefully as on clothing or other products, and learn what the labels mean (Figure 20–3). Some of the information there is required by law: the *identity* of the food, the *weight* or *volume* of the contents, and the *name and address* of the manufacturer or distributor. Other information, such as nutritional value or grade, may be there only if the manufacturer chooses to put it on the label.

9. Don't be overly eager for "high grade" food. All foods which are sold are legally required to meet the same standards of purity and wholesomeness, so in these important regards Grade A (Fancy) is no better than Grade B (Choice or Extra Standard) or Grade C (Standard). Higher-grade foods are superior only in qualities such as tenderness (in meat), and in appearance or uniformity of size (in canned fruits and vegetables). They are neither more nutritious nor safer than lower-grade foods.

10. Recognize that many convenience foods, such as cake mixes, frozen orange juice concentrates, instant potatoes, canned vegetables and fruits, and certain types of frozen dinners, are as inexpensive as their made-from-scratch counterparts. Others, such as frozen vegetables in special sauces, are considerably more expensive. However, the choice of whether or not to use convenience foods often depends on factors other than price, such as the need to save time and effort, or the family's categorical statement that instant mashed potatoes taste like papier-mâché.

11. Try to buy only the amounts needed. Ideally, meals could be planned so accurately that there are no unexpected leftovers. In reality, however, leftover food is depressingly predictable, and deciding what to do with it can be a problem. From the point of view of economy, leftovers should be carefully stored and used in the near future. Many women prefer not to bother, especially if the amount left over is small, but feel guilty about throwing food away. The result may be a habit commonly known as the "human garbage-disposal syndrome," in which somebody (usually the homemaker) disposes of all leftovers by eating them. Overweight women sometimes state that this is the single greatest factor in their failures to lose weight. It may help to remember that overbuying and then overeating by a guilt-ridden American never helped a hungry person anywhere.

12. Remember that if the cost of food you buy to prepare at home is high, the cost of eating out is usually even higher. Why deceive ourselves into thinking that the hamburger bought at a chain outlet is as cheap as one cooked at home? The meat patty in the hamburger bought away from home may weigh only $1\frac{1}{2}$ ounces; if it is as cheap as one cooked at home, it may well be because the home-cooked one is two or three times as large.

13. Keep in mind that consumers' decisions can affect prices, just as prices affect consumers' decisions. Buying a product is casting a vote for that product, indicating acceptance of the price. *Decreased* purchases of high-priced foods can have real impact on the market, forcing the prices down as supplies of unpurchased foods accumulate.

14. Recognize that, in the final analysis, the amount of economizing done is largely a matter of personal taste. Some people enjoy the challenge of getting maximal food value for the smallest amount of money; others would prefer to do without almost anything else rather than give up eating well, and "eating well" does not mean just meeting nutritional needs. These are the people who are happy only if they can have the most tender cuts of meat, the most expensive types of bread, the best wines and cheeses, and so on. To them, food is entertainment and enjoyment, and they would feel very unhappy if forced to decrease their food budget drastically.

FOOD PREPARATION AND SERVICE: WHAT IS REALLY IMPORTANT?

Some people (men as well as women) look upon preparing and serving food as a creative activity which they enjoy. They seek out new recipes, buy special equipment such as coffee grinders and garlic presses, and happily spend hours cooking, setting tables, and creating centerpieces. Others, however, consider cooking a necessary chore, about as creative as folding socks or cleaning up after the cat, and, despite sex-role stereotyping, women as well as men may feel this way. Some feel vaguely guilty about their lack of enthusiasm for cooking ("Women are the nurturing sex"; "Cooking is a natural feminine activity") but on sober thought there is no more reason for every woman to enjoy preparing food than for every man to enjoy making furniture. Cooking, canning, and otherwise working with food at home may, in the future, become a lost art, or at most a hobby occasionally indulged in. This will not necessarily mean that nutritional status will suffer—only that people will need to learn how to select and use commercially processed foods more intelligently.

A few requirements for food handling are certainly justified. First, food must be sufficient in quantity to satisfy hunger, and prepared and served well enough to be acceptable to those who eat it. Second, food must be clean and safe to eat, because food-borne illnesses become a problem if reasonable standards of hygiene are not applied, or if foods are held at a temperature at which bacteria flourish. Finally, of course, food must supply adequate amounts of essential nutrients; there is no point in selecting good nutrient sources and then destroying much of the value of food by overcooking or otherwise mishandling it. These minimum standards are necessary.

However, standards far above this level are so frequently presented in cookbooks, newspapers, and magazines that a comment about them seems needed. Homemakers are advised to cook waffles, pancakes, hot cereal, and sausage for breakfast; to never, but never, use the same ingredient twice in a meal (as, for example, tomato sauce on the meat loaf and sliced tomatoes in the salad); to consider the color, shape, texture, and flavor of each food in each meal; to invest considerable time in setting and decorating the table. There is nothing really wrong with these suggestions. What *is* wrong is the assumption that such factors are important to everybody. In fact, to some people such preoccupation with the niceties of dining represents an outmoded refinement which has little relevance to modern life. A breakfast of cold cereal, milk, and orange juice, although objectionable to some people, is perfectly acceptable to others, and unless a paper plate or a table devoid of tablecloth and centerpiece makes you lose your appetite, you can very safely choose to ignore standards regarding such matters.

FOOD ADDITIVES

A food additive is any substance put into food which becomes part of the food and has some effect on its characteristics; unintentional or incidental additives are those which were not deliberately added, as when substances in a plastic or paper container gets into packaged food, or when traces of pesticides appear as residues in foods.

Before any *intentional* additive can be used, it must be shown that it performs a useful purpose in food: preserving appearance, taste, or wholesomeness; improving flavor; increasing nutritional value; or producing an acceptable consistency. An additive that serves no such useful function is not approved for use in foods.

The manufacturer of any new additive must test the substance for toxicity in laboratory animals. The amounts fed to the animals are much higher than the amounts reasonably expected to be ingested by people eating the product. Further, it must be shown that it does not produce cancer in test animals, even at levels *far* above those which would be possible for a human to ingest. Any chemical which causes any form of cancer in any animal species is banned, even if the test conditions were such that no individual could possibly eat this amount of the substance in an entire lifetime.

Additives that have been tested for safety, or which have been in general use long enough to be known as nontoxic in reasonable use, are included in the GRAS (Generally Regarded As Safe) list, and are thereby approved by the Food and Drug Administration.

Control of *unintentional* additives, such as pesticide residues, is exerted in two ways. First, the firm promoting a chemical which may leave a residue on food must prove that the resulting expected levels are safe. Second, samples of food products are regularly inspected and tested to be certain that the chemical is being used properly and that residue levels are indeed within the established safe tolerance.

TABLE 20–1
Some natural toxins in foods

Toxin	Examples of foods in which the toxin is found
Hydrogen cyanide (the lethal agent in state gas chambers)	Lima beans
Arsenic (infamous as a poison)	Shellfish
Solanine (found in the deadly nightshade plant)	Potatoes
Oxalic acid (a chemical used as a rust-remover)	Spinach, rhubarb
Myristicin (capable of producing hallucinations)	Nutmeg

Note: Compared to foods obtained from vertebrates, foods from lower organisms contain more substances toxic to humans. This reflects our closer evolutionary relationship, and thus our greater similarity, to higher organisms than to plants and lower animals.

Because of the extensive legal restrictions on additives, individual decisions regarding them are restricted to choices among additives which are of proven safety and usefulness. However, consumers often fail to appreciate the amount of effort that goes into the testing of additives. They read a food label and see names like "monoglyceride," "butylated hydroxytoluene," or "lecithin," and recoil in horror from these sinister-sounding chemicals. Actually, all of these have been rigorously tested and proved to be considerably safer than many other food components. In fact, the only way to avoid ingesting any "poisonous chemicals" at all would be to stop eating completely, for many natural unprocessed foods contain minute amounts of toxins (Table 20–1).

Individual consumers are of course free to use food additives such as salt, sugar, and monosodium glutamate (MSG) in any amounts they please. The greatest possibility of excessive use of food additives therefore occurs *after* consumers purchase foods, rather than before.

INFORMATION ON NUTRITION: RELIABLE OR NOT?

Freedom of expression is a basic right of the citizens of a democracy, and we therefore would not want to have censorship of books and other publications even if it were possible. This right of free expression extends to material written about nutrition, regardless of whether the author is a qualified source of information.

How, then, can you decide whether to accept the statements in a given book? One way is to look for claims characteristic of the charlatan. Does the author claim to have effected miraculous cures with special diets and supplements, or state that the American food supply is inadequate to support health? Are unusual foods, usually more expensive than their ordinary counterparts, advocated? If so, it is very likely that the book is a useless or even potentially dangerous source of misinformation.

For people who need help in making a decision on whether to accept a specific statement on nutrition, there are numerous sources of assistance available to answer inquiries. Some of these are shown in Table 20–2.

WHAT LEGAL RESTRAINTS RESTRICT INDIVIDUAL CHOICES?

Although the ultimate responsibility for making decisions rests with the individual consumer, certain potentially dangerous choices are made impossible through the work of various governmental agencies. Federal agencies are generally concerned with food in interstate commerce, whereas state and local agencies, which may vary greatly from one state to another, are in charge of food produced and sold within the state.

The principal federal agencies involved in consumer protection, including regulation of the food supply, are the following:

Food and Drug Administration (FDA)

The Food and Drug Administration is involved in many aspects of consumer protection other than food regulation. Its main responsibilities with respect to food and nutrition include the following:

1. It sets standards of identity, which define the ingredients in certain types of foods; standards of quality for a number of foods; standards of fill of container, to prevent deception of the consumer; and standards of enrichment for foods which have been fortified or enriched with nutrients.
2. It requires proper labeling of foods. Unless information on the label is an accurate statement of the contents, the food can be considered misbranded.
3. It forbids adulteration. Foods can be adulterated in several ways: by the use of cheaper ingredients as a substitute for the more expensive ones that properly should have been used; by the presence of excessive amounts of unacceptable materials such as insect parts or animal hairs; or by the use of materials which constitute actual health hazards, such as chemicals that are unsafe or present in excessive amounts.

The Food and Drug Administration has legal authority to seize any food product which does not comply with any of these regulations; however, it is still the individual consumer's responsibility to report any foods found to be mislabeled, unclean, spoiled, or otherwise in violation of federal regulations.

TABLE 20–2

Some sources of reliable nutrition information

Source	Examples of activities
The American Dietetic Association 620 N. Michigan Avenue Chicago, Illinois 60611	Answers general questions through publications; may refer specific questions to local ADA chapter or other nearby sources.
American Medical Association 535 N. Dearborn Street Chicago, Illinois 60610	Informs the public through publications, including the magazine, *Today's Health,* and through a question and answer service.
Chicago Nutrition Association 8158 S. Kedzie Avenue Chicago, Illinois 60652	Provides "Nutrition References and Book Reviews," which classes various nutrition books as "Recommended," "Recommended for Special Purposes," or "Not Recommended."
National Academy of Sciences—National Research Council 2101 Constitution Avenue Washington, D.C. 20418	Publishes the Recommended Dietary Allowances; furnishes information through numerous other publications.
Council of Better Business Bureaus 1150 17th Street N.W. Washington, D.C. 20036	Answers queries on the accuracy of nutrition information obtained from business firms and on the value of products such as vitamin supplements.
National Dairy Council 111 N. Canal Street Chicago, Illinois 60606	Provides excellent films for use in nutrition education.
National Meat and Livestock Board 33 S. Wabash Avenue Chicago, Illinois 60603	Informs consumers on the selection and use of meats.
The Nutrition Foundation, Inc. 99 Park Avenue New York, N.Y. 10016	Supports basic research in nutrition; publishes materials suitable for nutrition education at various levels.
Superintendent of Documents U.S. Government Printing Office Washington, D.C. 20402	Provides information on documents available, as well as the documents themselves.
U.S. Department of Agriculture Washington, D.C. 20250	Publishes handbooks and bulletins on nutrient content of foods and on new food products.
Universities and colleges: Extension services Departments of nutrition, food science and food technology Colleges of medicine	Staff members answer specific questions, including those in letters, or refer the questioner to other appropriate sources. Cornell University, Ithaca, New York, offers Extension Bulletin 1158, "Nutrition Books: A Guide to Their Reliability."

The United States Department of Agriculture (USDA)

The U. S. Department of Agriculture insures wholesomeness of foods through its food inspection program, on a voluntary basis for processed fruits and vegetables, but required for meats. A label, stamped on fresh meats with a harmless purple dye or printed on the labels of processed meats, indicates that the foods meet USDA standards. Grade standards for qualities other than wholesomeness are also set by USDA. Canned fruits, for example, may be graded A, B, C, or Substandard. Even the substandard grade, however, is wholesome and nutritious; the various grades merely indicate qualities such as uniformity of size, and not any characteristic that could represent a hazard to health.

Public Health Service

The U. S. Public Health Service, which is in the Department of Health, Education and Welfare, is concerned with the prevention of food-borne diseases. For example, its recommendations are incorporated into present law regarding the pasteurization of milk. Sanitation standards for commercial food handlers, such as in restaurants, were also developed by the Public Health Service, although the responsibility of administering the regulations on sanitation falls to state and local departments of health. If an individual consumer finds violations of these regulations, he or she should register a complaint with the local or state health department; merely deciding to avoid a given restaurant in the future does not protect other members of the public.

Federal Trade Commission (FTC)

A major function of the Federal Trade Commission is to protect consumers from false or misleading advertising. If advertisers refuse to comply voluntarily with the commission's advertising guides, court action can be used to stop deceptive advertising, and a company may be ordered to pay a severe penalty for failing to comply with the commission's orders. However, the individual's decisions on advertising must be based on the recognition that clever advertising can mislead the uninformed consumer even though it is within the strict letter of the law. People should also realize that, in the end, the costs of even the most honest advertising are passed on to the consumer, and that advertised brands consequently may cost much more than retailer brands of the same quality. "Let the buyer beware" is an old warning which people are well advised to keep in mind. The more well-informed people are, the more able they are to "beware" in their own best interests.

SUGGESTED READINGS

"A Complete Summary of the Iowa Breakfast Studies." Chicago, Cereal Institute, Inc., 1962.

Davis, C. M. "Results of the Self-Selection of Diets by Young Children." *Canadian Medical Association Journal* 41 (1939):257.

Food and Nutrition Board. "General Policies in Regard to Improvement of Nutritive Values of Foods." Washington, D.C., Food and Nutrition Board, NAS-NRC, 1975.

Gray, G. A. "Metabolic Factors in the Control of Energy Stores." *Metabolism* 24 (1975):99.

Hall, R. L. "Food Additives." *Nutrition Today* 8 (1973):20.

Hall, R. L. GRAS—Concept and Application. *Food Technology* 29 (1975):48.

"Home and Garden Bulletin No. 183: Your Money's Worth in Foods." Washington, D.C., *USDA*, 1970.

Janssen, W. F. and E. P. Waters. "What Some Food Labels Don't Tell." *FDA Consumer:* July–August, 1972.

Kermode, G. O. "Food Additives." *Scientific American* 226 (1972):15.

Nutrition Foundation. *Index of Nutrition Education Materials.* New York: The Nutrition Foundation, Inc., 1974.

Thatcher, F. S. and D. S. Clark, eds. *Microorganisms in Foods.* Toronto: University of Toronto Press, 1968.

White, P. L. "A Brief History of the AMA's Council on Foods and Nutrition." *Nutrition Today* 10 (1975):10.

21

remaining problems: some proposed solutions

The twentieth century has seen an impressive amount of growth and development in the young science of nutrition. This past progress is often cited as evidence that the world has the capacity to deal effectively with the formidable nutritional problems yet to be solved. However, many of the most difficult problems in the past lay in the areas of science and technology. In contrast, most of the obstacles which now must be overcome before the gap can be closed between the actual and the ideal are not primarily scientific and technical. Rather, they are social, political, economic, educational, and administrative problems, many of which urgently require international cooperation of a scope never previously known in the history of humanity.

In this chapter, the main issues in nutrition today are outlined and some of the broad strategies that have been proposed for the future are set forth. Naturally a single chapter cannot pretend to describe the full scope of present problems; nor, without a crystal ball, would it be possible to predict with certainty future trends.

The urgent problem of feeding the world's population adequately is actually a whole spectrum of problems, many of which are linked to each other. Four would appear to be especially crucial:

1 Increasing the amount and nutritional quality of food produced and establishing a system of world food reserves.
2 Controlling population growth and eventually stabilizing the size of the world population.
3 Educating people with respect to nutrition.
4 Accomplishing the research yet needed for rational solutions to all nutrition-related problems.

INCREASING AND IMPROVING FOOD SUPPLIES

And he gave it for his opinion, that whoever could make two ears of corn or two blades of grass to grow upon a spot of ground where only one grew before, would deserve better of mankind, and do more essential service to his country, than the whole race of politicians put together.

–Jonathan Swift, *Gulliver's Travels,* Voyage to Brobdingnag, chap. 6.

Although inequitable distribution has resulted in an excess of food for some of the world's people, current worldwide food consumption per person does not represent an adequate intake even of energy, not to mention essential nutrients. One reason for this is that existing knowledge is not being applied effectively in the form of action-oriented food production programs. Even in the developed countries, crop yields are considerably lower than the theoretical maximum productivity of the land. In developing countries, yields of basic food crops such as grains may be only one-fourth of the yields in the developed countries.

Horizontal expansion of crop production—bringing new lands under cultivation—has been suggested as a way of increasing food supplies. However, there are several reasons why we should not be too optimistic about this approach. One is that heavy capital investment would be required for inputs such as farm machinery, irrigation systems, and fertilizers. These the peoples of developing countries can ill afford. Another is that enormous damage may be done to the environment when land is converted from forests or grasslands to agricultural land. The main problem, however, is that vast expanses of unexploited potentially productive land simply do not exist in the world today; much of the world's land area is not being used for food production for the simple reason that it is of little value for this purpose. There are no continents, or even sizable parts of continents, remaining to be discovered and exploited as there were until just a few centuries ago.

Vertical expansion of food production—increasing the yield on lands already under cultivation—probably represents the chief practical means of alleviating food shortages. The difficulties lie in applying the enormous amount of scientific knowledge and agricultural technology which we already have.

Irrigation is an obvious necessity for raising crops in very arid regions, where nature leaves people high and dry (Figure 21–1). More recently, the possibilities of supplemental irrigation in areas with fair amounts of rainfall have been realized; where people have been persuaded that the amount of water supplied to crops can be determined by humans rather than by the whims of nature, production has been increased substantially. By replacing the muscle power otherwise needed to pump the water to the fields, mechanical pumps make irrigation vastly more easy and efficient. However, the cost of the pumps and fuel to operate them is often beyond the means of the people of developing countries.

Fertilizers offer enormous potential for increasing crop yields. Traditionally, human and animal wastes have been used to enrich soils in the developing countries. Chemical fertilizers offer definite advantages over wastes; they can be made available in much larger quantities, and they are free of the infectious microorganisms with which feces are commonly contaminated. However, unlike human and animal wastes, chemical fertilizers must be purchased, and many farmers in the developing countries cannot afford to buy them. Thus a vicious cycle is set up (Figure 21–2). A system of credit, which would allow the farmer to borrow money to buy fertilizers, may be the only practical means of breaking this cycle.

Pesticides could increase food availability in two leading ways. They could vastly increase the amount of food obtained at harvest by controlling pests which damage or destroy living plants and animals. In addition, they could prevent much of the enormous waste which

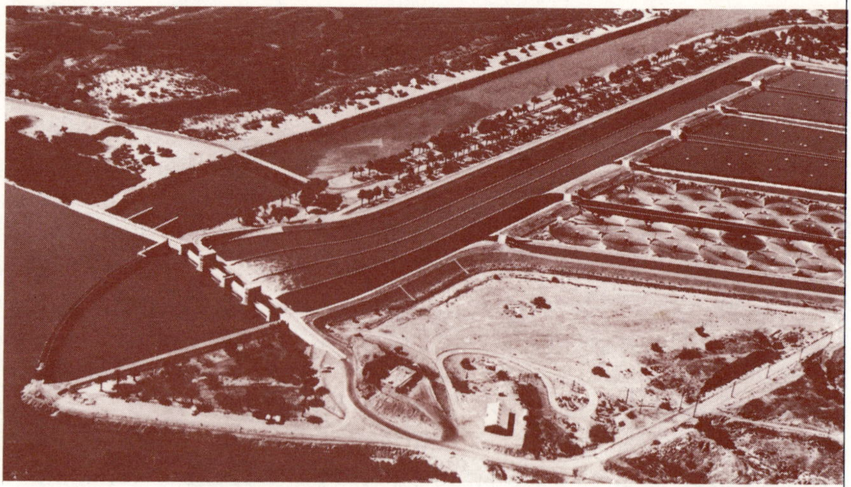

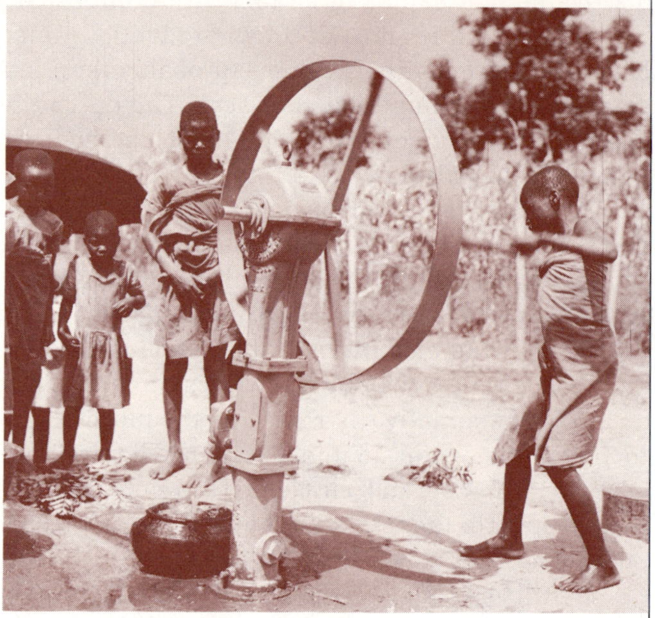

FIGURE 21–1

The complex system that includes the Imperial Dam (above) makes California's Imperial Valley one of the world's richest agricultural areas, although it would be as barren as a desert without irrigation. More than 30 crops with an annual value of over $1 million are produced in the Valley. (Photo courtesy Dow Chemical Company.) By contrast, water must be pumped from wells by human muscle power in many developing countries (below), making potentially productive land valueless because of lack of water. (UNICEF photo by Alistair Matheson.)

occurs after food is harvested. In some developing countries, more than one-fourth of the food harvested may be lost to insects, rats, monkeys, birds, molds, and other forms of life. To decrease these losses, pesticides, as well as modern storage facilities and efficient distribution systems which protect food from pests, are urgently needed. Religious objections to the killing of any form of life may inhibit the use of pesticides in some areas, but the foremost problem in most developing countries is a lack of pesticides rather than an excess of concern for the pests.

Genetic improvement—alteration of the inherited characteristics of plants and animals themselves rather than manipulation of the environmental conditions under which they grow—is another promising approach. Changing the genetic characteristics of organisms can increase the amount of food obtained, or it can improve its nutritional value. A new strain of rice, optimistically called "miracle rice," has been developed; compared to traditional varieties, it responds better to fertilizers and produces much greater yields. "Miracle wheat," suited to the conditions of soil and climate found in many developing countries, may allow these countries to achieve self-sufficiency in grain production. The protein in a new type of corn has an amino acid pattern so superior to that of ordinary corn that its quality is comparable to that of milk protein. Also, domestic animals can, through selective breeding, be improved in a variety of ways. Thus the application of modern knowledge of genetics can result in increased quantities of meat, milk, and eggs or in improved quality of products (Figure 21–3).

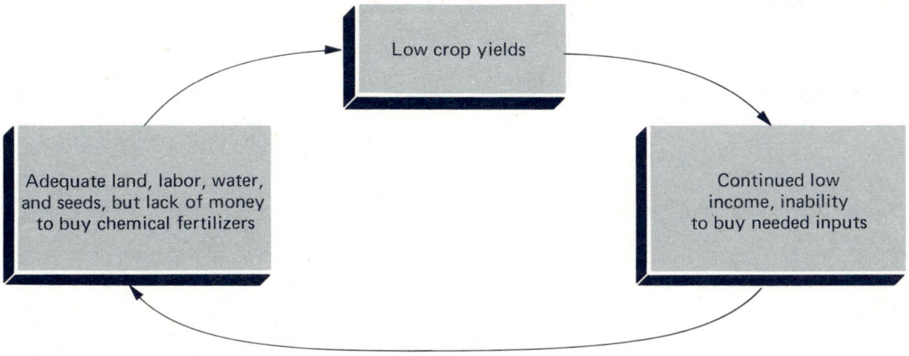

FIGURE 21–2. A vicious cycle that limits food production in many developing areas.

However, unexpected health hazards may be inadvertently created by the very methods responsible for agricultural expansion. An example is the painful and sometimes fatal disease known as *schistosomiasis,* caused by small parasitic worms known as *schistosomes.* These worms develop in snails, after which they may find their way into the body of a human, where they cause extensive damage to blood vessels and many organs. The disease became a major public health problem in Egypt after the Aswan Dam was built. The dam, which provides much-needed water for irrigation, at the same time provides ideal breeding grounds for snails. Thus, the great gains in health which resulted from increased agricultural productivity were at least partially offset by the increased spread of disease caused by the parasitic schistosomes.

Fertilizers also may have undesirable consequences. High-yield varieties of cereals commonly require the use of much greater quanti-

FIGURE 21-3

Foods can be improved by altering the genetics of plants and animals as well as by manipulating their environments. Pork from three genetic strains of hogs, bred to convert feed to different proportions of lean meat and fat, shows that "breeding lean" offers an alternative to "feeding lean." (USDA photo by Murray Lemmon.)

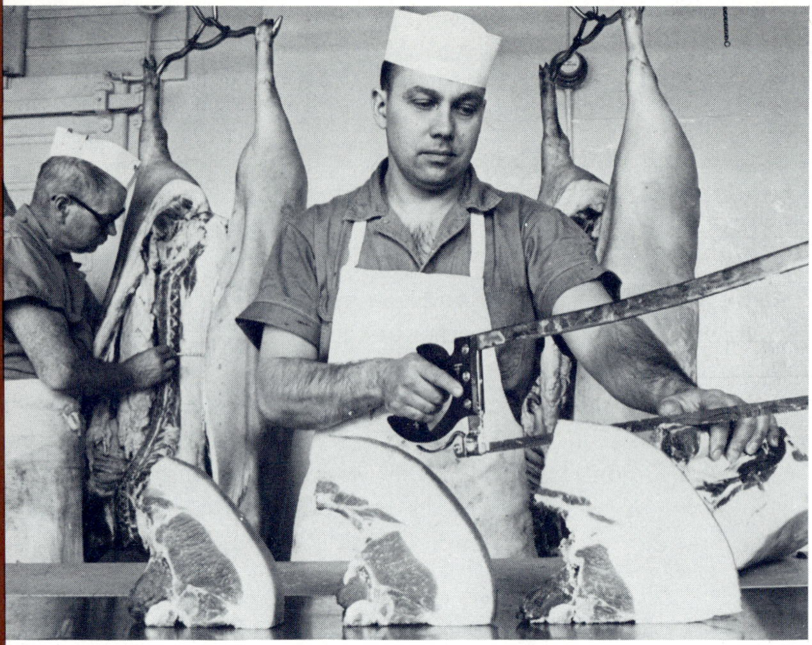

ties of fertilizers than did the traditional varieties they replaced. When fertilizers are applied heavily, chances are great that some of these chemicals will find their way into streams and ponds. Here they may promote excessive growth of algae, making the water unfit for drinking, and killing the fish which are an important protein source in many developing countries. Although weekend fishers in the United States may find it merely annoying when fish disappear from their former haunts, people in some developing countries may, when this happens, lose a leading, or perhaps their only, source of high quality protein.

Unorthodox foods

People generally like and accept the foods with which they are familiar, and resist those that are strange to them. "Unnatural" foods developed through modern technology may therefore be regarded with particular suspicion, even by those who accept the fact that we are committed to technology and cannot return completely to nature for such products as fabrics, housing materials, and medicine. Those living in poverty, who are the very people who would benefit most from these nutritious, inexpensive new foods, may be even more resistant to changing their food habits than are the more affluent people who can afford a conventional nutritious diet. Consumer acceptance thus constitutes a formidable barrier to the use of many valuable products that have been developed recently. Studies of cultural habits and attitudes, followed by application of proven advertising techniques, will probably be necessary for successful promotion of foods such as the following:

Vegetable protein blends. Plant proteins can be combined so that the amino acids lacking in one plant are supplied by another plant in the mixture. Incaparina, made from cottonseed, corn, and soy, was one of the earliest such mixtures developed. Similar products include Pro Nutro, used in Africa, and Multiple Purpose Food in India. These blends are used chiefly as milk substitutes for feeding infants and children, but other children and adults have been enticed into using flavored, soft drink-like soy beverages, such as Vitasoy and Saci, through advertising techniques that emphasize pleasure and popularity rather than nutrient content.

Leaf proteins. The leaves of the cassava, a staple plant in large parts of Africa, actually have a higher protein concentration than the tubers which the people use as food. Furthermore, the nutritional quality of leaf proteins is better than that of some seed proteins, and as good as that of many animal proteins. Leaf proteins therefore probably could be used to improve the nutrition of people living in certain wet tropical countries which, although unsuited to the production of crops such as grains, are ideal for lush growth of leafy plants. Leaf proteins initially have little appeal to many people, being dark green in color and having a faint flavor of spinach or tea. However, people often accept the novel color and flavor in time, especially if the product is mixed with other ingredients which mask its unusual qualities.

Oilseed meals. The chief advantage of using oilseed meals as protein sources lies in the amounts available, which are so vast that no other single source of unconventional high-protein food available at present could contribute so much towards ameliorating protein deficiency. This is because crops such as peanuts (or "groundnuts"), cotton, sesame, soybeans, and coconut are grown partly or entirely for the oil which is extracted from their seeds. The protein-rich solid material which remains is commonly used as fertilizer or in animal feed. In these ways, then, oilseed meals already contribute indirectly to human diets by increasing the amounts of plants and animals produced. However, *direct* consumption of oilseed meals by people is much more efficient than channeling the protein through plants and animals before it is finally available to humans. Used as an ingredient in various foods, including breads and similar cereal products, the oilseed meal yields a food with greatly improved nutritional value compared to the same food prepared without the added seed meal.

Isolated Soy Proteins (ISP). Soy protein has been available in relatively pure form since the 1930s, when it was used for industrial purposes, such as serving as a pigment binder in paper coatings. The same methods used to isolate soy proteins for industrial purposes can be used to obtain the proteins for use in making foods such as artificial meats. These meat analogs, or textured protein products (TPP) (Figure

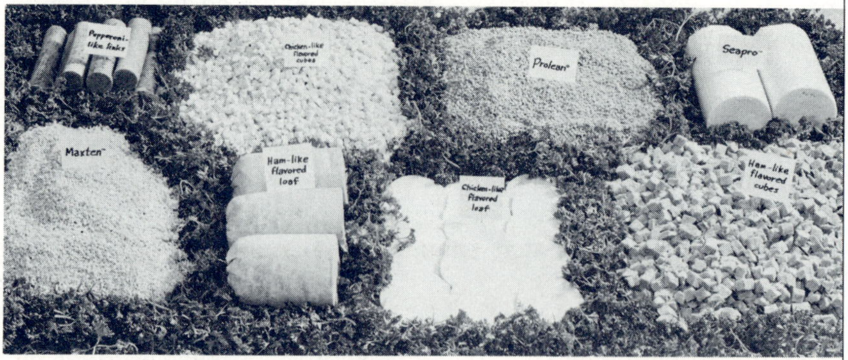

FIGURE 21–4
A starting material such as soybean protein can be used to produce an array of foods. (Photo courtesy of Miles Laboratories, Inc.)

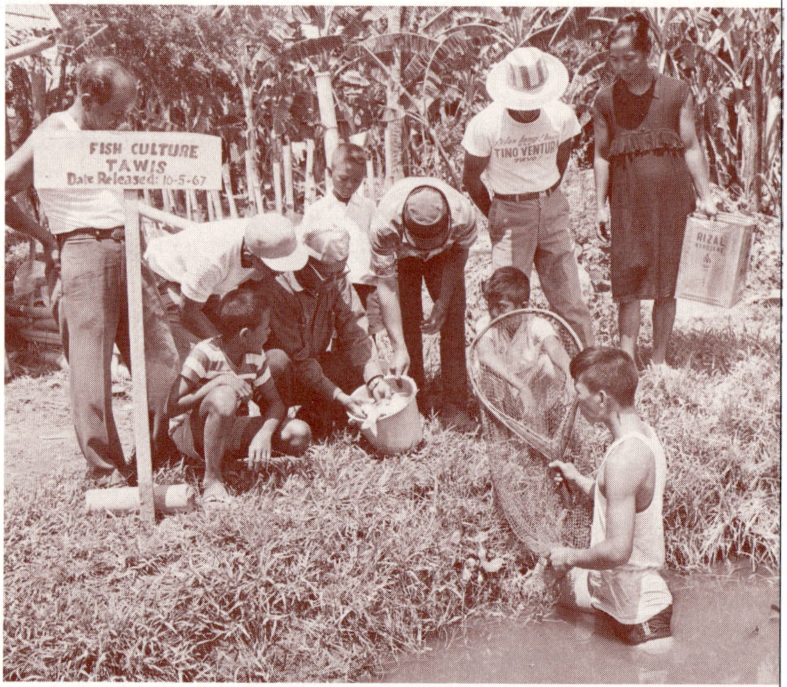

FIGURE 21–5
Fish grown in ponds furnish high quality protein, as in this fish culture project in the Philippines. (UNICEF photo by Mallica Vajrathon.)

21–4), are made by spinning soy proteins into fibers—just as textile fibers are spun. The fibers are then shaped and flavored to make products that resemble foods such as beef, chicken, and bacon. Isolated soy protein (ISP) can also be added to breads, meat patties, and other foods, just as soy meal and flour are. Because ISP has a milder flavor than the meal or flour, a large amount can be added and still be acceptable to consumers. Also, ISP is approximately 90 percent protein whereas soy meal or flour generally contain approximately 50 percent protein. A given amount of ISP therefore increases the protein content of foods much more than would the same amount of the other soy products.

Fish Protein Concentrate (FPC). "Trash" fish, otherwise unacceptable to humans, can be made into an inexpensive, tasteless, odorless powder which is 80 to 90 percent protein of high nutritional value. Water and fat are removed from the fish, but otherwise the whole animals, including bones, fins, heads, and entrails, are used. Understandably, some people have objected to this method of preparation, on the basis of esthetics as well as safety. However, the Food and Drug Administration has approved FPC as being both wholesome and nutritious, and it is now allowed for domestic use as well as for use in international food-assistance programs. When even small amounts are incorporated into staple foods such as breads, FPC greatly increases the nutritional value of the foods without adding a detectable fishy odor or taste, which would undoubtedly result in consumer rejection.

Hunting and harvesting the seas

On land, humans have gone beyond the stage of hunting and finding food and have developed complex systems of agriculture and animal husbandry. Why, it may be asked, could this not also be done in the seas? Aquatic plants such as seaweeds could then be harvested as wheat is on land, and fish and other aquatic animals could be confined and fed as hogs and cattle are. The result, some optimists believe, could be a veritable feast of loaves and fishes for the hungry people of the world.

To a limited extent, *aquaculture,* or the raising of aquatic organisms for food, is already practiced. In some countries, fish are commonly grown in ponds, (Figure 21–5), and it is economically feasible to raise luxury items such as lobsters and prawns (Figure 21–6). Kelp, a type of seaweed, is an example of a marine plant which is grown as food; unfortunately, however, humans cannot digest most of the carbohydrates found in sea plants, which are therefore of very limited value in human diets.

Even if farming the seas should not prove feasible on a large-scale basis, it is sometimes argued, more efficient fishing methods should result in enormously increased catches. Oceans and seas, after all, cover almost three-fourths of the earth's surface. In these waters there may be as much as 700 billion tons of phytoplankton, the microscopic forms of plant life which constitute the bottom of the food chain for aquatic life. This phytoplankton, it has been estimated, should be sufficient to support a "world biomass" of up to two billion tons of fish yearly, or some forty times the current level.

There are, however, several reasons why such speculations should be considered cautiously. Many areas of the ocean are far from teeming with life; in fact, these areas are similar to the deserts of land. This can be explained in terms of the two factors which largely determine the biological productivity of a given part of the oceans: the supply of dissolved nutrients and the amount of light available to support growth of phytoplankton. Most of the nutrients in ocean waters are found in

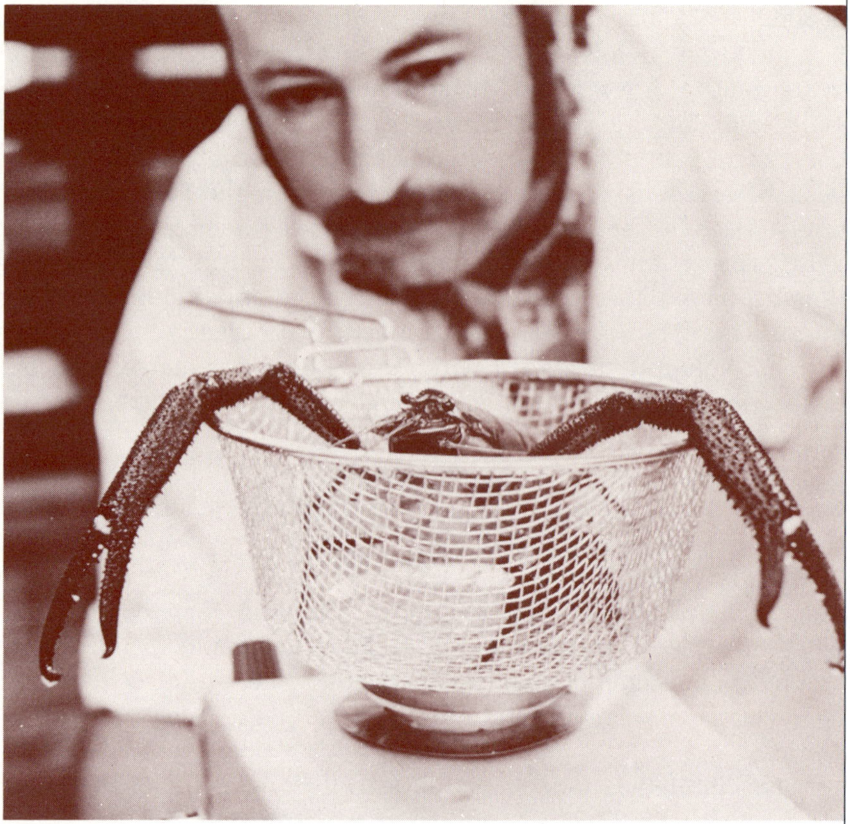

FIGURE 21–6
Marine animals such as this giant prawn sell at such high prices that they can profitably be raised for food. However, such luxuries are economically beyond the reach of most of the world's people. (Photo courtesy Syntex Corporation.)

deeper waters, because of the continuous slow downward movement of plankton and their dead remains. These nutrients can be returned to the surface if the water below is warmer than the water above, conditions which promote vertical mixing. Unfortunately this is more likely to occur in temperate and polar regions (where illumination is worst) than in warmer zones. Therefore, unlike the situation on land, where many areas have both adequate nutrients and adequate light, rather seldom are nutrients and light present at the same time in optimal amounts in the oceans.

Another problem is that food chains tend to be longer for the aquatic animals desired as food than for most of the land animals used as food (Figure 21–7). Except for a few species, such as the anchovy, food fish are carnivores. This means that most of the plant life in the oceans is used to support the lives of enormous numbers of aquatic animals which humans consider inedible; these animals in turn nourish a comparatively small number of edible fish. The demand for fish is, after all, not just for any kind of aquatic animal, any more than the demand for land animals is. Marine plants mainly support the lives of organisms which are underutilized as food, for the very good reason

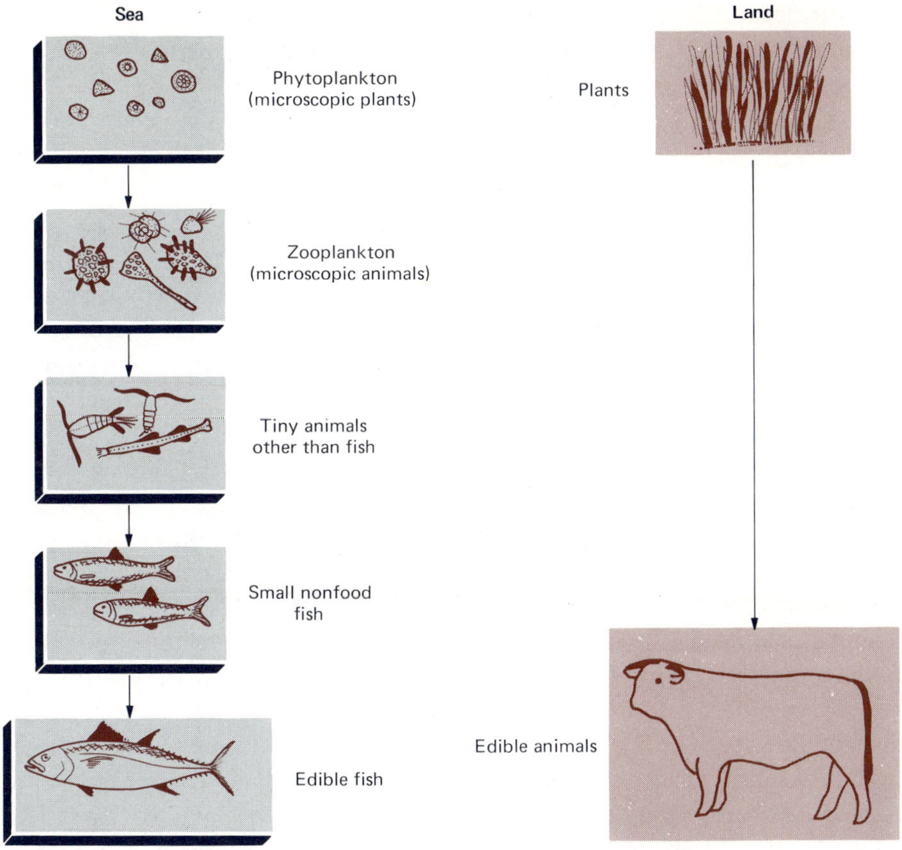

FIGURE 21–7. Compared to the food chains on land, those in the seas are much longer. Thus most of the living things in the sea are eaten, not by humans, but by animals that people reject as food.

that people do not wish to eat them. In contrast, land plants are likely to be consumed directly by the herbivorous animals such as cattle, which are widely accepted as food by humans.

Of the aquatic species which people *do* want to eat, many stocks have already been seriously depleted by overfishing. Because no country has exclusive rights to the sea, controls to avoid overfishing are difficult to enforce. It is possible to establish international agreements to set a limit on the amount of a given type of fish that can be caught before closing the season. However, this often causes each fisher to increase the rate of catch so that the season lasts for only a very short time. This can put a severe stress on the facilities for storing, processing, and marketing the catch, and because fish are highly perishable, the end result may be great waste of the fish.

All in all, the potential of the oceans to supply adequate food for the earth's expanding population remains unknown. Hopefully, humanity will have the wisdom to control its own needs and greed so that the tragic misuse of much of the planet's lands and inland waters will not be repeated in the oceans. Otherwise, we could lose forever all chance of benefitting from whatever the oceans may have to offer for humans in the future.

CONTROLLING POPULATION GROWTH

As recently as 1900, a newborn baby in a country such as the United States had the same slim chance of surviving for the next week as a man of 90 had. High birth rates were thus balanced by high death rates, particularly among the young, and population growth was therefore controlled largely by nature.

During the twentieth century, however, effective treatments have been found for all of the diseases that had previously taken a heavy toll of the young. In the developed countries today, over 97 percent of newborn infants survive to adulthood. Even in developing countries, although death rates among infants and children are still high compared to those of developed countries, they have been drastically lowered in recent decades. Birth rates, however, remain high. The net result is a rate of population growth more rapid than ever before in history, approaching 4 percent per year in some developing countries. Worldwide, the population growth rate is approximately 2 percent per year—enough to double the world's population in thirty-five years. Although the United Nations established a Population Commission as early as 1946, it was not until the 1960s that large numbers of people became convinced that active population policies were urgently needed, particularly by the developing countries.

Uncontrolled excessive human fertility has numerous detrimental effects on human health. By offsetting gains in food production, population growth keeps at a low figure the amount of food available per person. Indeed, in some parts of the world increased food production has been more than offset by increased numbers of people, so that per capita food availability has actually fallen during the period when total agricultural productivity increased (Figure 21–8). Repeated pregnancies and lactations also constitute an almost continuous nutritional drain on women of reproductive age, affecting the health of both the mother and the large number of children she must care for. The common practice of early curtailment of breast feeding, by reason of another pregnancy, contributes significantly to the high infant mortality rate typical of developing countries, where the choice is often not between human milk or cow's milk but between human milk or no milk at all.

Methods of preventing excess fertility have been used since antiquity. However, until fairly recently the available methods were crude, unreliable, unpleasant, or dangerous. *Abstinence*—restraint of sexual activity—is 100 percent effective, but psychologically unacceptable to the vast majority of people. *Rhythm*—periodic abstinence during the

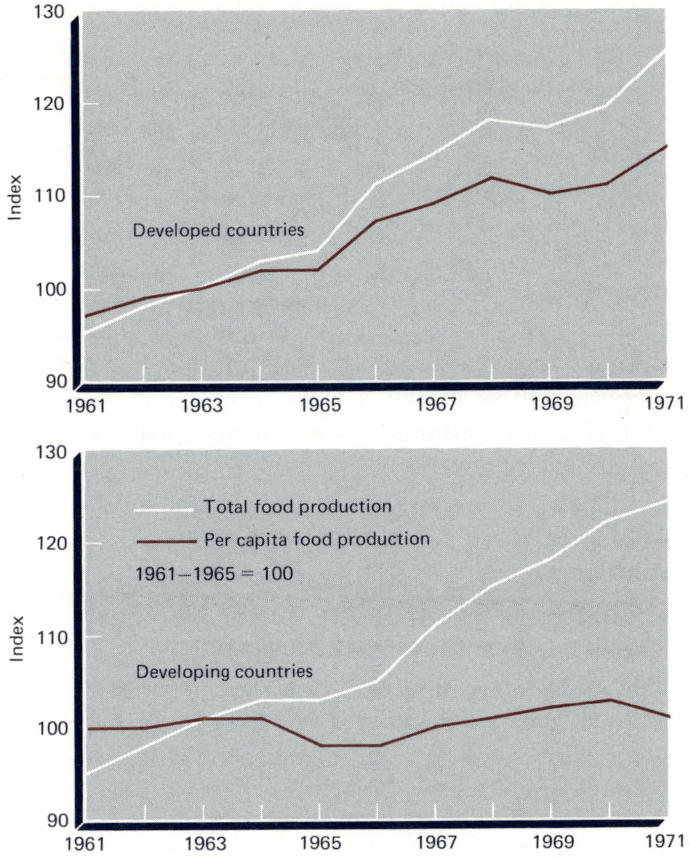

FIGURE 21–8. In some areas, rapid population growth has offset increased food production. (From Population Bulletin, Vol. 29, 1973.)

time when the woman is most likely to conceive—is only slightly more acceptable than total abstinence for many people, and, moreover, it is not very effective because of variations in the reproductive cycle. *Coitus interruptus,* in which sexual intercourse is purposely interrupted by the man prior to ejaculation, is commonly very unsatisfactory to both partners, and it is often ineffective. *Abortion,* the termination of a pregnancy before the fetus is mature enough to survive outside the uterus, is safe only if performed by a qualified person. But despite strong social pressures and considerable danger, abortion, whether legal or not, has been used extensively in many cultures. And if births cannot be prevented by any available means, infanticide may be used as a last resort.

Two modern methods of fertility control that have gained tremendous acceptance in developed countries are the *oral contraceptive agents* (OCA) and the *intrauterine device* (IUD), both of which are 100 percent effective, or virtually so. Oral contraceptives contain female sex hormones that interfere with the release of mature ova by the ovaries.

The IUD may interfere with fertilization of the ovum by the sperm, or it may prevent implantation of the fertilized ovum in the uterus. Although neither of the two methods is ideal for all (oral contraceptives cause unpleasant side effects in some women, and the IUD sometimes causes slight bleeding at about the middle of the menstrual cycle), practically all women can use either one or the other. Scientifically and technically, therefore, the problem of controlling human fertility has been solved.

However, the psychological, social, economic, and cultural factors that influence reproductive behavior are another matter altogether. People sometimes assume that the population problem would be solved if effective contraceptive methods were to be made available throughout the world. However, although both contraceptives and the information on how to use them are necessary, they are not in themselves sufficient to insure population control; no contraceptive is effective unless it is used, and the startling fact is that the vast majority of the people of the world want more offspring than the number which the world can support.

The religious influence against birth control is extremely strong in some areas. A church may teach that contraception is a sin because sexual activity is "intended" for procreation. Some religions object to certain specific aspects of birth control; for example, the IUD is unacceptable to many Hindus and Moslems because they believe that the slight midcycle bleeding renders the female "unclean," just as menstruation is thought to. Because an "unclean" female is considered unfit for intercourse as well as for handling food for two weeks after the bleeding occurs, men understandably object to a method which forces them to forego intercourse, and perhaps even to cook their own food, for an additional two weeks each month.

However, the influence of religion on reproductive behavior should not be exaggerated. In some countries, the birth rate among those whose religion officially forbids "artificial" birth control is as low as among those of other religions; and although some of the world's highest birth rates are found in Catholic countries in South America, some of the lowest are found in Catholic countries of Europe. Also, unwillingness to accept birth control because of religious teachings is often strongest among the older, more conservative members of the population, many of whom are beyond childbearing age anyway.

Cultural factors other than religion also may discourage the use of contraceptives. For example, high status may be attached to a large number of children, so that a man who fails to impregnate his wife every year or two may find his virility seriously questioned and his wife regarded with pity and ridicule. In cultures which have an extended family organization, the prestigious older members often resist limitation of family size, as they resist social changes in general, or they may specifically disapprove of birth control because they consider it their personal right to enjoy having many grandchildren in their old age.

Fatalism is another cultural phenomenon that hampers the practice of fertility control. Fatalism is not, as is sometimes believed, necessarily a lack of concern about the events in one's life. Rather it is the belief that all events are predetermined by fate and therefore cannot be altered by human activity. The idea that they can take the initiative in determining the direction of their lives is so foreign to many people that they may literally be unable to conceive of choosing not to conceive.

Socioeconomic class differences in the use of contraceptives are also important. Compared to the very poor, people in the more favored classes can more easily afford to buy contraceptives, and are more likely to have the knowledge and motivation to use them. This is true in developed as well as developing countries. However, the social structure of most developing countries consists of a relatively small upper class and middle class, and a disproportionately large lower class. Thus the rejection of birth control by those in the lower socioeconomic strata has much more impact on birth rates in the developing countries than in the developed ones.

The status of women, which has recently become a major issue in developed countries, has probably been a contributing factor in the dramatic decline of fertility in these countries. In many traditional societies, however, the status of women depends primarily upon their ability to bear children. Improved opportunities for education and for employment of women could allow them to achieve status by means other than childbirth (Figure 21–9).

Population control, motivated by the needs of society, will undoubtedly be necessary in addition to family planning, which is based on the perceived needs of individuals. For this reason, vigorous governmental and international promotion of social changes is increasingly being recognized as essential in bringing the reproductive behavior of individuals into accord with the defined objective of world population control (Figure 21–10). Prohibition of child labor would make large numbers of children an economic liability, rather than a temporary asset in the food–population race, as they are when children contribute to family income by working the land. Social security programs would decrease the need to have many children to insure economic support in old age. Bonuses for child spacing offer a tangible immediate reward to those who agree to control their own fertility; in India, for example, bonuses have been offered to women who agree to the use of the IUD and to men who agree to the sterilizing operation, vasectomy. Unfortunately, people often accept these procedures only after they have already had four, six, or more children, and although this is somewhat better than no control at all, it is far from the replacement level of reproduction actually needed to eventually stabilize the world population size.

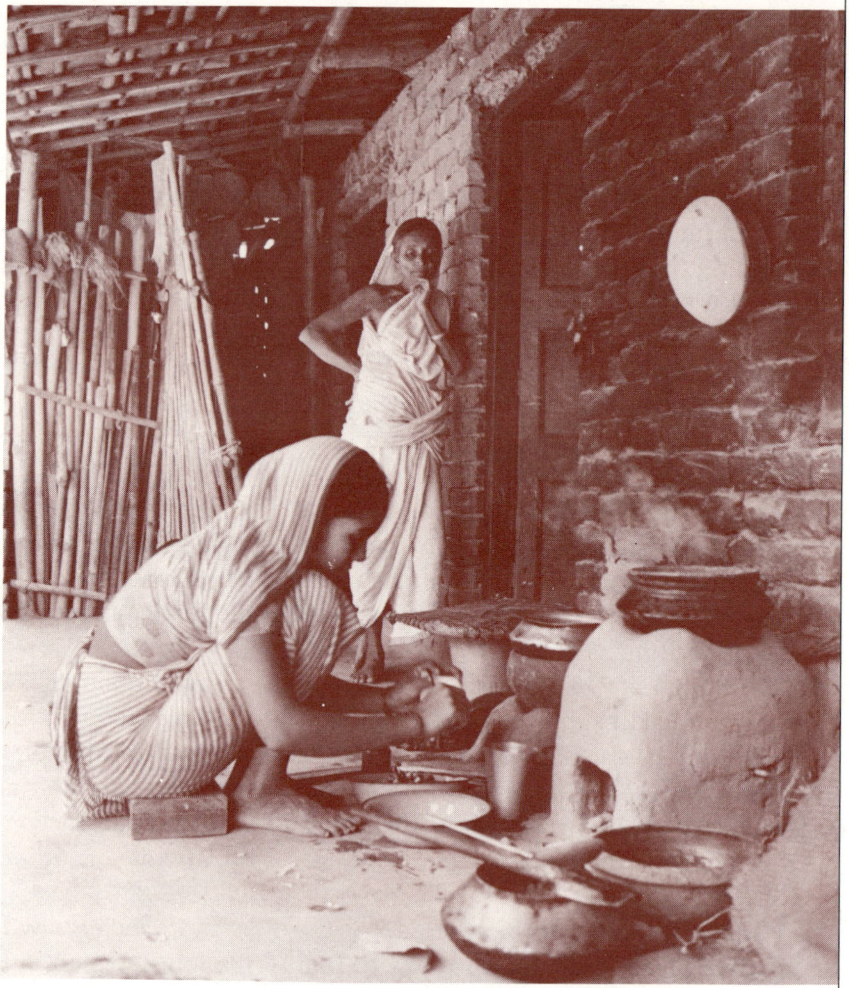

FIGURE 21–9

How can birth rates decline if a woman's status is determined by her roles as mother, grandmother, and mother-in-law? Improved educational and work opportunities for women could provide status by means other than reproduction. (UNICEF photo by Abigail Heyman.)

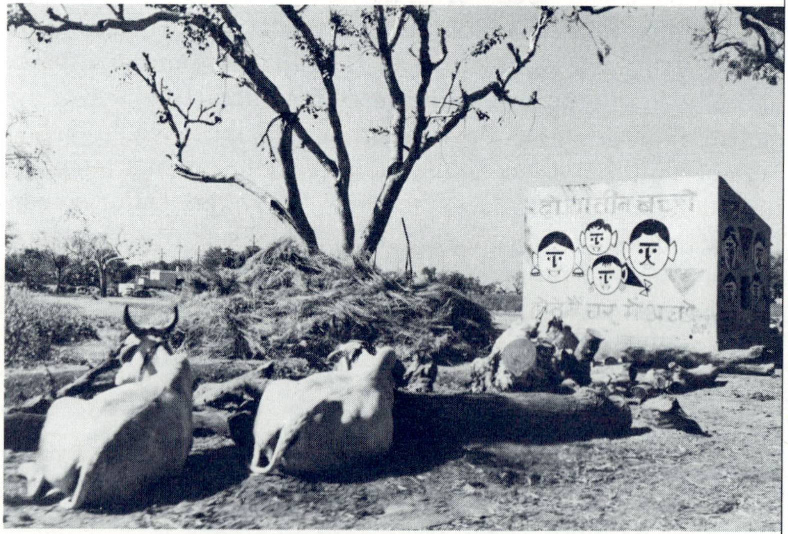

FIGURE 21–10

In India, a widely-used birth-control poster suggests that "a small family is a happy family." Sacred cows, which are not eaten and that compete with humans for food, browse contentedly nearby. (UNICEF/ Abigail Heyman.)

Paradoxically, improved nutrition may eventually be instrumental in lowering the birth rate, as it has been instrumental in lowering the death rate. One reason for the high birth rates in developing countries is that a large number of births has traditionally been necessary to insure the survival of one or two male offspring to adulthood. As people gradually learn that many children need not be born only to die early in life from malnutrition and infection, they become willing to have fewer children. However, because attitudes toward reproduction change very slowly, results should not be expected within the next decade or so. Increased food production is the only realistic short-term goal for dealing with the food supply–population race, although, on a long-term basis, control of population growth is the only possible solution.

EDUCATING PEOPLE WITH REGARD TO NUTRITION

Will the availability of more and better food automatically assure better nutritional status for most of the people of the world? It is commonplace to assume so. However, against this view are a number of counterarguments, the most compelling of which is that there is no assurance that more and better food will be used by those who need it most unless active educational programs are also provided.

To some extent, education in general is associated with nutritional status. Compared to poorly educated people, the well-educated are more likely to have the income necessary to purchase enough food (although this does not always insure that it is of high quality nutritionally); they are more likely to be aware of the relationships of nutrition to health, and to be skeptical of superstitions and taboos that are not supported by the facts; and they are more able to obtain the medical and dental care necessary to treat underlying diseases that could interfere with normal utilization of nutrients.

Even in highly literate countries, however, ignorance regarding nutrition and health may abound. A study conducted for the Food and Drug Administration revealed that the health practices and beliefs of many Americans are fallacious or questionable. The most common misconception was the belief that extra vitamins provide more pep and energy; three-fourths of the subjects questioned agreed with this. Twenty-six percent of the sample reported having used nutrient supplements (pills or liquids containing vitamins and/or minerals) with the expectation of observing actual benefits, and without a physician's advice. One-fifth agreed that diseases such as cancer and arthritis are caused at least partly by deficiencies of vitamins and minerals.

Fortunately, however, questionable health *practices* were not consistently related to questionable *beliefs*. Many who held questionable beliefs did not act upon these, or acted upon them as something "worth a try" rather than because of any strong conviction that the results would be satisfactory. More educated and affluent respondents were somewhat more likely to have used special "health foods," but were less likely than others to be motivated by a belief that these foods would actually improve their health; rather, they gave reasons such as liking the taste or wishing to be socially agreeable. In contrast, people with less education and income tended to express beliefs related to health; they imagined that "health foods" contain more vitamins, are purer than ordinary foods, and so on.

Nutrition education is specifically concerned with trying to inform people about nutrition and to persuade them to modify their nutritional practices. Patterns of human behavior are always in the process of change; nutrition education simply seeks to direct this change toward improvement, and to speed up the process. Individual food habits, patterns of infant and child care, and food production practices are all of concern to the nutrition educator; and because such aspects of life are as deeply imbedded in the cultural pattern of many communities as religion is, they may be as resistant to change.

For example, in many developing countries the best food and the largest quantity of food is reserved for the male head of the family; women and older children (especially male children) come next; last on the list is the preschool child. Lacking the protection afforded the infant at the mother's breast, the recently weaned young child is therefore nutritionally the least favored member of the society. Often this is not primarily because food is lacking, but rather because of deeply held beliefs regarding the feeding of children. Foods such as meat and eggs may be considered "too strong" for a child, so that even if these foods were available in abundance, parents might continue to withhold them from young children because of the mistaken belief that they are harmful. Nutrition education as well as food is therefore needed, especially for vulnerable groups such as young children, whose nutrition may be adversely affected more by customs and traditions than by the limitations of the food supply.

Traditional nutrition education has frequently failed in the past, largely because it has often been, to put it bluntly, boring. A passive, uninvolved captive audience can be forced to commit certain information to memory, especially if they know that they are later to be tested on the material. This, however, is not effective nutrition education, unless the acquired knowledge has some effect on the attitudes and behavior of the learner. The ability to list the major food sources of each essential nutrient, for example, has little impact on people's lives unless it motivates the individuals to accept those food sources.

Because education is an art rather than an exact science, not all educators would agree on a given method of achieving the desired goal. The following steps are therefore presented as *one* way in which a nutrition educational program might proceed:

1. Find out as much as possible about the people who are to be

taught: income, present food habits, cooking practices, religious beliefs, superstitions, total health status. Although asking questions is the most rapid method of getting information, observation is more accurate; many people (consciously or not) do not give accurate answers to personal questions. Most importantly, determine the needs of the learners as they themselves perceive their needs. For example, if people wish above all that their children attain a higher level of education than the parents did, a program that concentrates on convincing the parents that well-nourished children have a better chance of succeeding in school would probably be more effective in motivating parents toward improved child feeding than a program that emphasizes other benefits of improved diet.

2. Plan an educational program that concentrates on important points which actually need improvement. Beneficial or innocuous practices may be best left alone, even if based on erroneous beliefs. For example, many people believe that a late evening feeding of a solid food, such as cereal, causes a baby to sleep through the night; some think that apples eaten in the evening cause bed wetting. Although beliefs such as these are not based on fact, they are harmless to nutritional status. Attacking them therefore serves no useful purpose, and may detract from more important issues.

3. Adjust the subject matter to the people—not the people to the program. The material suitable for a group of middle-class Americans may be totally inappropriate for people in a developing country. An outstanding example is seen in the case of methods recommended for feeding infants. Lessons on formula preparation are perfectly suitable in developed countries, where the milk supply is safe, plentiful, and inexpensive and where almost everybody has facilities for sterilizing and refrigerating the formula. In a developing country, advice on formula feeding may serve only to erode the practice of breast feeding, which is unquestionably superior to formula feeding when milk and adequate facilities are lacking. Under these conditions, education regarding formula feeding is probably best omitted, except, of course, for those women unable to breast-feed their infants. In such situations, prolonged breast feeding—at least for a year, and possibly up to two years or even longer—is unquestionably the most appropriate course to stress in an educational campaign.

4. Select methods appropriate to the learners (Figure 21–11). Lectures and textbooks are not always the only, or even the best, techniques available. Drawings and posters, for example, can often communicate more than words can; if the learners themselves create these, the results may be even more effective than if pictures drawn by others are merely viewed by the learners. A demonstration of procedures, such as food preparation, leads to better audience retention than does a step-by-step oral recitation. In many developing countries, school gardens grown as part of applied nutrition programs allow children to "learn by

FIGURE 21–11
How **subject matter is taught is as important as** *what* **is taught. Methods appropriate to the the learners are essential to a successful nutrition education program. (Photos courtesy UNICEF/Alastair Matheson and CARE.)**

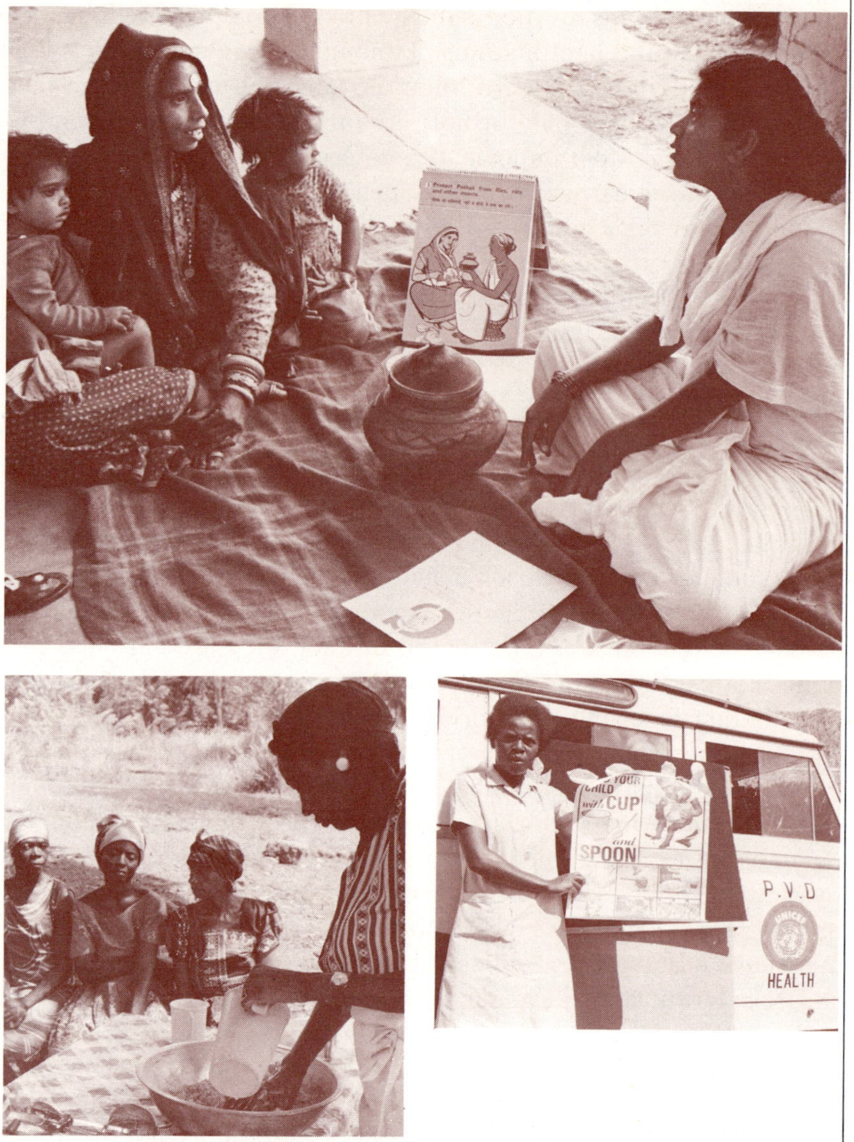

doing," a very effective technique (Figure 21–12). Films, realistic models of materials such as foods, and actual samples of the material to be discussed are additional possibilities. All of these can be useful even in working with the highly literate; for people who are not literate, they may be absolutely essential to learning.

5. Evaluate the effectiveness of the program frequently, and use praise lavishly when desirable changes occur. Too often, nutrition education programs have not been evaluated at all; the assumption has simply been made that the program must somehow be accomplishing

its intended purpose. Although this has undoubtedly brought about a sense of gratification in the educators, it has not always resulted in an improvement in the conditions they sought to change.

RESEARCH: QUESTIONS AND ANSWERS, NOW AND FOR THE FUTURE

What relationships of nutrition to human health remain to be discovered? Which food aid programs and nutrition education programs will be most effective for different groups of people? What motivates people to change their ways of eating, of producing food, of determining family size? How can food be produced and processed so as to obtain maximum yields with a minimum of damage to the environment?

These are just a few of the nutrition-related questions which remain largely unanswered. Their importance is so obvious that, despite the already uncomfortably large disparity between what is known and what is practiced, most people would agree that we need even more research in nutrition and related disciplines. People therefore generally approve of *applied* research, which is directed toward solving specific recognized problems.

Less often recognized is the value of *basic* research, which seeks answers to questions whether or not the answers are of any apparent practical use. Basic research is sometimes thought to be ivory tower, removed from reality, useful only in "satisfying private curiosity at public expense," and therefore perhaps an esoteric luxury which might well be suspended in favor of other more serious activities.

However, the duality between applied and basic research is often more apparent than real. Research has a way of yielding unexpected results, and a project not designed to solve any particular practical problem may nevertheless point the way to a solution. A discovery may lie fallow for years or even decades, to emerge in the future as the answer to a question not even anticipated at the time the discovery was made.

An unusual but actual example: The vampire bat is one of the greatest threats to the South American cattle industry, drinking the blood of cattle as well as of humans. This not only weakens the animals by causing anemia, but also may cause the fatal disease, rabies, with which bats are often infected. However, an ingenious method of controlling the bat population has recently been developed. Cattle are given an anticoagulant, a drug which counteracts the effects of vitamin K. Bats that drink the cattle's blood receive a fatal dose of the anticoagulant, and subsequently die of internal hemorrhage.

This method of pest control may seem simple, but it was made possible only through an enormous body of knowledge gained from basic as well as applied research. After vitamin K was discovered, its structure and functions were thoroughly studied. Antivitamins, com-

FIGURE 21–12
School gardens have educational value, as well as providing nutritious foods for children. (UNICEF photo by Ling.)

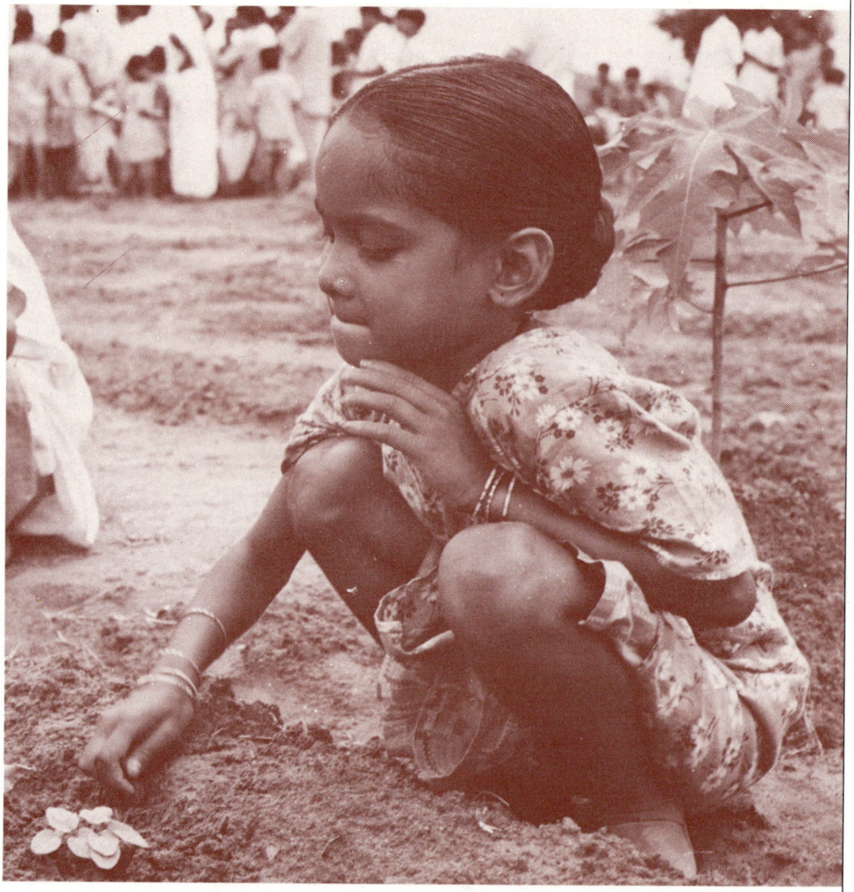

pounds with structures similar enough to vitamin K to block the function of the vitamin itself, could then be developed. Finally, animals were tested in order to determine the effects of a given concentration of the antivitamin in the bodies of various species. In this way, it was eventually learned that the level of antivitamin K that is harmless in the blood of cattle is fatal to the bat which drinks the cattle's blood.

Because the answers to today's questions will not necessarily be relevant in the future, both applied and basic research must be endless processes. Indeed, the answers to one question may themselves lead to further questions. For example, the genetic research which led to the Green Revolution not only showed that high-yielding strains of wheat and rice could be created, but stimulated further questions: Can plants other than grains be improved to the same degree? Will the high-yielding strains prove to be susceptible to diseases that the "inferior" strains could resist? If so, can ways be found to speed up the evolutionary process so as to obtain strains that are both high-yielding and resistant to disease? How can the Green Revolution benefit the 30 percent of the population of developing countries who exist outside the cash economy, as well as the commercial farmers with relatively large land holdings? What kinds of government commitments at the policy-making level are needed to bring the advantages of agricultural development to all of the people? What undesirable as well as beneficial changes in the structure of society can be anticipated when agricultural advances such as the Green Revolution are introduced? The answers to all of these questions may be involved in making farreaching decisions about human destiny.

However, even if both basic and applied nutrition research were inconsequential in solving practical problems, they could be defended as valuable. All organisms must be nourished; only humans have the capacity to wonder how and why. In understanding the processes involved in nutrition in the broadest sense, it is possible to gain a view of ourselves as parts of a complex ecosystem in which all other lives are linked to our own, and life itself is linked to the nonliving world. In this way, we may acquire significant insights into our own biological, psychological, and social natures. Surely this in itself is enough to justify research in nutrition as in any other area of human knowledge.

SUGGESTED READINGS

Agricultural Information Bulletin No. 355: Consumer Products by Design. Washington, D.C., *USDA,* 1973.

The American Assembly, Columbia University. *Uses of the Seas.* Englewood Cliffs, N. J.: Prentice-Hall, 1968.

Berelson, B. "World Population: Status Report 1974." New York: The Population Council, Inc., 1974.

Ehrlich, P. R., A. H. Ehrlich, and J. P. Holdren. *Human Ecology.* San Francisco: W. H. Freeman and Company, 1973.

Ennis, W. B., Jr., W. M. Dowler, and W. Klassen. "Crop Protection to Increase Food Supplies." *Science* 188 (1975):593.

Jukes, T. H. "Chemical Residues in Foods." *Journal of the American Dietetic Association* 59 (1971):203.

Latham, M. C. "Nutrition and Infection in National Development." *Science* 188 (1975):561.

National Analysts, Inc. A Study of Health Practices and Opinions. Springfield, Va., National Technical Information Service, June 1972.

Thompson, R. D., G. C. Mitchell, and R. J. Burns. "Vampire Bat Control by Systemic Treatment of Livestock with an Anticoagulant." *Science* 177 (1972):806.

Todhunger, E. N. "Food Habits, Food Faddism, and Nutrition." *World Review of Nutrition and Dietetics* 16 (1973):287.

Tydings, J. D. *Born to Starve.* New York: Morrow, 1970.

United Nations, "Human Fertility and National Development." New York, 1971.

Wittwer, S. H. "Food Production: Technology and the Resource Base." *Science* 188 (1975):579.

index

76 77 78 79 80 9 8 7 6 5 4 3 2 1